# HIV-associated Hematological Malignancies

Marcus Hentrich • Stefan K. Barta
Editors

# HIV-associated Hematological Malignancies

Springer

*Editors*
Marcus Hentrich
Department of Hematology and Oncology
Red Cross Hospital
University of Munich
Munich
Germany

Stefan K. Barta
Department of Medical Oncology
Fox Chase Cancer Center
Philadelphia, PA
USA

ISBN 978-3-319-26855-2    ISBN 978-3-319-26857-6 (eBook)
DOI 10.1007/978-3-319-26857-6

Library of Congress Control Number: 2016931558

Springer Cham Heidelberg New York Dordrecht London


Printed on acid-free paper

Springer International Publishing AG Switzerland is part of Springer Science+Business Media (www.springer.com)

# Foreword

During the first decade of the AIDS epidemic in the USA, it was hard to imagine that the nightmare would ever end; death surrounded us, both professionally and personally, as friends, family, and patients alike died, despite any or all of our efforts as physicians. Hematologists and oncologists played an important role in those early days, as we were among the first of specialists who were willing to commit ourselves to the care of these patients and to the challenge of treating those who were not only severely immunosuppressed by HIV but were also afflicted by opportunistic malignancies, which were remarkably aggressive, widespread, and clearly different from our experience with other, HIV-uninfected patients. We became the support for these patients, not only in the medical sense but also in terms of dealing with truly marginalized individuals, who had to endure the prejudice and fear of the world around them and, to some extent, around us as well.

But we persisted, and slowly, progress was made. We found that these patients could simply not tolerate the dosages of chemotherapy that were routinely employed with curative intent in uninfected persons and were forced to use suboptimal dosing and scheduling, which allowed some patients to survive, though the vast majority did not. The advent and widespread use of combination antiretroviral therapy (cART) in 1996 brought about what might be considered one of the medical miracles of our time, with the death rate from AIDS decreasing by approximately 75 % within the first year of their use. The risk of new opportunistic infections among HIV-infected persons also declined dramatically during this time, as did the incidence of Kaposi's sarcoma; lymphoma, however, did not decrease as dramatically, thereby becoming one of the more common of initial AIDS-defining diagnoses.

Nonetheless, cART also provided the mechanism by which patients with AIDS-related lymphoma (ARL) and other malignancies could and would survive, for when used with standard doses of chemotherapy, or with novel regimens of infusional chemotherapy, response rates and even overall median survival now approach that of HIV-uninfected patients with the same tumor types. Stem cell transplantation, once deemed thoroughly impossible in the setting of ARL, has also been proven safe and effective in HIV-infected patients, including those with lymphoma, Hodgkin lymphoma, and other hematologic malignancies. In fact, the only patient in the world known to have been cured of HIV infection (the "Berlin patient") accomplished this feat by receipt of an allogeneic stem cell transplant from an HIV-negative donor with homozygous deletion of CCR4 Δ 32, inhibiting the entry of HIV virions into the patient's newly generated donor CD4+ cells, while also curing his acute myeloblastic leukemia. This discovery, in itself, has now led to a series of experiments which attempt to cure not only the underlying hematologic malignancy but the HIV infection itself, by means of various gene therapy approaches.

The years have been long, and the suffering will remain imprinted in our memories, but in the past 30 years, we have come a long, long way. The various chapters in this book will document in great detail just how far and remarkable that path has become. By presenting information on the full range of hematologic malignancies seen in the setting of HIV, in terms of epidemiology, pathogenesis, factors predictive of development of disease, prognostic factors at diagnosis and at time of treatment, as well as optimal therapeutic approaches including newly developed targeted therapies, the reader will be rewarded by a concise yet comprehensive review of the past, present, and future of this remarkably challenging and fascinating field.

Alexandra M. Levine, MD, MACP
Chief Medical Officer
Dr. Norman and Melinda Payson Professor in Medicine
Deputy Director of Clinical Affairs, Comprehensive Cancer Center
Professor, Department of Hematology & Hematopoietic Cell Transplantation
City of Hope National Medical Center
Duarte, CA, USA
May 9, 2015

# Preface

With the advent of potent combination antiretroviral therapy (cART), incidence and mortality rates of HIV-associated non-Hodgkin lymphomas (HIV-NHL) have decreased. By contrast, the incidence of Hodgkin lymphoma in HIV-infected patients (HIV-HL) has remained unchanged or even increased. Both HIV-NHL and, to a lesser extent, HIV-HL remain a major cause of morbidity and mortality in HIV-infected patients. Furthermore, although the absolute rates for other hematological malignancies such as acute leukemias and myeloproliferative disorders in people living with HIV (PLWH) are low, incidence appears to be higher when compared to the general population.

In the context of relatively sparse prospective randomized trials, the optimal treatment of hematological malignancies remains a challenge, particularly in patients with severe immunosuppression.

This book will present a general introduction to and review of HIV-associated hematological malignancies, with a special focus on practical management issues. Many book chapters are written by colleagues who have been instrumental in shifting the balance for PLWH with blood cancers. While two decades ago this diagnosis meant a death sentence, advances in treatment have transformed these cancers into often curable conditions.

The Editors

Philadelphia, PA, USA

Stefan K. Barta
Marcus Hentrich

# Acknowledgments

This textbook was conceived as a collaborative effort between the editors and Springer International Publishing AG.

We are greatly indebted to Isabel Arnold who initiated this textbook and shared the editors' commitment and determination to make this project a success.

The expert support provided by Meike Stoeck and Rosemarie C. Unger is also greatly appreciated.

Finally, we are profoundly grateful to all the contributing authors whose efforts define this work.

## Contents

# Pathology

**1**

Ethel Cesarman and Amy Chadburn

## Contents



E. Cesarman, MD (✉) • A. Chadburn, MD
Department of Pathology and Laboratory Medicine, Weill Cornell Medical College, 1300 York Yve, New York, NY 10065, USA
e-mail: ecesarm@med.cornell.edu; achadbur@med.cornell.edu



M. Hentrich, S.K. Barta (eds.), *HIV-associated Hematological Malignancies*,
DOI 10.1007/978-3-319-26857-6_1

Non-Hodgkin B-cell lymphomas (B-NHL) are greatly increased in incidence in people with HIV with high-grade lymphomas considered an AIDS-defining condition. NHLs are the second most common malignancy in individuals with HIV infection globally, following Kaposi sarcoma (KS). However, this trend has changed in developed countries as a result of widespread use of combined antiretroviral therapy (CART), where B-NHL has surpassed KS as the most common malignancy in individuals with HIV infection [117, 118]. One epidemiologic study found that NHL comprises 53 % of all AIDS-defining cancers and that it is the most common cancer-related cause of death in HIV-infected individuals (36 % of deaths during 1996–2006) [118]. While AIDS-related B-NHL has decreased in incidence since the introduction of CART, classical Hodgkin lymphoma (cHL), other non-AIDS-defining types of non-Hodgkin lymphoma and multicentric Castleman disease have been increasing. In the United States, cHL is still less frequently reported than NHL in HIV-infected patients [117], but in Europe it appears to be more common; the Swiss Cohort Study found a standardized incidence ratio (SIR) of 35 for cHL, which was higher than that of KS (SIR = 25) and B-NHL (SIR = 24) [30]. In addition, as people with AIDS survive longer, a wide range of non-AIDS-related cancers are emerging in HIV-infected individuals, including leukemias and myelodysplastic syndrome (MDS) [94, 102, 116, 122].

The role of HIV infection in the pathogenesis of hematological malignancies is clearly multifactorial and involves disrupted immune surveillance to tumor antigens, viral infection, genetic alterations, chronic antigenic stimulation, and cytokine dysregulation [15, 48, 70]. While HIV has been considered a biological carcinogen by the IARC [1], it does not infect the lymphoma cells and is therefore thought to act as an indirect carcinogen (via immune suppression, inflammation, etc.). However, possible direct effects through secreted or transmitted viral proteins may also play a role, and there is experimental evidence supporting oncogenic functions of HIV Tat [73, 80]. While the role of HIV appears to be indirect, the specific and direct role of the two human gammaherpesviruses is well documented. These two viruses are Epstein-Barr virus (EBV/HHV-4) and Kaposi sarcoma herpesvirus (KSHV/HHV-8). Regarding the specific immunological alterations that are related to lymphoma development, several B-cell stimulatory cytokines are increased in HIV-infected people prior to a diagnosis of lymphoma, namely, IL6, IL10, CRP, sCD23, sCD27, and sCD30 [11]. Increased serum levels of the CXCL13 chemokine have also been noted in HIV-infected individuals before a diagnosis of lymphoma, and specific alleles of CXCL13 or its receptor CXCR5 are associated with these increased CXCL13 levels, implying a possible genetic predisposition [63]. These studies have suggested that evaluation of serum levels of these cytokines may identify HIV-positive patients at highest risk for B-NHL and possibly earlier diagnosis.

## 1.1 AIDS-Related Lymphomas

AIDS-related lymphomas (ARLs) are almost always of B-cell origin, and some specific lymphoma types are more common in HIV-infected patients. Some of these lymphoma types can occur in both HIV uninfected and infected patients, while others preferentially develop in the context of AIDS or in patients with other immunodeficiencies, and the WHO classification has used this distinction [103]. Lymphomas that are more commonly associated with AIDS tend to have more frequent viral associations. HIV-related lymphomas were initially classified by morphology and/or by primary site of presentation (i.e., systemic, primary central nervous system, body cavity) [70]. Now, these lymphomas have been classified according to the WHO classification as distinct disease entities based on morphology, immunophenotype, and sometimes, molecular alterations [6, 103, 110]. The distribution of these subtypes and association with EBV, and latency pattern as determined on analysis of 212 cases, was recently published and is shown in Table 1.1 [3].

The following paragraphs list the lymphoma subtypes most frequently seen in HIV-infected individuals, in approximate order of frequency and their main pathological diagnostic features.

**Table 1.1** Pathological subclassification and EBV assessment by EBER-ISH and immunohistochemistry for LMP1 and EBNA2 in AIDS-related lymphoma

| AIDS lymphoma subtype | No. | EBV positive (%) EBER-ISH | Immunophenotype | | |
|---|---|---|---|---|---|
| | | | Latency I $LMP1^{-}EBNA^{-}$ (% of $EBV^{+}$) | Latency II $LMP1^{+}EBNA2^{-}$ (% of $EBV^{+}$) | Latency III $LMP1^{+}EBNA2^{+}$ (% of $EBV^{+}$) |
| DLBCL non-GC | 48 | 27 (56 %) | 10 (37 %) | 8 (30 %) | 8 (30 %) |
| DLBCL GCB | 98 | 25 (25 %) | 19 (76 %) | 3 (12 %) | 3 (12 %) |
| DLBCL null | 13 | 4 (31 %) | | 1 (25 %) | 3 (75 %) |
| BL | 19 | 10 (53 %) | 9 (90 %) | 1 (10 %) | |
| PBL | 9 | 8 (89 %) | 8 (100 %) | | |
| PEL (solid variant) | 14 | 12 (86 %) | 11 (92 %) | 1 (8 %) | |
| BCL-U | 4 | 3 (75 %) | 3 (100 %) | | |
| Polymorphic LPD | 7 | 5 (71 %) | 1 (20 %) | 1 (20 %) | 3 (60 %) |
| Total | 212 | 94 (44 %) | 61 (65 %) | 15 (16 %) | 17 (18 %) |

Published in Arvey et al. [3]

These 212 cases were classified as latency I in EBER1 cases when no LMP1 or EBNA2 was expressed, as latency II when these were positive for LMP1 but negative for EBNA2 and as latency III where there was expression of both EBNA2 and LMP1

*BCL-U* B-cell lymphoma, unclassifiable, with features of DLBCL and BL, *DLBCL null* negative for CD10, BCL6, and MUM1, *LPD* lymphoproliferative disorder, *PEL* primary effusion lymphoma

### 1.1.1 Diffuse Large B-Cell Lymphomas (DLBCL)

These are the most common AIDS-related lymphomas and occur in both HIV-infected and HIV-uninfected individuals. In patients with HIV infection, DLBCLs were originally divided based on cellular morphology into centroblastic (Fig. 1.1a) and immunoblastic (Fig. 1.1b) categories and based on location into systemic and primary central nervous system lymphomas (CNS). The immunoblastic type is mostly seen in people with AIDS and is more frequently associated with EBV infection, with reported rates of positivity by this virus as high as 80–90 % [17]. Immunoblastic lymphomas have also been shown to frequently have an unrestricted EBV latency (type III) [17, 105]. This subtype includes most AIDS-related primary CNS lymphomas. However, immunoblastic lymphomas are less frequently seen in the era of CART, at least in the US and Europe, as this type of DLBCL occurs in the context of severe immunodeficiency, because the EBV proteins expressed in these tumors are not only oncogenic but also immunogenic [20, 75]. EBV is most commonly detected in diagnostic pathology laboratories using in situ hybridization for EBERs (Fig. 1.1c), which are abundantly expressed, noncoding viral RNAs. Cases with centroblastic morphology occur regardless of HIV infection. These lymphomas are subdivided into germinal center and non-germinal center subtypes (non-GC or ABC) in both HIV-positive and HIV-negative patient populations. However, in people with AIDS, the clinical significance of this subclassification is more controversial and may be dependent of treatment [23, 25, 40]. DLBCLs in patients with

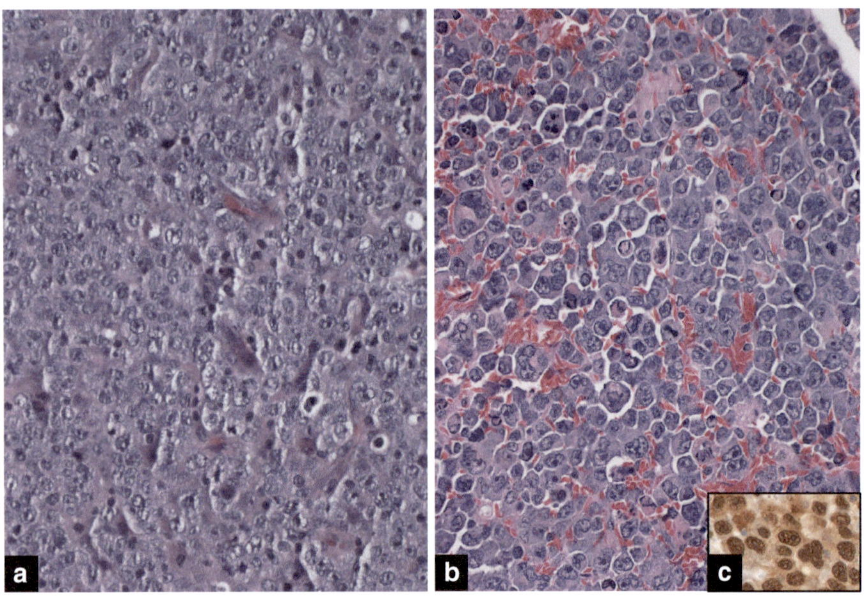

**Fig. 1.1** Diffuse large cell lymphoma (DLBCL). HIV-DLBCLs morphologically are either “centroblastic” (**a**) or “immunoblastic” (**b**) in appearance. The “immunoblastic”-appearing lesions are more frequently EBV positive (**c**) (**a**, **b**: hematoxylin and eosin, 40× original magnification; **c**: In situ hybridization; 40× original magnification)

AIDS more frequently have an extranodal presentation, a larger proportion are of the germinal center subtype, and there is a more common association with EBV (30 % in AIDS vs. <5 % in HIV-). One study of 70 AIDS-related DLBCL showed that EBV positivity was independently associated with a higher 2-year overall mortality and recommended incorporating EBV status with IPI in prognostication [26], although this association has not been found in other studies [23]. In terms of EBV latency, the GC subtype of AIDS DLBCL is less frequently EBV positive than the non-GC subtype (25 % vs. 56 %) and more frequently exhibits type I latency (76 % of EBV+ cases), in contrast to a fairly even distribution in latency profiles in the non-GC subtype, at least as assessed by immunohistochemistry (Table 1.1) [3].

A diagnosis of DLBCL can be made by morphologic evaluation of hematoxylin and eosin (H&E)-stained tissue sections based on a loss of normal tissue architecture and sheets of large cells of B-cell origin, as determined by immunohistochemistry for B-cell antigens, such as PAX5 or CD20. Classification into the main cell of origin subtypes can be made using molecular approaches such as gene expression profiling and RNA sequencing. Although these are the most reliable methods of cell of origin subclassification, they are not yet available as part of routine patient care. Thus, surrogate immunohistochemistry studies are used by the majority of clinical laboratories [28, 60, 131]. Newer technologies and classifiers that allow analysis of gene expression using formalin-fixed paraffin embedded samples have been reported to be better at subclassification than immunohistochemistry. These include a 21-gene QuantiGene Plex Assay [59], a LIMD1-MYBL1 two-gene index [135], a 14-gene reverse transcriptase multiplex ligation-dependent probe amplification assay, and a 30-gene panel using digital multiplexed gene expression (DMGE; Nanostring) [84]. These methods remain to be validated by more investigators and have not been tested in AIDS-related lymphomas. Immunohistochemistry with Ki67 is also useful in AIDS-related lymphomas to evaluate the proliferation index, which can have prognostic significance as individuals with tumors with a higher proliferation index have been found to respond better to aggressive chemotherapy regimens [23]. Proliferation rate assessment may also help differentiate DLBCL from Burkitt lymphoma, although many DLBCLs in HIV+ patients can have very high proliferation rates.

### 1.1.2 Burkitt Lymphomas (BL)

Three epidemiologic subtypes of BL are recognized: endemic, sporadic, and AIDS related. The typical histological appearance of BL is the presence of cohesive sheets of malignant cells that are small to intermediate in size and contain moderately abundant basophilic cytoplasm and round, regular nuclei possessing two to five distinct nucleoli. The presence of abundant mitotic figures, and numerous, evenly distributed tingible body macrophages with abundant clear cytoplasm are characteristic and have led to a description of BL having a “starry-sky” appearance (Fig. 1.2). However, BL occurring in individuals with AIDS may have atypical features, such as some cases showing plasmacytoid differentiation and others exhibiting greater nuclear polymorphism [103]. The immunophenotype of BL includes positivity for

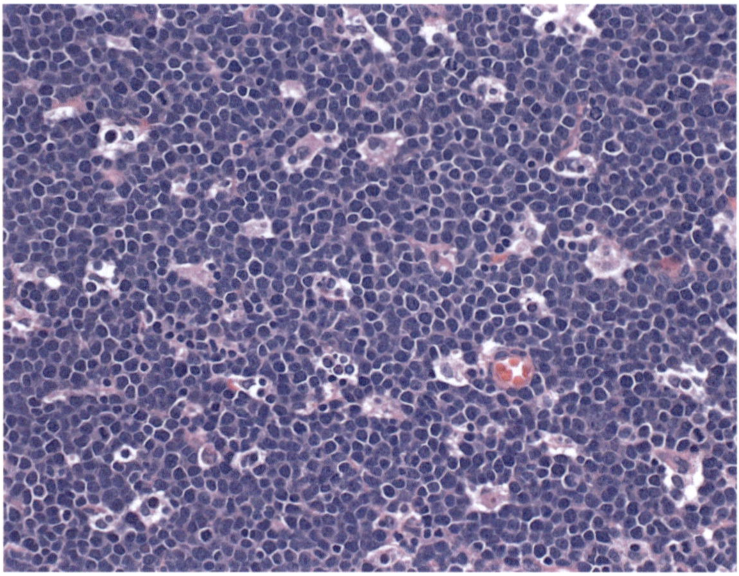

**Fig. 1.2** Burkitt lymphoma. Note the "starry-sky" appearance with numerous tingible body macrophages. Scattered mitotic figures are seen. The cells are medium in size with scant cytoplasm and squared-off cytoplasmic borders (hematoxylin and eosin; 40× original magnification)

B-cell antigens, CD10, and BCL6 and negativity or only weak positivity for BCL2. Ki67 immunohistochemistry will be positive in >95 % of the tumor cells, as BL is one of the fastest growing tumors in humans.

The molecular hallmark of BL is the translocation of the *MYC* oncogene into one of the immunoglobulin (Ig) loci. The t(8;14), involving the *MYC* and immunoglobulin heavy chain (*IGH*) genes, is the most common, but approximately 10 % of the cases have a *MYC* translocation to one of the Ig light chain genes. The clinical method most commonly used to assess the presence of this translocation is fluorescent in situ hybridization (FISH) using a break-apart probe, which will show a split signal independent of the translocation partner. The consequence of this translocation is thought to be a deregulated expression of *MYC*. Mutations in the *MYC* regulatory and coding regions also occur in BL [8, 13, 22, 101, 112] and have been shown to contribute to abnormal expression or prolonged protein stability. In the absence of a demonstrable *MYC* translocation, the histology and phenotype must be otherwise completely typical for a diagnosis of BL.

### 1.1.3 B-Cell Lymphoma, Unclassifiable, with Features Intermediate between DLBCL and BL (BCL-U)

This designation has been given to high-grade lymphomas that do not fit cleanly into the DLBCL or BL categories [69]. Some of these cases used to be classified as atypical or Burkitt-like lymphoma. Unfortunately, the criteria for this designation are not always completely objective, and thus this nomenclature is used for a heterogeneous group of cases. A molecular designation cannot be made, because the presence or absence of *MYC* translocations is not sufficient as it can be seen in otherwise typical cases of BL or DLBCL. Rather, this category should be used for cases with unusual morphology or phenotype. Some of these cases may belong to a separate molecular category ascribed to lymphomas with *MYC* translocations and a complex karyotype, including additional translocations in oncogenes such as BCL-6 and/or BCL-2 (double- or triple-hit lymphomas). Others may correspond some cases classified by histology as BL but upon gene expression profiling do not have a Burkitt signature [35, 62] or express the classic immunophenotypic profile. BCL-U may be EBV positive or negative, but the true proportion is not clear, as these rare cases were only recently recognized by the WHO.

### 1.1.4 Classical Hodgkin Lymphoma (CHL)

While not considered an AIDS-defining malignancy, AIDS-CHL is increased in incidence in HIV-infected individuals and may be surpassing AIDS-NHL in frequency in some populations [30, 54]. The proportion of AIDS-CHL appears to have been increasing as individuals with HIV infection experience longer life expectancies and better immunological control with CART [54]. While CHL occurs in both HIV-infected and HIV-uninfected individuals, there are some important differences in these two patient populations. In particular, AIDS-CHL is accompanied by EBV infection in close to 90 % of cases, while only approximately one third of CHLs are positive for EBV in immunocompetent individuals. In addition, the mixed cellularity or lymphocyte-depleted forms of CHL comprise a larger number of cases in HIV+ patients, while the nodular sclerosis subtype is more common in the general population [16, 103].

### 1.1.5 Primary Effusion Lymphoma (PEL)

PEL is a rare lymphoma subtype, accounting for less than 5 % of all HIV-related NHLs. It can also occur in individuals without HIV infection but is extremely rare in this latter context. PEL is characterized by the presence of KSHV (also called HHV-8) within the tumor cells, and this virological association is considered a diagnostic criterion [21, 88, 103]. It presents most commonly as a lymphomatous effusion involving one or more of the pleural, peritoneal, and pericardial spaces. However, about one third of the cases can show dissemination to extracavitary sites. Some rare cases of AIDS-related NHL are associated with KSHV infection but without evidence of body cavity involvement. These have been designated solid or extracavitary PEL and represent approximately 5 % of all AIDS-NHLs. They typically have the morphology of DLBCL, frequently with immunoblastic features, but like PELs, they frequently lack of expression of B-cell antigens and are commonly co-infected with EBV [24].

In addition to the presence of KSHV, the vast majority of PEL cases are co-infected with EBV. While PEL is a tumor of B-cell origin, it is characterized by the lack of expression of B-cell-associated antigens and immunoglobulins (Ig). This lack of B-cell antigens in a neoplastic cell of B-cell origin is not unique to PEL and can be seen in other B-cell malignancies, such as the Reed-Sternberg cells of CHL. Morphologically, it is composed of large tumor cells, with features that can be immunoblastic or anaplastic. However, the lack of B-cell antigen expression can make these difficult to identify by immunohistochemistry, and a tumor other than lymphoma may be suspected (Fig. 1.3), particularly since PELs are often positive for antigens such as CD138 and EMA (epithelial membrane antigen), which can be seen in other entities including plasma cell myeloma and some carcinomas. The presence of KSHV is most easily assessed by immunohistochemistry for the KSHV nuclear antigen LANA (encoded by ORF73), which is commercially available (Fig. 1.3).

Patients presenting with a primary lymphomatous effusion that lacks KSHV have been reported, but these appear to be a different disease entity, which have been referred to by some investigators as KSHV- or HHV-8-negative PEL [5, 85, 93, 127]. A recent paper described two cases of KSHV-negative PEL with a review of the literature including 48 additional cases. Among these, 21 % were positive for

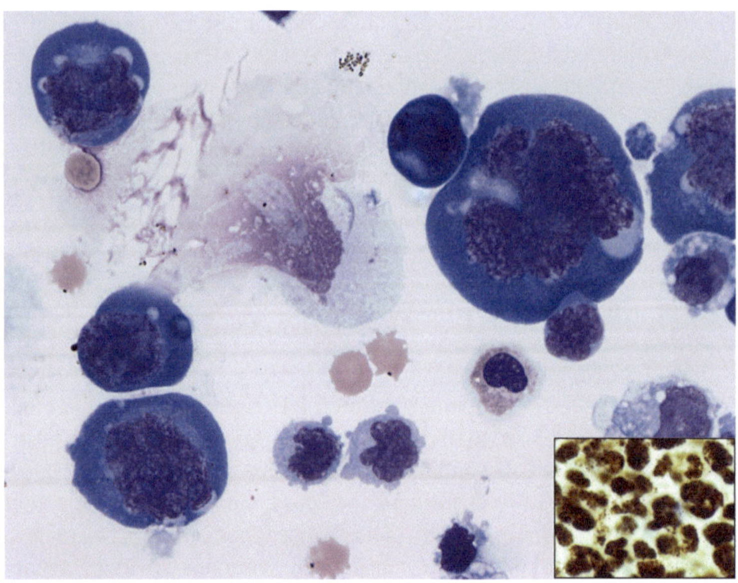

**Fig. 1.3** Primary effusion lymphoma (PEL). The neoplastic cells are large (see red cells and granulocyte in comparison) and pleomorphic, prominent large nucleoli, and abundant cytoplasm (Giemsa; 100× original magnification). The insert shows positivity for KSHV LANA by immunohistochemistry in a cell block

EBV and 22 % for hepatitis C virus (HCV). Where clinical information was available, all of these KSHV-negative cases occurred in HIV-negative individuals, and the patients had a median age at diagnosis of 74 years [111], consistent with the notion that that this is a different disease entity than PEL.

### 1.1.6 Plasmablastic Lymphoma (PBL)

This is a very aggressive malignancy that was first reported in the oral cavity of HIV-infected individuals [37] but subsequently was shown to occur in other sites, as well as in conjunction with other immunodeficient states [31]. This lymphoma subtype seems to be particularly common in HIV-infected patients in India, so there may be a particular geographic distribution [57]. The vast majority of cases in the oral cavity are EBV positive, but in other sites, up to 25 % of cases are EBV negative. The immunophenotype of these lymphomas resembles that of plasma cells, with expression of plasma cell antigens including MUM1 and CD138, but usually no expression of B-cell antigens like CD20 and CD79a. There is expression of monotypic cytoplasmic immunoglobulin in the majority of cases, which can be useful to distinguish PBL from PEL. The stringency of the criteria used for classification of these lesions has varied over time, with some studies using a very strict definition (such as presentation in the oral cavity and presence of EBV), which results in PBL being an extremely rare entity. However, a more general definition, provided by the 2008 WHO, includes both EBV-negative cases and extraoral presentation, as long as the morphology (as illustrated in Fig. 1.4) and immunophenotype are that of B immunoblasts or plasma cells [120], and thus according to these criteria, PBL is less rare. A recent report of five cases with a review of the literature identified 248 PBL cases, out of which 157 were in HIV-positive patients, 43 % were outside the oral cavity, and 86 % were EBV positive [33]. This is a highly aggressive tumor that responds poorly to all available therapies, with a median survival of around 14 months in HIV-positive patients. Approximately half of the cases have been shown to have a *MYC* translocation [129], and, at least according to this molecular study, there are no translocations as evidenced by fluorescent in situ hybridization (FISH) in the other common lymphoma-associated genes (*BCL2*, *BCL6*, *MALT1*, *PAX5*), although gains of some of these loci were found in over a third of the cases.

### 1.1.7 Polymorphic B-Cell Lymphoid Proliferations (Poly-LPDs)

These are very rare lesions that morphologically resemble the polymorphic post-transplantation lymphoproliferative disorders (PTLDs) seen in solid organ and bone marrow transplant recipients [88, 103]. HIV-poly-LPDs have been diagnosed in both HIV-positive adults and children [55, 89, 123, 133]. They are composed of a heterogeneous mixture of cells including lymphocytes, plasmacytoid lymphocytes, plasma cells, epithelioid histiocytes, and immunoblasts, the latter of which exhibit

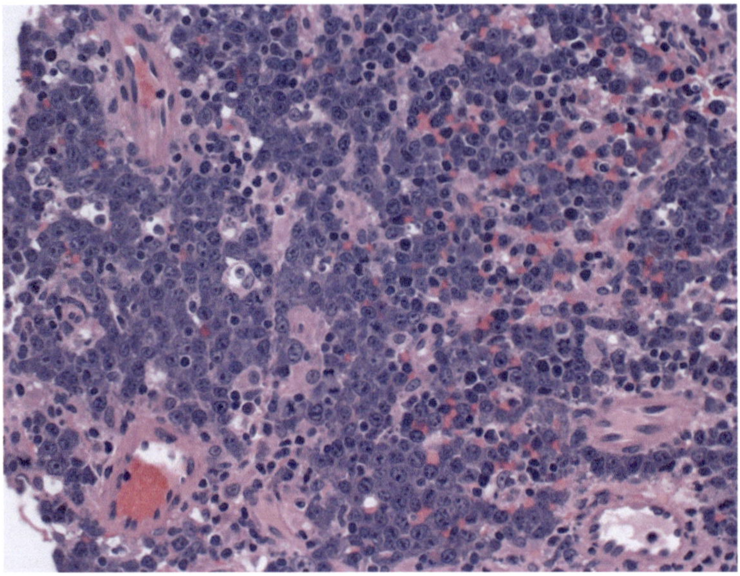

**Fig. 1.4** Plasmablastic lymphoma. This example plasmablastic lymphoma was from the anal region and shows sheets of cells with plasma cell features (hematoxylin and eosin, 40× original magnification)

a variable degree of cytologic atypia (Fig. 1.5). Foci of necrosis can also be seen within the lesions. In most cases, B cells account for the majority of the cells. Although in some cases contain polytypic B cells, most show a predominance of either kappa- or lambda-positive cells, while in some the B cells aberrantly express CD43 indicating the presence of an abnormal B-cell population. As with polymorphic PTLDs, most HIV-poly-LPDs are EBV positive [55, 83, 89, 123, 133]. Molecular genetic studies show that the vast majority of the HIV-poly-LPD cases are monoclonal based on either the presence of an immunoglobulin gene rearrangement or clonal EBV infection. In general structural alterations in oncogenes and tumor suppressor genes are rare but if present are associated with more aggressive disease behavior [89]. Although only limited clinical outcome information has been reported, patients who experienced regression of their HIV-poly-LPD following antiviral therapy have been reported [14, 83].

### 1.1.8 Lymphoma Arising in KSHV-Associated Multicentric Castleman Disease (MCD)

These are very rare lymphomas that mainly occur in HIV-positive patients [41]. Their original designation was of plasmablastic lymphoma [41], but they are a different disease entity from plasmablastic lymphomas associated with EBV infection

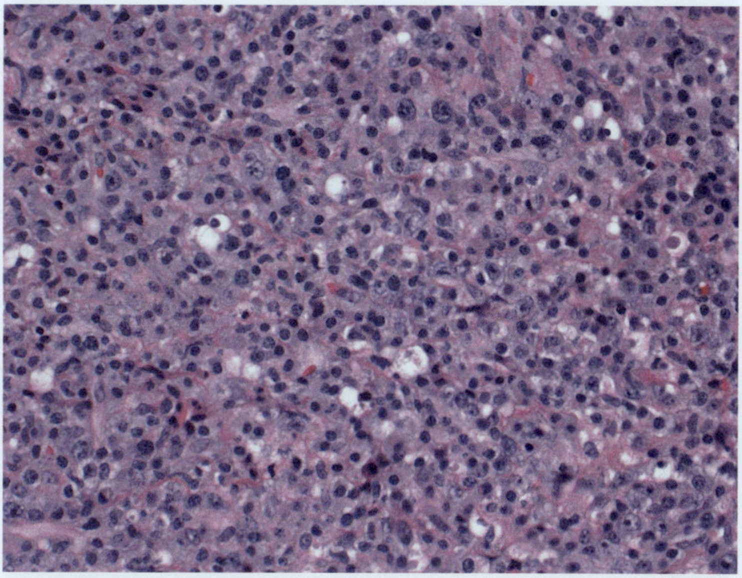

**Fig. 1.5** HIV-associated polymorphic lymphoproliferative disorder. Note the heterogeneous or polymorphic cell population which is composed of a mixture of cells including cells with plasmacytic differentiation and cells which are Reed-Sternberg like in appearance (hematoxylin and eosin, 40× original magnification)

(described above) as they are KSHV positive but EBV negative. Lymphomas arising in KSHV-associated MCD also have characteristics that differentiate them from PEL (and solid/extracavitary PEL): (i) they are KSHV+ but EBV negative; (ii) they express IgMλ cytoplasmic immunoglobulin (while PELs do not express Ig); (iii) there is a background of MCD in the involved lymph nodes; and (iv) they do not contain mutations in the immunoglobulin genes and therefore are thought to arise from naïve B cells rather than from terminally differentiated B cells as in PEL. A separate KSHV-associated lesion has also been reported, called germinotropic lymphoproliferative disorder, in which germinal center B cells are co-infected with EBV and KSHV [39].

## 1.2 Other Non-Hodgkin Lymphomas also Occurring in Immunocompetent Patients

Recent epidemiological studies have shown that although the risk of developing AIDS-defining NHL subtypes is very high compared to the general population, the risk of developing other types of lymphomas, including some T-cell lymphomas (SIR = 3.6–14.2), marginal zone lymphoma (SIR = 2.4), lymphoplasmacytic lymphoma/Waldenstrom macroglobulinemia (SIR = 3.6), and lymphoblastic leukemia/lymphoma (SIR = 2.4) is also elevated in the HIV patient population [53].

### 1.2.1 Anaplastic Large Cell Lymphoma (ALCL)

This non-AIDS-defining lymphoma is associated with one of the highest risks of development in HIV-positive patients (SIR = 14.2). Furthermore, ALCL accounts for approximately 20–30 % of the T-cell lymphomas in HIV-infected individuals [4, 19]. These lymphomas in the HIV-positive population are morphologically similar to those seen in HIV-negative patients where the lesions are composed of large pleomorphic cells, including hallmark cells and are bright CD30 positive and usually express CD4 (Fig. 1.6). However, in comparison to the HIV-negative population where a large proportion of the cases are ALK1 positive and usually EBV negative, ALCL lesions in HIV-positive individuals are ALK-1 negative based on immunostaining, and approximately one third of cases are positive for EBV [98]. Although HIV-associated ALCL can occur in the lymph nodes, virtually all patients have extranodal disease, most frequently involving the lung, liver, and spleen, soft tissue, skin, and bone marrow. Lesions in unusual sites, such as the gingiva, have also been reported [50, 98, 108, 109].

The majority of the HIV-positive individuals who develop ALCL are men (ratio 3.5–4:1) with a mean age of 38 years (range of 1–76 years) [98, 109]. Most HIV-positive ALCL patients are significantly immunosuppressed with a mean CD4 count, based on a large review, of less than 100/dL [98]. The disease is aggressive with approximately 70–75 % of HIV-positive ALCL patients dying, usually of either lymphoma or infectious complications [98, 108, 109].

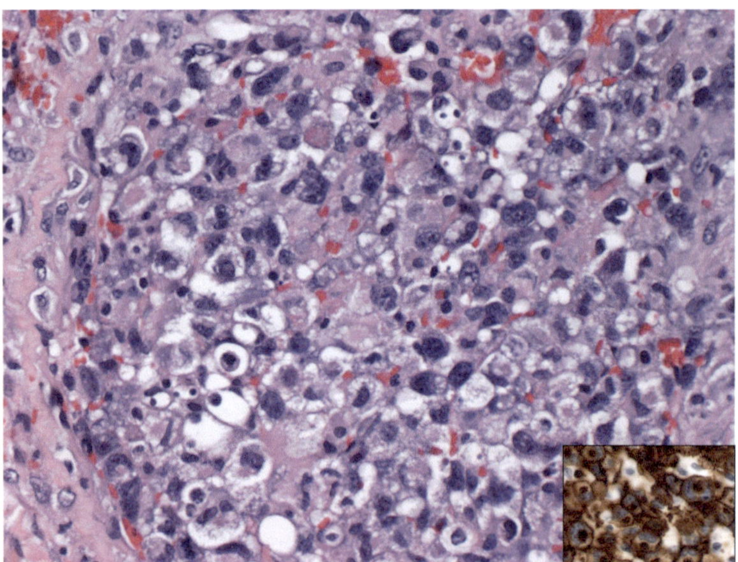

**Fig. 1.6** Anaplastic large cell lymphoma, ALK negative. Note the presence of "hallmark" cells and the bright CD30 expression (*inset*) by the neoplastic cells (hematoxylin and eosin, 40× original magnification; inset, immunoperoxidase, 40× original magnification)

## 1.3 Other Non-AIDS-Defining Hematological Malignancies

As patients are living longer with HIV infection, a number of malignancies in these patients are becoming more frequent, including carcinomas, such as the colon, breast, lung, and prostate [96]. Hematological malignancies not typically associated with AIDS have also been emerging, and HIV-infected patients with leukemias and CLL have been reported. A study in Japan identified 47 patients with non-AIDS-defining hematological malignancies [58], and these types of cases have also been reported in Africa [86]. However, the literature on these diseases in HIV+ patients is often limited to small series and case reports. The following paragraphs are an overview of the pathology of some of the most common myeloid disorders, leukemias and myeloma, and when available, specific characteristics of cases reported in patients with HIV infection.

### 1.3.1 Acute Myeloid Leukemia

Although epidemiologic studies in the United States and Italy do not indicate an increased standard incidence rate (SIR) of AML in HIV-infected persons, studies from France showed that the risk of AML in HIV-positive patients is twice that of the general population [43, 102, 121]. Acute myeloid leukemia can occur in patients of any HIV-risk group including sexually transmitted, transfusion-related, and drug use-risk groups and at any stage of HIV disease [2, 61]. AML can develop at any age in HIV-positive patients, including children; however, the mean and median age at diagnosis is approximately 40 years [2, 44, 61, 119, 121, 128]. Although many of the cases are classified as acute myeloid leukemia, not otherwise specified, cases of acute myeloid leukemia from all categories in the 2008 WHO classification, including cases of acute myeloid leukemia with recurrent genetic abnormalities, such as t(8;21), t(15;17), inv(16)(p13.1q22), and t(3;3), acute myeloid leukemia with myelodysplasia-related changes, and therapy-related myeloid neoplasms have been described (Fig. 1.7) [2, 10, 44, 61, 82, 121]. There appears, however, to be relatively large number of cases which are classified morphologically as acute myeloid leukemia with maturation (FAB M2) and acute myelomonocytic leukemia (FAB M4), with or without the associated genetic alterations of t(8;21) and inv(16) [2, 61, 121]. Cases of myeloid sarcoma have also been reported [32, 81, 107].

The majority of the HIV-positive patients with AML who are treated with induction chemotherapy go into clinical remission, but many subsequently relapse. Although in general the prognosis for HIV-positive AML patients is poor, long-term clinical remissions (approximately 10 years) have been reported in the literature. As with diffuse large B-cell lymphoma, the level of immunosuppression as reflected by the CD4 count appears to be an important prognostic indicator. Patients with CD4 counts less than 200/dL have much shorter survival times than those with a CD4 count greater than 200/dL at diagnosis [2, 44, 121]. In addition, AMLs with an unfavorable karyotype are associated with a worse prognosis [44].

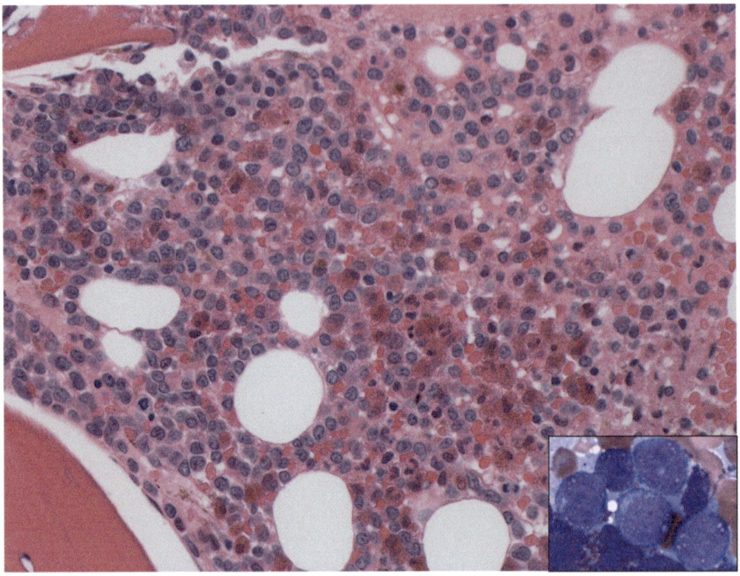

**Fig. 1.7** Acute myeloid leukemia. This acute myeloid leukemia in a HIV-positive patient was myeloperoxidase, CD13, CD33, CD15, CD34, and CD117 positive and exhibited a complex karyotype (hematoxylin and eosin, 40× original magnification; insert Giemsa 100× original magnification)

### 1.3.2 Chronic Myelogenous Leukemia

BCR-ABL-1 positive chronic myelogenous leukemia (CML) can occur in both HIV-positive children and adults with a median age at diagnosis in the mid-to-late 30s, although some studies, predominately in western countries, show it to be a more of a disease in older patients [61, 76, 78, 95, 114, 130]. Most case reports and small series from Europe and the United States show CML occurring predominately in HIV-positive men, while studies from South Africa show a male to female ratio in the HIV-positive patient population closer to that of HIV-negative individuals with CML [78, 95]. The occurrence of CML in HIV-positive patients is thought to be coincidental; in one large institution in South Africa, only 18 HIV-positive patients developed CML, representing only 7.5 % of all CML diagnoses, over a 20-year period, while in another institution in the United States, only three cases were diagnosed over a 6 year period [95, 114].

Morphologically, cases of CML, chronic phase, in HIV-positive patients show similar findings as seen in HIV-negative patients, both in the peripheral blood (including leukocytosis with a leftward shift and basophilia) and in the bone marrow (hypercellularity with myeloid hyperplasia, increased myeloblasts, and megakaryocytic hyperplasia) [114]. Conventional cytogenetics and/or FISH shows t(9;22) with or without additional abnormalities [61, 95, 114]. In most cases the HIV-positive patients are in the chronic phase at diagnosis; however, some are in the accelerated phase or blast phase at diagnosis [95]. It is thought that CML may behave more aggressively in HIV-positive patients, as reported in a relatively large series from South Africa, presenting with greater splenomegaly, more advanced disease based on the Sokal score and a higher incidence of accelerated/blast phase than their HIV-negative counterparts [95]. The treatment of CML in all patients, including those that are HIV positive, has been transformed with the introduction of tyrosine kinase inhibitors (TKIs). However, drug-drug interactions between antiretroviral medications and TKIs, therapies that may use the same enzymes in metabolism, are thought to be important [36]. Although TKIs have improved outcomes in HIV-positive patients with CML, there are reports of poorer responses to TKIs compared to HIV-negative patients as well as indications that some patients on CART and imatinib who have achieved a major response with respect to the their CML have experienced a decrease in their CD4 count [95, 114]. In addition, in some HIV+ patients on CART, TKIs can be associated with anemia [114].

### 1.3.3 Polycythemia Vera and Primary Myelofibrosis

The incidence of these diseases in the HIV+ patient population is very low [7, 34, 42, 72, 113, 134]. Many, but not all, of the reported HIV+ patients with polycythemia vera appear to have secondary polycythemia, whether due to smoking, testosterone administration, or, possibly, antiretroviral therapy [7, 34, 42, 61, 72, 113, 132, 134]. Thus, the incidence of primary polycythemia vera is exceedingly small, and the optimal treatment in HIV positive patients is not clear including the efficacy of CART [34, 42, 72, 113, 134]. There are, however, rare case reports of HIV-positive patients with polycythemia who have experienced transformation to acute leukemia [61]. In addition, primary myelofibrosis is very rare with only scattered case reports in the literature [34].

### 1.3.4 Myelodysplastic Syndrome (MDS)

Only a small number of well-documented cases of HIV myelodysplasia (HIV-MDS) are reported in the literature, and it is often difficult to determine which cases are MDS or HIV-related myelopathy (HIV-MP). Many of the morphologic changes seen in HIV bone marrows are reminiscent to the changes seen in MDS including megaloblastoid hematopoiesis, hypercellularity, and megakaryocytic dysplasia [66, 67]. However, several studies evaluating bone marrow samples from HIV-infected individuals in comparison to HIV-negative patients with MDS have shown that there are differences between the two clinical settings, including the presence of more atypical micromegakaryocytes in HIV-negative MDS and the lack of severe nuclear lobulation abnormalities (i.e. pseudo-Pelger forms) in mature neutrophils as well as the absence of nuclear bridging in erythroblasts in HIV-MP [67, 124, 125]. Furthermore, in HIV-negative MDS, an increase in blasts and cytogenetic abnormalities are often found which is usually not the case for HIV-MP [64, 67].

Clinically, the HIV-negative patients less often respond to erythropoietin administration and experience progression of their disease, while the opposite is true for the HIV-MP patients [67].

The clearly documented cases of HIV-MDS are clinically and pathologically different than HIV-MP [67, 106, 122]. Similar to their HIV-negative MDS counterparts, these myeloid neoplasms in HIV-positive patients usually have cytogenetic abnormalities (when examined) and, where there is sufficient follow-up, often progress to acute leukemia. However, in contrast to primary HIV-negative MDS, where the incidence of monosomy 7 or del(7q) is approximately 10 % [12], in HIV-MDS chromosome, 7 abnormalities have been seen in 9/13 (approximately 70 %) of the evaluated cases [106, 122]. In addition, one study showed that the mean age at presentation is younger (55 vs. 65 years), the incidence of progression to acute leukemia is higher (63 % vs. 26 %), and the median survival shorter (8 vs. 22 months) for the HIV-MDS patients compared to their HIV-negative counterparts [122].

### 1.3.5 Acute Lymphoblastic Leukemia

Although there appears to be no significant association between HIV infection and acute lymphoblastic leukemia in some countries where studies have been done, such as Uganda [90], in the United States the incidence of all precursor lymphoid neoplasms in HIV-positive individuals is increased (SIR = 2.4) compared to their immunocompetent counterparts [53]. Furthermore, a recent study from Japan showed that lymphoblastic leukemias account for approximately 15 % of non-AIDS-defining hematologic malignancies in HIV-positive patients [58]. Acute lymphoblastic leukemia can occur in both HIV-positive children and HIV-positive adults and can be of either B- or T-cell phenotype [29, 46, 51, 52, 68, 77, 79, 90, 99, 100, 119, 126]. In addition, a rare case of HIV-associated Ph + ALL has been also reported [126]. In most instances, these precursor lesions are composed of lymphoblasts with finely dispersed chromatin, inconspicuous nucleoli, and scant cytoplasm and, where reported, have been found to be TdT and/or CD34 positive [29, 46, 52, 68, 77, 79, 100, 126]. However, care must be taken when reading the literature as many of the B acute lymphoblastic leukemias reported during early in the AIDS epidemic were actually Burkitt lymphoma in the peripheral blood. Although many patients die of their disease or complications of treatment [46, 51, 77, 79, 99], some patients with multiagent chemotherapy with or without transplant can experience long-term survivals [119, 126].

### 1.3.6 Chronic Lymphocytic Leukemia/Small Lymphocytic Lymphoma (CLL/SLL)

CLL/SLL is an uncommon malignancy in the HIV patient population. In Japan, only one case of CLL in a HIV-positive individual was reported between 1991 and 2010, while in a single university teaching institution in Nigeria, only 4 % of all CLL cases between 1993 and 2008 occurred in HIV-positive persons [9, 58]. In the United States, only 1.1 % of all HIV-associated lymphomas diagnosed between 1996 and 2000 were CLL [53]. However, this is somewhat increased compared to a single-institution series between 1982 and 2000 where only 2 out of 410 (0.5 %) HIV-associated lymphomas were CLL/SLL [74]. Unfortunately, the CART status of the CLL patients in these studies from the United States is not reported [53, 74]. As the CLL patients are usually included in larger group studies, it is difficult to determine clinical characteristics and outcomes of the patients. However, the three patients reported from Nigeria were all females, median age of 56, who presented with high stage disease; all died within a few weeks of diagnosis. A well-documented case study from the United States, with phenotypic and genotypic data, described a 65-year-old man who initially presented with indolent disease, went untreated for 7 months, and subsequently developed aggressive disease, dying approximately 2.5 years after diagnosis [104]. A small number of CLL cases of T-cell phenotype have also been reported. All of these cases were found to be composed of suppressor/cytotoxic T cells [65, 71].

### 1.3.7 Plasma Cell Myeloma

The definition of plasma cell myeloma according to the 2008 WHO is "a bone marrow-based, multifocal plasma cell neoplasm associated with an M-protein in serum and/or urine" [87]. The diagnosis is based on a combination of pathological, radiological, and clinical features. These latter features include the presence of clonal plasma cells as well as related organ or tissue impairment such as hypercalcemia, renal insufficiency, anemia, and bone lesions [87]. Based on these criteria, the diagnosis of plasma cell myeloma in HIV-positive patients can be difficult as some to many of the diagnostic findings in this clinicopathologic entity can be also seen as a secondary events due to HIV infection, opportunistic infection, or therapy [45]. For example, studies have found that 23–83 % of HIV patient bone marrow samples exhibit plasmacytosis [18, 66, 92], and between 2.5 and 56 % of all HIV patients have monoclonal or mono-/oligoclonal serum proteins (MGUS) [27, 45]. Furthermore, many HIV-positive patients are anemic or have renal insufficiency secondary to HIV infection or other causes [45, 92].

Plasma cell myeloma is thought to account for approximately 0.01–0.03 % of all neoplasms in HIV-infected individuals [47, 49, 56]. However, it is not clear if the risk or incidence of plasma cell myeloma in HIV-positive patients is increased [27, 38, 47, 49, 56]. It does appear that the median age at diagnosis of plasma cell myeloma/plasmacytoma in the HIV patient population is significantly lower, approximately 32 years [45, 91, 97], compared to HIV-negative individuals where the median age at diagnosis of plasma cell myeloma is about 70 years [87]. The relative risk of patients with HIV and plasma cell myeloma dying is threefold that of HIV-negative patients [115].

## References

1. A review of human carcinogens, Part B: Biological agents. IARC Monographs on the evaluation of carcinogenic risks to humans. Lyon: World Health Organization International Agency for Research on Cancer; 2012.
2. Aboulafia DM, Meneses M, Ginsberg S, Siegel MS, Howard WW, Dezube BJ. Acute myeloid leukemia in patients infected with HIV-1. AIDS. 2002;16:865–76.
3. Arvey A, Ojesina AI, Pedamallu CS, Ballon G, Jung J, Duke F, Leoncini L, de Falco G, Bressman E, Tam W, Chadburn A, Meyerson M, Cesarman E. The tumor virus landscape of AIDS-related lymphomas. Blood. 2015;125:e14–22.
4. Arzoo KK, Bu X, Espina BM, Seneviratne L, Nathwani B, Levine AM. T-cell lymphoma in HIV-infected patients. J Acquir Immune Defic Syndr. 2004;36:1020–7.
5. Ashihara E, Shimazaki C, Hirai H, Inaba T, Hasegawa G, Mori S, Nakagawa M. Human herpes virus 8-negative primary effusion lymphoma in a patient with a ventriculoperitoneal shunt tube. Int J Hematol. 2001;74:327–32.
6. Asou H, Said JW, Yang R, Munker R, Park DJ, Kamada N, Koeffler HP. Mechanisms of growth control of Kaposi's sarcoma-associated herpes virus-associated primary effusion lymphoma cells. Blood. 1998;91:2475–81.
7. Battan R, Ottaviano P, Porcelli M, Distenfeld A. Polycythaemia in patient with AIDS. Lancet. 1990;335:1342–3.
8. Bhatia K, Huppi K, Spangler G, Siwarski D, Iyer R, Magrath I. Point mutations in the c-Myc transactivation domain are common in Burkitt's lymphoma and mouse plasmacytomas. Nat Genet. 1993;5:56–61.
9. Bolarinwa RA, Ndakotsu MA, Oyekunle AA, Salawu L, Akinola NO, Durosinmi MA. AIDS-related lymphomas in Nigeria. Braz J Infect Dis. 2009;13:359–61.
10. Breccia M, Gentile G, Martino P, Petti MC, Russo E, Mancini M, Alimena G. Acute myeloid leukemia secondary to a myelodysplastic syndrome with t(3;3) (q21;q26) in an HIV patient treated with chemotherapy and highly active antiretroviral therapy. Acta Haematol. 2004;111:160–2.
11. Breen EC, Hussain SK, Magpantay L, Jacobson LP, Detels R, Rabkin CS, Kaslow RA, Variakojis D, Bream JH, Rinaldo CR, Ambinder RF, Martinez-Maza O. B-cell stimulatory cytokines and markers of immune activation are elevated several years prior to the diagnosis of systemic AIDS-associated non-Hodgkin B-cell lymphoma. Cancer Epidemiol Biomarkers Prev. 2011;20:1303–14.
12. Brunning RD, Orazi A, Germing U, Le Beau MM, Porwit A, Baumann I, Vardiman J, Hellstrom-Lindberg E. Myelodysplastic syndromes/neoplasms. In: Swerdlow SH, Campo E, Harris NL, Jaffe ES, Pileri SA, Stein H, Thiele J, editors. WHO classification of tumours of haematopoietic and lymphoid tissues. Lyon: IARC Press; 2008.
13. Burns BF, Wood GS, Dorfman RF. The varied histopathology of lymphadenopathy in the homosexual male. Am J Surg Pathol. 1985;9:287–97.
14. Buxton J, Leen C, Goodlad JR. Polymorphic lymphoid proliferations occurring in HIV-positive patients: report of a case responding to HAART. Virchows Arch. 2012;461:93–8.
15. Carbone A. Emerging pathways in the development of AIDS-related lymphomas. Lancet Oncol. 2003;4:22–9.
16. Carbone A, Gloghini A, Serraino D, Spina M. HIV-associated Hodgkin lymphoma. Curr Opin HIV AIDS. 2009;4:3–10.
17. Carbone A, Tirelli U, Gloghini A, Volpe R, Boiocchi M. Human immunodeficiency virus-associated systemic lymphomas may be subdivided into two main groups according to Epstein-Barr viral latent gene expression. J Clin Oncol. 1993;11:1674–81.
18. Castella A, Croxson TS, Mildvan D, Witt DH, Zalusky R. The bone marrow in AIDS. A histologic, hematologic, and microbiologic study. Am J Clin Pathol. 1985;84:425–32.
19. Castillo JJ, Beltran BE, Bibas M, Bower M, Collins JA, Cwynarski K, Diez-Martin JL, Hernandez-Ilizaliturri F, Horwitz SM, Montoto S, Pantanowitz L, Ribera JM, Vose JM. Prognostic factors in patients with HIV-associated peripheral T-cell lymphoma: a multicenter study. Am J Hematol. 2011;86:256–61.

20. Cesarman E. Gammaherpesvirus and lymphoproliferative disorders in immunocompromised patients. Cancer Lett. 2011;305:163–74.
21. Cesarman E, Chang Y, Moore PS, Said JW, Knowles DM. Kaposi's Sarcoma-associated Herpesvirus-like DNA sequences in AIDS-related body cavity-based lymphomas. N Eng J Med. 1995;332:1186–91.
22. Cesarman E, Dalla-Favera R, Bentley D, Groudine M. Mutations in the first exon are associated with altered transcription of c-myc in Burkitt lymphoma. Science. 1987;238:1272–5.
23. Chadburn A, Chiu A, Lee JY, Chen X, Hyjek E, Banham AH, Noy A, Kaplan LD, Sparano JA, Bhatia K, Cesarman E. Immunophenotypic analysis of AIDS-related diffuse large B-cell lymphoma and clinical implications in patients from AIDS Malignancies Consortium clinical trials 010 and 034. J Clin Oncol. 2009;27:5039–48.
24. Chadburn A, Hyjek E, Mathew S, Cesarman E, Said J, Knowles DM. KSHV-positive solid lymphomas represent an extra-cavitary variant of primary effusion lymphoma. Am J Surg Pathol. 2004;28:1401–16.
25. Chadburn A, Noy A, Lee JY, Hyjek E, Banham AH, Sparano JA, Bhatia K, Cesarman E. Reply to K Dunleavy et al. J Clin Oncol. 2010;28:e261–2.
26. Chao C, Silverberg MJ, Martinez-Maza O, Chi M, Abrams DI, Haque R, Zha HD, Mcguire M, Xu L, Said J. Epstein-Barr virus infection and expression of B-cell oncogenic markers in HIV-related diffuse large B-cell lymphoma. Clin Cancer Res. 2012;18:4702–12.
27. Chiao EY, Krown SE. Update on non-acquired immunodeficiency syndrome-defining malignancies. Curr Opin Oncol. 2003;15:389–97.
28. Choi WW, Weisenburger DD, Greiner TC, Piris MA, Banham AH, Delabie J, Braziel RM, Geng H, Iqbal J, Lenz G, Vose JM, Hans CP, Fu K, Smith LM, Li M, Liu Z, Gascoyne RD, Rosenwald A, Ott G, Rimsza LM, Campo E, Jaffe ES, Jaye DL, Staudt LM, Chan WC. A new immunostain algorithm classifies diffuse large B-cell lymphoma into molecular subtypes with high accuracy. Clin Cancer Res. 2009;15:5494–502.
29. Ciobanu N, Andreeff M, Safai B, Koziner B, Mertelsmann R. Lymphoblastic neoplasia in a homosexual patient with Kaposi's sarcoma. Ann Intern Med. 1983;98:151–5.
30. Clifford GM, Polesel J, Rickenbach M, Dal Maso L, Keiser O, Kofler A, Rapiti E, Levi F, Jundt G, Fisch T, Bordoni A, de Weck D, Franceschi S. Cancer risk in the Swiss HIV Cohort Study: associations with immunodeficiency, smoking, and highly active antiretroviral therapy. J Natl Cancer Inst. 2005;97:425–32.
31. Colomo L, Loong F, Rives S, Pittaluga S, Martinez A, Lopez-Guillermo A, Ojanguren J, Romagosa V, Jaffe ES, Campo E. Diffuse large B-cell lymphomas with plasmablastic differentiation represent a heterogeneous group of disease entities. Am J Surg Pathol. 2004;28:736–47.
32. Colovic N, Jurisic V, Terzic T, Jevtovic D, Colovic M. Alveolar granulocytic sarcoma of the mandible in a patient with HIV. Onkologie. 2011;34:55–8.
33. Corti M, Villafane MF, Bistmans A, Campitelli A, Narbaitz M, Bare P. Oral cavity and extra-oral plasmablastic lymphomas in AIDS patients: report of five cases and review of the literature. Int J STD AIDS. 2011;22:759–63.
34. Darne C, Solal-Celigny P, Herrera A, Ramond MJ, Brun-Vezinet F, Brousse N, Boivin P. Acute myelofibrosis and infection with the lymphadenopathy-associated virus/human T-lymphotropic virus type III. Ann Intern Med. 1986;104:130–1.
35. Dave SS, Fu K, Wright GW, Lam LT, Kluin P, Boerma EJ, Greiner TC, Weisenburger DD, Rosenwald A, Ott G, Muller-Hermelink HK, Gascoyne RD, Delabie J, Rimsza LM, Braziel RM, Grogan TM, Campo E, Jaffe ES, Dave BJ, Sanger W, Bast M, Vose JM, Armitage JO, Connors JM, Smeland EB, Kvaloy S, Holte H, Fisher RI, Miller TP, Montserrat E, Wilson WH, Bahl M, Zhao H, Yang L, Powell J, Simon R, Chan WC, Staudt LM. Molecular diagnosis of Burkitt's lymphoma. N Engl J Med. 2006;354:2431–42.
36. Deeken JF, Pantanowitz L, Dezube BJ. Targeted therapies to treat non-AIDS-defining cancers in patients with HIV on HAART therapy: treatment considerations and research outlook. Curr Opin Oncol. 2009;21:445–54.
37. Delecluse HJ, Anagnostopoulos I, Dallenbach F, Hummel M, Marafioti T, Schneider U, Huhn D, Schmidt-Westhausen A, Reichart PA, Gross U, Stein H. Plasmablastic lymphomas

of the oral cavity: a new entity associated with the human immunodeficiency virus infection. Blood. 1997;89:1413–20.
38. Dezube BJ, Aboulafia DM, Pantanowitz L. Plasma cell disorders in HIV-infected patients: from benign gammopathy to multiple myeloma. AIDS Read. 2004;14:372–4, 377–9.
39. Du MQ, Diss TC, Liu H, Ye H, Hamoudi RA, Cabecadas J, Dong HY, Harris NL, Chan JK, Rees JW, Dogan A, Isaacson PG. KSHV- and EBV-associated germinotropic lymphoproliferative disorder. Blood. 2002;100:3415–8.
40. Dunleavy K, Wilson WH. Role of molecular subtype in predicting outcome of AIDS-related diffuse large B-cell lymphoma. J Clin Oncol. 2010;28, e260.
41. Dupin N, Diss TL, Kellam P, Tulliez M, Du MQ, Sicard D, Weiss RA, Isaacson PG, Boshoff C. HHV-8 is associated with a plasmablastic variant of Castleman disease that is linked to HHV-8-positive plasmablastic lymphoma. Blood. 2000;95:1406–12.
42. Edwards TB, Nelson RP, Ballester OF, Saba HI, Lockey RF. Polycythemia as a complication of human immunodeficiency virus infection. South Med J. 1993;86:686–8.
43. Engels EA, Biggar RJ, Hall HI, Cross H, Crutchfield A, Finch JL, Grigg R, Hylton T, Pawlish KS, Mcneel TS, Goedert JJ. Cancer risk in people infected with human immunodeficiency virus in the United States. Int J Cancer. 2008;123:187–94.
44. Evans MW, Sung AD, Gojo I, Tidwell M, Greer J, Levis M, Karp J, Baer MR. Risk assessment in human immunodeficiency virus-associated acute myeloid leukemia. Leuk Lymphoma. 2012;53:660–4.
45. Fiorino AS, Atac B. Paraproteinemia, plasmacytoma, myeloma and HIV infection. Leukemia. 1997;11:2150–6.
46. Flanagan P, Chowdhury V, Costello C. HIV-associated B cell ALL. Br J Haematol. 1988;69:287.
47. Frisch M, Biggar RJ, Engels EA, Goedert JJ, Group, A. I.-C. M. R. S. Association of cancer with AIDS-related immunosuppression in adults. JAMA. 2001;285:1736–45.
48. Gaidano G, Carbone A, Dalla-Favera R. Genetic basis of acquired immunodeficiency syndrome-related lymphomagenesis. J Natl Cancer Inst Monogr. 1998;23:95–100.
49. Gallagher B, Wang Z, Schymura MJ, Kahn A, Fordyce EJ. Cancer incidence in New York State acquired immunodeficiency syndrome patients. Am J Epidemiol. 2001;154:544–56.
50. Genet P, Chaoui D, Masse V, Al Jijakli A, Arakelyan N, Sutton L. Anaplastic large cell lymphoma occurring in an HIV-positive patient. Case Rep Hematol. 2012;2012:180204.
51. Geriniere L, Bastion Y, Dumontet C, Salles G, Espinouse D, Coiffier B. Heterogeneity of acute lymphoblastic leukemia in HIV-seropositive patients. Ann Oncol. 1994;5:437–40.
52. Ghosh M, Banerjee M, Chakraborty S, Bhattacharyya S. Successful outcome in a HIV infected child presenting with Pre-B Acute Lymphoblastic Leukemia. Indian J Pediatr. 2012;79:267–9.
53. Gibson TM, Morton LM, Shiels MS, Clarke CA, Engels EA. Risk of non-Hodgkin lymphoma subtypes in HIV-infected people during the HAART era: a population-based study. AIDS. 2014;28:2313–8.
54. Glaser SL, Clarke CA, Gulley ML, Craig FE, Digiuseppe JA, Dorfman RF, Mann RB, Ambinder RF. Population-based patterns of human immunodeficiency virus-related Hodgkin lymphoma in the Greater San Francisco Bay Area, 1988–1998. Cancer. 2003;98:300–9.
55. Grogg KL, Miller RF, Dogan A. HIV infection and lymphoma. J Clin Pathol. 2007;60:1365–72.
56. Grulich AE, Wan X, Law MG, Coates M, Kaldor JM. Risk of cancer in people with AIDS. AIDS. 1999;13:839–43.
57. Gujral S, Shet TM, Kane SV. Morphological spectrum of AIDS-related plasmablastic lymphomas. Indian J Pathol Microbiol. 2008;51:121–4.
58. Hagiwara S, Yotsumoto M, Odawara T, Ajisawa A, Uehira T, Nagai H, Tanuma J, Okada S. Non-AIDS-defining hematological malignancies in HIV-infected patients: an epidemiological study in Japan. AIDS. 2013;27:279–83.
59. Hall JS, Usher S, Byers RJ, Higgins RC, Memon D, Radford JA, Linton KM. QuantiGene plex represents a promising diagnostic tool for cell-of-origin subtyping of diffuse large B-cell lymphoma. J Mol Diagn. 2015;17:402–11.

60. Hans CP, Weisenburger DD, Greiner TC, Gascoyne RD, Delabie J, Ott G, Muller-Hermelink HK, Campo E, Braziel RM, Jaffe ES, Pan Z, Farinha P, Smith LM, Falini B, Banham AH, Rosenwald A, Staudt LM, Connors JM, Armitage JO, Chan WC. Confirmation of the molecular classification of diffuse large B-cell lymphoma by immunohistochemistry using a tissue microarray. Blood. 2004;103:275–82.
61. Hentrich M, Rockstroh J, Sandner R, Brack N, Hartenstein R. Acute myelogenous leukaemia and myelomonocytic blast crisis following polycythemia vera in HIV positive patients: report of cases and review of the literature. Ann Oncol. 2000;11:195–200.
62. Hummel M, Bentink S, Berger H, Klapper W, Wessendorf S, Barth TF, Bernd HW, Cogliatti SB, Dierlamm J, Feller AC, Hansmann ML, Haralambieva E, Harder L, Hasenclever D, Kuhn M, Lenze D, Lichter P, Martin-Subero JI, Moller P, Muller-Hermelink HK, Ott G, Parwaresch RM, Pott C, Rosenwald A, Rosolowski M, Schwaenen C, Sturzenhofecker B, Szczepanowski M, Trautmann H, Wacker HH, Spang R, Loeffler M, Trumper L, Stein H, Siebert R. A biologic definition of Burkitt's lymphoma from transcriptional and genomic profiling. N Engl J Med. 2006;354:2419–30.
63. Hussain SK, Zhu W, Chang SC, Breen EC, Vendrame E, Magpantay L, Widney D, Conn D, Sehl M, Jacobson LP, Bream JH, Wolinsky S, Rinaldo CR, Ambinder RF, Detels R, Zhang ZF, Martinez-Maza O. Serum levels of the chemokine CXCL13, genetic variation in CXCL13 and its receptor CXCR5, and HIV-associated non-hodgkin B-cell lymphoma risk. Cancer Epidemiol Biomarkers Prev. 2013;22:295–307.
64. Kaloutsi V, Kohlmeyer U, Maschek H, Nafe R, Choritz H, Amor A, Georgii A. Comparison of bone marrow and hematologic findings in patients with human immunodeficiency virus infection and those with myelodysplastic syndromes and infectious diseases. Am J Clin Pathol. 1994;101:123–9.
65. Kaplan MH, Susin M, Pahwa SG, Fetten J, Allen SL, Lichtman S, Sarngadharan MG, Gallo RC. Neoplastic complications of HTLV-III infection. Lymphomas and solid tumors. Am J Med. 1987;82:389–96.
66. Karcher DS, Frost AR. The bone marrow in human immunodeficiency virus (HIV)-related disease. Morphology and clinical correlation. Am J Clin Pathol. 1991;95:63–71.
67. Katsarou O, Terpos E, Patsouris E, Peristeris P, Viniou N, Kapsimali V, Karafoulidou A. Myelodysplastic features in patients with long-term HIV infection and haemophilia. Haemophilia. 2001;7:47–52.
68. Katzel JA, Kempin SJ, Lagmay-Fuentes P, Cook WA, Siegal FP, Henriquez LE, Lee MH, Vesole DH. Therapy-related leukemia in patients with human immunodeficiency virus infection after treatment for non-Hodgkin lymphoma. Am J Hematol. 2008;83:937–8.
69. Kluin PM, Harris NL, Stein H, Leoncini L, Raphael M, Campo E, Jaffe ES. B-cell lymphoma, unclassifiable, with features intermediate between diffuse large B-cell lymphoma and Burkitt lymphoma. In: Swerdlow SH, Campo E, Harris NL, Jaffe ES, Pileri SA, Stein H, Thiele J, editors. WHO classification of tumours of haematopoietic and lymphoid tissues. Lyon: IARC Press; 2008.
70. Knowles DM. Neoplastic hematopathology. Baltimore: Williams and Wilkins; 2001.
71. Knowles DM, Chamulak GA, Subar M, Burke JS, Dugan M, Wernz J, Slywitzky C, Pelicci P-G, Dalla-Favera R, Raphael B. Lymphoid neoplasia associated with the acquired immunodeficiency syndrome (AIDS). Ann Intern Med. 1988;108:744–53.
72. Koduri PR, Sherer R, Teter C. Polycythemia in patients infected with human immunodeficiency virus-1. Am J Hematol. 2000;64:80–1.
73. Kundu RK, Sangiorgi F, Wu LY, Pattengale PK, Hinton DR, Gill PS, Maxson R. Expression of the human immunodeficiency virus-Tat gene in lymphoid tissues of transgenic mice is associated with B-cell lymphoma. Blood. 1999;94:275–82.
74. Levine AM, Sadeghi S, Espina B, Tulpule A, Nathwani B. Characteristics of indolent non-Hodgkin lymphoma in patients with type 1 human immunodeficiency virus infection. Cancer. 2002;94:1500–6.
75. Liapis K, Clear A, Owen A, Coutinho R, Greaves P, Lee AM, Montoto S, Calaminici M, Gribben JG. The microenvironment of AIDS-related diffuse large B-cell lymphoma provides

insight into the pathophysiology and indicates possible therapeutic strategies. Blood. 2013;122:424–33.

76. Lorand-Metze I, Morais SL, Souza CA. Chronic myeloid leukemia in a homosexual HIV-seropositive man. AIDS. 1990;4:923–4.
77. Lorenzon D, Perin T, Bulian P, De Re V, Caggiari L, Michieli M, Manuele R, Spina M, Gattei V, Fasan M, Tirelli U, Canzonieri V. Human immunodeficiency virus-associated precursor T-lymphoblastic leukemia/lymphoblastic lymphoma: report of a case and review of the literature. Hum Pathol. 2009;40:1045–9.
78. Louw VJ. Chronic myeloid leukaemia in South Africa. Hematology. 2012;17 Suppl 1:S75–8.
79. Lum GH, Cosgriff TM, Byrne R, Reddy V. Primary T-cell lymphoma of muscle in a patient infected with human immunodeficiency virus. Am J Med. 1993;95:545–6.
80. Luzzi A, Morettini F, Gazaneo S, Mundo L, Onnis A, Mannucci S, Rogena EA, Bellan C, Leoncini L, de Falco G. HIV-1 Tat induces DNMT over-expression through microRNA dysregulation in HIV-related non Hodgkin lymphomas. Infect Agent Cancer. 2014;9:41.
81. Manfredi R, Sabbatani S, Chiodo F. Advanced acute myelogenous leukaemia (AML) during HAART-treated HIV disease, manifesting initially as a thyroid mass. Scand J Infect Dis. 2005;37:781–3.
82. Mani D, Dorer RK, Aboulafia DM. Therapy-related acute myeloid leukemia following HIV-associated lymphoma. Clin Lymphoma Myeloma. 2009;9:316–9.
83. Martin SI, Zukerberg L, Robbins GK. Reactive Epstein-Barr virus-related polyclonal lymphoproliferative disorder in a patient with AIDS. Clin Infect Dis. 2005;41:e76–9.
84. Masque-Soler N, Szczepanowski M, Kohler CW, Spang R, Klapper W. Molecular classification of mature aggressive B-cell lymphoma using digital multiplexed gene expression on formalin-fixed paraffin-embedded biopsy specimens. Blood. 2013;122:1985–6.
85. Matsumoto Y, Nomura K, Ueda K, Satoh K, Yasuda N, Taki T, Yokota S, Horiike S, Okanoue T, Taniwaki M. Human herpesvirus 8-negative malignant effusion lymphoma: a distinct clinical entity and successful treatment with rituximab. Leuk Lymphoma. 2005;46:415–9.
86. Mbanya DN, Minkoulou EM, Kaptue LN. HIV-1 infection in adults with haematological malignancies in Yaounde, Cameroon. West Afr J Med. 2002;21:183–4.
87. Mckenna RW, Kyle RA, Kuehl WM, Grogan TM, Harris NL, Coupland RW. Plasma cell neoplasms. In: Swerdlow SH, Campo E, Harris NL, Jaffe ES, Pileri SA, Stein H, Thiele J, editors. WHO classification of tumours of haematopoietic and lymphoid tissues. Lyon: IARC Press; 2008.
88. Nador RG, Cesarman E, Chadburn A, Dawson DB, Ansari MQ, Said J, Knowles DM. Primary effusion lymphoma: a distinct clinicopathologic entity associated with the Kaposi's sarcoma-associated herpesvirus. Blood. 1996;88:645–56.
89. Nador RG, Chadburn A, Gundappa G, Cesarman E, Said JW, Knowles DM. Human immunodeficiency virus (HIV)-associated polymorphic lymphoproliferative disorders. Am J Surg Pathol. 2003;27:293–302.
90. Newton R, Ziegler J, Beral V, Mbidde E, Carpenter L, Wabinga H, Mbulaiteye S, Appleby P, Reeves G, Jaffe H, Uganda Kaposi's Sarcoma Study, G. A case-control study of human immunodeficiency virus infection and cancer in adults and children residing in Kampala, Uganda. Int J Cancer. 2001;92:622–7.
91. Nogues X, Supervia A, Knobel H, Lopez-Colomes JL, Serrano S, Abella E. Multiple myeloma and AIDS. Am J Hematol. 1996;53:210–1.
92. Pande A, Bhattacharyya M, Pain S, Samanta A. Study of bone marrow changes in antiretroviral naive human immunodeficiency virus-infected anemic patients. Indian J Pathol Microbiol. 2011;54:542–6.
93. Paner GP, Jensen J, Foreman KE, Reyes CV. HIV and HHV-8 negative primary effusion lymphoma in a patient with hepatitis C virus-related liver cirrhosis. Leuk Lymphoma. 2003;44:1811–4.
94. Park LS, Tate JP, Rodriguez-Barradas MC, Rimland D, Goetz MB, Gibert C, Brown ST, Kelley MJ, Justice AC, Dubrow R. Cancer incidence in HIV-infected versus uninfected vet-

erans: comparison of cancer registry and ICD-9 code diagnoses. J AIDS Clin Res. 2014;5:1000318.
95. Patel M, Philip V, Fazel F, Lakha A, Vorog A, Ali N, Karstaedt A, Pather S. Human immunodeficiency virus infection and chronic myeloid leukemia. Leuk Res. 2012;36:1334–8.
96. Patel P, Hanson DL, Sullivan PS, Novak RM, Moorman AC, Tong TC, Holmberg SD, Brooks JT. Incidence of types of cancer among HIV-infected persons compared with the general population in the United States, 1992–2003. Ann Intern Med. 2008;148:728–36.
97. Patra SK, Soren M, Das AK, Mangal S. A rare case of multiple myeloma (Mm) presented with pancytopaenia in a patient of HIV – at very early age. J Clin Diagn Res. 2015;9:ED07–8.
98. Perez K, Castillo J, Dezube BJ, Pantanowitz L. Human immunodeficiency virus-associated anaplastic large cell lymphoma. Leuk Lymphoma. 2010;51:430–8.
99. Polizzotto MN, Skinner M, Cole-Sinclair MF, Opat SS, Spencer A, Avery S. Allo-SCT for hematological malignancies in the setting of HIV. Bone Marrow Transplant. 2010;45:584–6.
100. Presant CA, Gala K, Wiseman C, Kennedy P, Blayney D, Sheibani K, Winberg CD, Rasheed S. Human immunodeficiency virus-associated T-cell lymphoblastic lymphoma in AIDS. Cancer. 1987;60:1459–61.
101. Rabbitts TH, Hamlyn PH, Baer R. Altered nucleotide sequences of a translocated c-myc gene in Burkitt lymphoma. Nature. 1983;306:760–5.
102. Raffetti E, Albini L, Gotti D, Segala D, Maggiolo F, Di Filippo E, Saracino A, Ladisa N, Lapadula G, Fornabaio C, Castelnuovo F, Casari S, Fabbiani M, Pierotti P, Donato F, Quiros-Roldan E, Cohort M. Cancer incidence and mortality for all causes in HIV-infected patients over a quarter century: a multicentre cohort study. BMC Public Health. 2015;15:235.
103. Raphaël M, Said J, Borisch B, Cesarman E, Harris NL. Lymphomas associated with HIV infection. In: Swerdlow SH, Campo E, Harris NL, Jaffe ES, Pileri SA, Stein H, Thiele J, editors. WHO classification of tumours of haematopoietic and lymphoid tissues. 4th ed. Lyon: IARC Press; 2008.
104. Ravandi F, Verma A, Ridgeway J, Pursell K. Chronic lymphocytic leukemia (B-CLL) occurring with human immunodeficiency virus (HIV) infection: implications. Leuk Res. 2003;27:853–7.
105. Rea D, Delecluse HJ, Hamilton-Dutoit SJ, Marelle L, Joab I, Edelman L, Finet JF, Raphael M. Epstein-Barr virus latent and replicative gene expression in post-transplant lymphoproliferative disorders and AIDS-related non-Hodgkin's lymphomas. French Study Group of Pathology for HIV-associated Tumors. Ann Oncol. 1994;5 Suppl 1:113–6.
106. Rieg S, Lubbert M, Kern WV, Timme S, Gartner F, Rump JA. Myelodysplastic syndrome with complex karyotype associated with long-term highly active antiretroviral therapy. Br J Haematol. 2009;145:670–3.
107. Rizzo M, Magro G, Castaldo P, Tucci L. Granulocytic sarcoma (chloroma) in HIV patient: a report. Forensic Sci Int. 2004;146(Suppl):S57–8.
108. Rozza-De-Menezes RE, Jeronimo Ferreira S, Lenzi Capella D, Schwartz S, Willrich AH. Gingival anaplastic large-cell lymphoma mimicking hyperplastic benignancy as the first clinical manifestation of AIDS: a case report and review of the literature. Case Rep Dent. 2013;2013:852932.
109. Saggini A, Anemona L, Chimenti S, Sarmati L, Torti C, Di Stefani A, Bianchi L. HIV-associated primary cutaneous anaplastic large cell lymphoma: a clinicopathological subset with more aggressive behavior? Case report and review of the literature. J Cutan Pathol. 2012;39:1100–9.
110. Said J, Cesarman E, Knowles D. Lymphadenopathy and the lymphoid neoplasms associated with HIV infection and other causes of immunosuppression. In: Orazzi AWL, Foucar K, Knowles DM, editors. Knowles' neoplastic hematopathology. 3rd ed. Baltimore: Wolters Kuwer/Williams and Wilkins; 2014.
111. Saini N, Hochberg EP, Linden EA, Jha S, Grohs HK, Sohani AR. HHV8-negative primary effusion lymphoma of B-cell Lineage: two cases and a comprehensive review of the literature. Case Rep Oncol Med. 2013;2013:292301.

112. Sander CA, Yano T, Clark HM, Harris C, Longo DL, Jaffe ES, Raffeld M. p53 mutation is associated with progression in follicular lymphomas. Blood. 1993;82:1994–2004.
113. Sassaki MG, Souza CA, Siciliano RF, Leite AG, Padilha SL. Polycythemia vera in a patient with the human immunodeficiency virus: a case report. Braz J Infect Dis. 2000;4:204–7.
114. Schlaberg R, Fisher JG, Flamm MJ, Murty VV, Bhagat G, Alobeid B. Chronic myeloid leukemia and HIV-infection. Leuk Lymphoma. 2008;49:1155–60.
115. Selik RM, Rabkin CS. Cancer death rates associated with human immunodeficiency virus infection in the United States. J Natl Cancer Inst. 1998;90:1300–2.
116. Shiels MS, Engels EA. Increased risk of histologically defined cancer subtypes in human immunodeficiency virus-infected individuals: clues for possible immunosuppression-related or infectious etiology. Cancer. 2012;118:4869–76.
117. Shiels MS, Pfeiffer RM, Gail MH, Hall HI, Li J, Chaturvedi AK, Bhatia K, Uldrick TS, Yarchoan R, Goedert JJ, Engels EA. Cancer burden in the HIV-infected population in the United States. J Natl Cancer Inst. 2011;103:753–62.
118. Simard EP, Pfeiffer RM, Engels EA. Spectrum of cancer risk late after AIDS onset in the United States. Arch Intern Med. 2010;170:1337–45.
119. Stefan DC, Dippenaar A, de Bruin G, Uys R, van Toorn R. Challenges to treatment of leukemia in HIV-positive children. J Trop Pediatr. 2012;58:521–2.
120. Stein H, Harris NL, Campo E. Plasmablastic lymphoma. In: Swerdlow SH, Campo E, Harris NL, Jaffe ES, Pileri SA, Stein H, Thiele J, editors. WHO classification of tumours of haematopoietic and lymphoid tissues. Lyon: IARC Press; 2008.
121. Sutton L, Guenel P, Tanguy ML, Rio B, Dhedin N, Casassus P, Lortholary O, French Study Group on Acute Myeloid Leukaemia in, H. I. V. I. P. Acute myeloid leukaemia in human immunodeficiency virus-infected adults: epidemiology, treatment feasibility and outcome. Br J Haematol. 2001;112:900–8.
122. Takahashi K, Yabe M, Shapira I, Pierce S, Garcia-Manero G, Varma M. Clinical and cytogenetic characteristics of myelodysplastic syndrome in patients with HIV infection. Leuk Res. 2012;36:1376–9.
123. Tao J, Valderrama E. Epstein-Barr virus-associated polymorphic B-cell lymphoproliferative disorders in the lungs of children with AIDS: a report of two cases. Am J Surg Pathol. 1999;23:560–6.
124. Thiele J, Titius BR, Quitmann H, Fischer R, Salzberger B, Dienemann D, Stein H. Megakaryocytopoiesis in bone marrow biopsies of patients with acquired immunodeficiency syndrome (AIDS). An immunohistochemical and morphometric evaluation with special emphasis on myelodysplastic features and precursor cells. Pathol Res Pract. 1992;188:722–8.
125. Thiele J, Zirbes TK, Bertsch HP, Titius BR, Lorenzen J, Fischer R. AIDS-related bone marrow lesions – myelodysplastic features or predominant inflammatory-reactive changes (HIV-myelopathy)? A comparative morphometric study by immunohistochemistry with special emphasis on apoptosis and PCNA-labeling. Anal Cell Pathol. 1996;11:141–57.
126. Tomonari A, Takahashi S, Shimohakamada Y, Ooi J, Takasugi K, Ohno N, Konuma T, Uchimaru K, Tojo A, Odawara T, Nakamura T, Iwamoto A, Asano S. Unrelated cord blood transplantation for a human immunodeficiency virus-1-seropositive patient with acute lymphoblastic leukemia. Bone Marrow Transplant. 2005;36:261–2.
127. Tsagarakis NJ, Argyrou A, Gortzolidis G, Kentrou N, Papadhimitriou SI, Tzanetou K, Kakiopoulos G, Papadimitriou KA, Skoumi D, Paterakis G. Report of an HIV and HHV-8 negative case of primary effusion lymphoma with idiopathic T4 lymphocytopenia. Int J Hematol. 2009;90:94–8.
128. Tullu MS, Date NB, Ghildiyal RG, Modi CJ. Acute myelogenous leukemia in a child with HIV infection. Eur J Pediatr. 2010;169:629–31.
129. Valera A, Balague O, Colomo L, Martinez A, Delabie J, Taddesse-Heath L, Jaffe ES, Campo E. IG/MYC rearrangements are the main cytogenetic alteration in plasmablastic lymphomas. Am J Surg Pathol. 2010;34:1686–94.

130. Verneris MR, Tuel L, Seibel NL. Pediatric HIV infection and chronic myelogenous leukemia. Pediatr AIDS HIV Infect. 1995;6:292–4.
131. Visco C, Li Y, Xu-Monette ZY, Miranda RN, Green TM, Li Y, Tzankov A, Wen W, Liu WM, Kahl BS, D'amore ES, Montes-Moreno S, Dybkaer K, Chiu A, Tam W, Orazi A, Zu Y, Bhagat G, Winter JN, Wang HY, O'neill S, Dunphy CH, Hsi ED, Zhao XF, Go RS, Choi WW, Zhou F, Czader M, Tong J, Zhao X, van Krieken JH, Huang Q, Ai W, Etzell J, Ponzoni M, Ferreri AJ, Piris MA, Moller MB, Bueso-Ramos CE, Medeiros LJ, Wu L, Young KH. Comprehensive gene expression profiling and immunohistochemical studies support application of immunophenotypic algorithm for molecular subtype classification in diffuse large B-cell lymphoma: a report from the International DLBCL Rituximab-CHOP Consortium Program Study. Leukemia. 2012;26:2103–13.
132. Vorkas CK, Vaamonde CM, Glesby MJ. Testosterone replacement therapy and polycythemia in HIV-infected patients. AIDS. 2012;26:243–5.
133. Wang X, Nathan S, Catchatourian R, Richter 3rd H, Kovarik P. Polymorphic lymphoid proliferation presenting as ileocecal intussusception. Ann Hematol. 2007;86:453–4.
134. Willocks L, Ludlam CA, Welsby PD. Polycythaemia and HIV infection. Lancet. 1990;336:812–3.
135. Xu Q, Tan C, Ni S, Wang Q, Wu F, Liu F, Ye X, Meng X, Sheng W, Du X. Identification and validation of a two-gene expression index for subtype classification and prognosis in diffuse large B-cell lymphoma. Sci Rep. 2015;5:10006.

# 2 Epidemiology

Diego Serraino and Luigino Dal Maso

## Contents



## 2.1 Epidemiological Background

The International Agency for Research on Cancer (IARC) has recognized that several infectious agents are carcinogenic to humans (Group 1), as summarized in Table 2.1 [22]. In particular, the IARC Working Group on Biological Agents has determined that there is sufficient evidence in humans for the carcinogenicity of infection with HIV-1 (thereafter, HIV) as a cause of Kaposi's sarcoma (KS), non-Hodgkin's lymphoma (NHL), Hodgkin's lymphoma (HL), and cancers of the cervix, anus, and conjunctiva.

HIV increases the cancer risk in humans indirectly, primarily by immunosuppression. Many of the AIDS-defining malignancies have an infectious primary cause, e.g., EBV, HPV, and KSHV. In addition to HIV-mediated immunosuppression, other aspects of the HIV biology contribute to the increased incidence of lymphomas and of other cancers in individuals infected with HIV. Suggested mechanisms include HIV-mediated immune dysregulation, in particular the hyperactivation of B


D. Serraino (✉) • L. Dal Maso
Unit of Epidemiology and Biostatistics, CRO Aviano National Cancer Institute, IRCCS, via F. Gallini, 2, Aviano, PN 33081, Italy
e-mail: serrainod@cro.it





M. Hentrich, S.K. Barta (eds.), *HIV-associated Hematological Malignancies*,
DOI 10.1007/978-3-319-26857-6_2

**Table 2.1** Infectious agents for which there is a sufficient evidence of carcinogenicity for hematological malignancies

| Group 1 infectious agent | Lymphomas for which there is sufficient evidence in humans |
|---|---|
| Epstein-Barr virus (EBV) | Burkitt lymphoma, immunosuppression-related non-Hodgkin's lymphoma, extranodal NK/T-cell lymphoma (nasal type), Hodgkin's lymphoma |
| Hepatitis C virus (HCV) | Non-Hodgkin's lymphoma[a] |
| Kaposi's sarcoma herpes virus (KSHV) | Primary effusion lymphoma[a] |
| Human immunodeficiency virus, type 1 (HIV-1) | Non-Hodgkin's lymphoma, Hodgkin's lymphoma[a] |
| Human T-cell lymphotrophic virus, type-1 (HTLV-1) | Adult T-cell leukemia and lymphoma |
| Helicobacter pylori | Low-grade B-cell mucosa-associated lymphoid tissue (MALT) gastric lymphoma[a] |

Modified from IARC [22]

[a]Newly identified link between virus and cancer as of 2009

cells. However, unlike what is known about other cancer-associated viruses, there is no evidence that HIV infection by itself leads to cell transformation or immortalization [22].

In this chapter, the main epidemiological aspects of HIV-associated NHL and HL in the era of combination antiretroviral therapy (cART) will be briefly discussed, in addition to available data on leukemias and other hematological conditions.

## 2.2 Incidence and Excess Risk

NHL has been part of the AIDS case definition since the first years of the epidemic. In particular, three types of lymphoma were recognized in HIV patients and included as AIDS-defining illnesses since the beginning of the 1980s [9]. They are primary CNS lymphoma and large-cell immunoblastic lymphoma, which occur in severely immunodeficient patients, and Burkitt lymphoma that can occur at any stage of immune deficiency [14]. The relative contribution of diffuse large B-cell lymphoma (e.g., the most common subtype, including immunoblastic lymphomas) to all HIV-associated lymphomas increased in Italy from 36 % during 1986–1995 to 46 % in 2001–2005 [11]. However, a nonsignificant decrease emerged thereafter in the USA, from 46 % during 2001–2005 to 36 % in 2006–2010 [18].

The frequency of NHL varies by a small amount among HIV exposure groups [10]. This consistency suggests that cofactors for AIDS-related NHL are unlikely to be as important, or as unevenly distributed, as those for Kaposi's sarcoma (e.g., Kaposi herpes virus) or anal cancer (e.g., human papillomavirus), which are much more common among homosexual and bisexual men than in any other transmission group [10].

Improvements in immune function attributable to cART, widely available in industrialized countries since 1996, have led to a substantial decline in the incidence of most AIDS-defining conditions. The incidence of NHL declined approximately 80 % in the cART period [4, 14, 29], a substantial reduction that was, however, less marked than the incidence recorded for KS or other AIDS-defining conditions. As a consequence, after 1996, NHL became the most frequent cancer type in people diagnosed with HIV/AIDS (PWA), with incidence rates ranging from 1/1000 person years in HIV patients [15] to 3/1000 person years in AIDS patients [30, 32] (Table 2.2). In addition, a wide range of increased risks has been reported in population-based studies, mainly depending on the population under observation and the calendar years examined (Table 2.2). For instance, PWA in Italy from 1997 to 2004 showed an approximately 90-fold higher risk than the general population – such risk was 500-fold elevated for those diagnosed with NHL in the pre-cART era (i.e., 1986–1996) [10]. In the latest studies conducted in PWA, the relative increase appears much lower, ranging between 10- and 20-fold higher than in the general population in Switzerland [15] and the USA [17].

The pattern of risk for HIV-associated cancers in the cART era turned out to be similar to the one recorded in people iatrogenically immunosuppressed after organ transplantation [34]. A clinical-based cohort study conducted in Italy and France among HIV-infected people – with or without known dates of seroconversion – and among recipients of kidney or liver transplants, showed that the risk of NHL, as compared to the corresponding general population, was twofold lower in HIV-infected people treated with cART (i.e., SIR = 35) than in HIV-positive people who did not undergo cART (SIR = 72). Similarly, kidney transplant recipients who received mTOR inhibitors (i.e., a less immunodepressant antirejection regimen) showed a 70 % reduced risk of NHL, as compared to transplant recipients who underwent standard antirejection therapies [28]. These clinical-based data are in agreement with results from population-based studies, and they indicate a similar pattern of risk for lymphomas in immunosuppressed people, a pattern which does not seem to depend on the cause of immune deficiency [19, 34]. In particular, these observations point to the role of EBV as a causal factor for lymphomagenesis in the setting of acquired immune deficiencies [22].

The excess risk for Hodgkin's lymphoma in HIV-infected people was documented later than for NHL [33], because HL is one of the commonest cancers recorded among young adults in the general population, i.e., the individuals most heavily affected in the first decade of the HIV/AIDS epidemic. Over time, the contribution of HL increased during 1986–1995 to 2001–2005, from 4.8 % to 10.3 % of all HIV-associated lymphomas [11]. Incidence rates of HL in patients with HIV/AIDS ranged between 0.5 and 0.8/1000 person years [15, 30], with a 10- to 20-fold higher risk in comparison with the general population (Table 2.2).

As seen in HIV-associated NHL since the beginning of the epidemic, the excess risk for HIV-associated HL was not consistently observed across HL types [33, 36]. A very highly increased risk was observed for mixed cellularity HL, whereas a less pronounced excess risk was demonstrated for other subtypes [16, 33]. Interestingly, studies with a longer follow-up period have documented that, in the course of the HIV/AIDS epidemic, age-standardized incidence rates and excess risks for HL were consistently stable in HIV-infected people [6, 30, 40]. This observation suggests that cART has a limited impact on the development of HL.

**Table 2.2** Incidence rates (IR, per 100,000 person years), relative risk (RR) in comparison with the general population, and corresponding 95 % confidence interval (CI) of hematologic cancers in people with HIV/AIDS from population-based registry-linkage studies in the cART era (After 1996)

| Type of cancer | Study, year | Country | Cohort | *N* | IR | RR (95 %CI) |
|---|---|---|---|---|---|---|
| All cancer types | Engels et al. 2008 [14] | USA | HIV/AIDS | 871 | 468 | 2.1 (2.0–2.3) |
| | Polesel et al. 2010 [30] | Italy | AIDS | 375 | 1081 | – |
| | Franceschi et al. 2010 [15] | Switzerland | HIV/AIDS | 140 | 487 | 3.0 (2.6–3.6) |
| Non-Hodgkin's lymphoma | Grulich et al. 2007 [19] | *Meta-analysis* | | *5295* | | *77 (39–149)* |
| | Gibson et al. 2014 [17] | USA | HIV/AIDS | 2828 | 194 | 11 (10–11) |
| | Dal Maso et al. 2009 [10], Polesel et al. 2010 [30] | Italy | AIDS | 352 | 343 | 93 (84–104) |
| | Van Leeuwen et al. 2009 [43] | Australia | HIV/AIDS | 121 | | 13 (10–15) |
| | Franceschi et al. 2010 [15] | Switzerland | HIV/AIDS | 32 | 98 | 16 (11–23) |
| Hodgkin's lymphoma | Grulich et al. 2007 [19] | *Meta-analysis* | | *802* | | *11 (8–14)* |
| | Engels et al. 2008 [14] | USA | HIV/AIDS | 36 | 19 | 5.6 (3.9–7.8) |
| | Dal Maso et al. 2009 [10], Polesel et al. 2010 [30] | Italy | AIDS | 37 | 82 | 21 (15–29) |
| | Van Leeuwen et al. 2009 [43] | Australia | HIV/AIDS | 11 | | 7 (4–13) |
| | Franceschi et al. 2010 [15] | Switzerland | HIV/AIDS | 13 | 53 | 28 (15–48) |
| Multiple myeloma | Grulich et al. 2007 [19] | *Meta-analysis* | | *76* | | *2.7 (2.1–3.4)* |
| | Engels et al. 2008 [14] | USA | HIV/AIDS | 8 | 4 | 1.4 (0.6–2.7) |
| | Dal Maso et al. 2009 [10], Polesel et al. 2010 [30] | Italy | AIDS | 4 | 8 | 3.9 (1.0–10.0) |
| | Franceschi et al. 2010 [15] | Switzerland | HIV/AIDS | 2 | – | 5.1 (0.5–18.9) |
| Leukemias | Grulich et al. 2007 [19] | *Meta-analysis* | | *235* | | *3.2 (2.5–4.1)* |
| | Engels et al. 2008 [14] | USA | HIV/AIDS | 7 | 4 | – |
| | Dal Maso et al. 2009 [10], Polesel et al. 2010 [30] | Italy | AIDS | 3 | 5 | 1.1 (0.2–3.3) |
| | Van Leeuwen et al. 2009 [43] | Australia | HIV/AIDS | 9 | | 1.9 (0.9–3.6) |
| | Franceschi et al. 2010 [15] | Switzerland | HIV/AIDS | 1 | | 1.1 (0.0–6.5) |

*N* number of cancer cases

The occurrence of leukemia and of multiple myeloma was also documented in people with HIV/AIDS in Europe, the USA, and Australia [22], with incidence rates lower than ten cases per 100,000 years of observation. In Italy, the risk of leukemias (all types) in people with HIV/AIDS was nearly fivefold higher before cART, whereas it was similar to the one recorded in the general population (RR = 1.1) thereafter [10] and consistently in different countries (Table 2.2). Similar incidence rates in PWA have been reported for multiple myeloma and plasma cell neoplasms, for which elevated rates in people with HIV/AIDS before and after the widespread use of cART [10] were reported less consistently [14, 15, 43].

Excess cancer incidence among HIV-infected people has been recently estimated also in absolute terms in the USA. Robbins and colleagues [32] reported that 88 % of NHL and approximately 50 % of HL cancer cases (i.e., 1440 and 290 cases, respectively), in HIV-infected patients in 2010, were related to HIV infection. It was also estimated that, during 1992–2009 in the USA, 5.9 % of all NHL cases occurred in HIV-positive patients, 9.6 % in men and 1.3 % in women [38]. These proportions were highest for Burkitt (27 %), diffuse large B-cell (8 %), and peripheral T-cell (3 %) lymphomas, with proportions below 1 % in the other subtypes [38]. Overall, similar data for NHL were reported in the pre-cART period (8 %) among Italian PWA aged 15–49 years [8].

The contribution of HIV infection impact on the burden of HL is smaller than that for NHL. In the USA, it was estimated that 3.8 % of all HL cases diagnosed in 2000–2010 (8 % in men and 1.5 % in women) occurred in HIV-positive patients, with proportions >10 % for lymphocyte-depleted and mixed cellularity HL [39].

## 2.3 Survival and Risk of Death

The life expectancy of PWA has dramatically increased in high-resource countries during the cART era, though it remains still lower than that of the general population [2, 20, 37]. The survival of PWA after a diagnosis of cancer, especially KS and NHL, has been explored by several clinical-based investigations [5, 27, 42]. However, population-based studies on cancer survival in PWA are few [18] and so are the comparisons of cancer survival with the general population (thereafter referred to as non-PWA) [3, 7, 11].

Figure 2.1 and Table 2.3 report the results of a population-based record linkage study of the Italian National AIDS Registry with the database of all Italian cancer registries [11]. The aim was to provide population-based estimates of PWA cancer survival in Italy, and to compare such estimates with those recorded in persons of the same age and sex affected by the same cancer but without AIDS (non-PWA).

As shown in Figure 2.1, also in the cART era, people with AIDS and NHL or HL had a significantly reduced survival, in comparison with non-PWA, at both one and 5 years after diagnosis. A 5-year survival of 64 % at 5 years was registered among non-PWA with NHL from Italian cancer registries, but only 25 % of PWA were alive 5 years after the diagnosis of NHL. Similarly, 42 % of PWA were alive after the diagnosis of HL, as compared to 86 % of matched non-PWA from Italian cancer

**Table 2.3** Comparison of the risk of death (hazard ratios HR; and 95 % confidence intervals CI) at 5 years from cancer diagnosis in people with AIDS (PWA) *versus* non-PWA. Italy, 1996–2005

| | PWA | | | Non-PWA | | | |
|---|---|---|---|---|---|---|---|
| ICD10; cancer type | Cases | Deaths | Overall survival (%) | Cases | Deaths | Overall survival (%) | HR (95 % CI) |
| All cancer patients | 1297 | 751 | (42) | 2935 | 1042 | (65) | 2.9 (2.6–3.3) |
| C82-C85,C88,C96; NHL | 561 | 418 | (25) | 1122 | 402 | (64) | 3.4 (2.9–4.1) |
| NHL, brain | 47 | 43 | (9) | 94 | 67 | (29) | 3.1 (1.6–6.2) |
| NHL, DLBC, and immunoblastic | 264 | 187 | (29) | 528 | 180 | (66) | 3.0 (2.3–3.8) |
| NHL, Burkitt | 39 | 29 | (26) | 78 | 43 | (45) | 1.2 (0.7–2.2) |
| NHL, follicular and SLL/CLL | 11 | 8 | (27) | 22 | 2 | (91) | 27.4 (1.1–757) |
| NHL, T cell | 13 | 8 | (38) | 26 | 3 | (88) | 20.9 (1.6–268) |
| NHL, other specified histology | 7 | 5 | (29) | 14 | 5 | (64) | 15.6 (1.3–186) |
| NHL, NOS | 180 | 138 | (23) | 360 | 102 | (72) | 5.3 (3.8–7.5) |
| C81; Hodgkin's lymphoma | 36 | 21 | (42) | 180 | 25 | (86) | 5.9 (3.1–11.2) |
| HL, mixed cell | 17 | 7 | (59) | 85 | 14 | (84) | 2.7 (1.0–7.3) |
| HL, nodular sclerosis | 9 | 7 | (22) | 45 | 5 | (89) | 19.9 (3.6–109) |
| HL, NOS | 10 | 7 | (30) | 50 | 6 | (88) | 8.8 (2.5–30.9) |
| C91-C95; leukemias | 6 | 6 | (0) | 30 | 13 | (57) | 6.5 (1.7–24.2) |

Modified from Dal Maso et al. [11]

*NOS* not otherwise specified, *CLL/SLL* chronic lymphocytic leukemia/small lymphocytic lymphoma, *NHL* non-Hodgkin's lymphoma

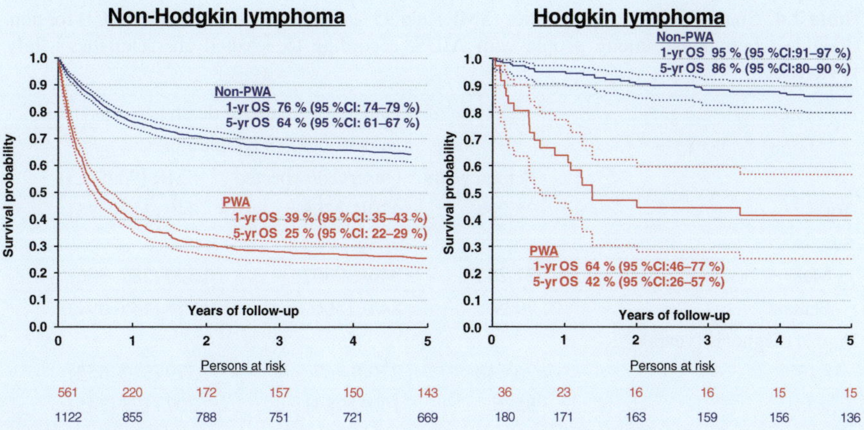


**Fig. 2.1** Observed survival (OS) after cancer in persons with AIDS (PWA)[a] and non-PWA[b] in NHL and HL. Italy, 1996–2005. *Dotted lines* represent 95 % confidence intervals (95 % CI). [a]Patients aged 16–74 years. [b]Matched (1:2 for NHL, 1:5 for HL) by histology, sex, age, period of diagnosis, and Italian area (Modified from Dal Maso et al. [11])

registries. In the same period, PWA had a 3.4-fold elevated risk of death for all NHLs combined than non-PWA (Table 2.3). The risk of death for PWA was particularly elevated for follicular NHL (HR = 27.4) and T-cell NHL (HR = 20.9). Similarly, the risk of death for PWA and HL was about sixfold higher than among non-PWA and HL (HR = 5.9), with a very elevated risk emerging for the nodular sclerosis type of HL (HR PWA vs. non-PWA = 19.9) (Table 2.3).

A recent population-based record linkage study evaluated the effect of HIV on overall and on cancer-specific mortality, in six areas of the USA [7]. When all-cause mortality was considered as outcome, the US study showed risks of death similar to the Italian ones. HIV patients with diffuse large B-cell lymphomas displayed HR of death of 3.6 (3.0 in Italy) while for HL patients the HR was 4.2. However, the study showed that HIV was not associated with increased mortality when only cancer-specific mortality was used as outcome [7].

Cancer continues to be an important cause of mortality in PWA in high-resource countries during the cART era [12, 21, 37]. It was estimated that NHL and KS represented 15–18 % of all deaths with several hundredfold higher risks of death than in the general population [1, 35]. In addition, non-AIDS-defining cancers (i.e., cancers other than KS, NHL, and invasive cervical cancer) caused approximately 10–15 % of all deaths in PWA [1, 24, 25, 31, 35, 41], with a sevenfold higher risk of death than that of the general population [44].

In comparison with the general population of the same sex and age, Italian PWA diagnosed in the early years of the cART era had an approximately 350-fold elevated risk of death for NHL and of about 150-fold elevated risk for HL [35, 44]. The median age of PWA and HL was 41 years, and the median time from HL to death was only 4 months [44]. Data regarding selected variables of PWA and NHL, with corresponding standardized mortality ratios (SMR), are listed in Table 2.4 [35].

**Table 2.4** Standardized mortality ratios (SMR) and 95 % confidence intervals (95 % CI) for non-Hodgkin's lymphoma among people with AIDS, according to selected characteristics.[a] Italy, 1999–2006

| | | Underlying cause of death | |
|---|---|---|---|
| | | Non-Hodgkin's lymphoma | |
| | Person years | Observed/expected | SMR (95 % CI) |
| Total | 35,224 | 430/1.2308 | 349 (317–384) |
| Sex | | | |
| Male | 27,285 | 346/1.0802 | 320 (287–356) |
| Female | 7939 | 84/0.1506 | 558 (445–691) |
| Age at diagnosis (years) | | | |
| <45 | 26,648 | 270/0.467 | 579 (512–652) |
| ≥45 | 8576 | 160/0.7641 | 209 (178–245) |
| HIV transmission category | | | |
| Intravenous drug user | 14,374 | 159/0.2961 | 537 (457–627) |
| Men having sex with men | 6602 | 90/0.3117 | 289 (232–355) |
| Heterosexual | 12,279 | 144/0.5188 | 278 (234–327) |
| Calendar year | | | |
| 1999–2000 | 3047 | 88/0.0842 | 1046 (839–1289) |
| 2001–2002 | 7467 | 109/0.2299 | 474 (389–572) |
| 2003–2004 | 11,046 | 122/0.3843 | 317 (264–379) |
| 2005–2006 | 13,663 | 111/0.5325 | 208 (171–251) |

Modified from check leading Serraino et al. [35]

[a]In some items, the sum does not add up to the total because of missing values

As it can be seen, particularly high risks of death for NHL were recorded among females (SMR = 558), intravenous drug users (SMR = 537), and in PWA with NHL diagnosed in 1999–2000 (SMR = 1046).

## Conclusions

Overall, three times as many cancers were observed among PWA, compared to the general population, with a more than tenfold increase for NHL and HL. NHL became, in the 2000s, the most common cancer type among HIV-infected patients in high-income countries. In addition, the observed pattern of lymphoid neoplasms in PWA did not substantially change in recent years. A persisting, although narrowing, gap in cancer survival between PWA and non-PWA is still observed. The combination of higher incidence of NHL and lower survival after diagnosis leads to more than a hundredfold higher risk of death for this neoplasm in HIV-infected patients.

Prevention programs for HIV-infected persons need to be enforced, particularly those aiming at smoking and alcohol cessations and at treating HCV infection and preneoplastic HPV-related lesions. Unfortunately, they may have only a limited impact on the incidence of lymphoid neoplasms.

The recent epidemiological evidence on HIV-associated lymphomas and hematological malignancies, summarized in this chapter, indicate a need to enhance the therapeutic approach to reduce mortality for these neoplasms in

PWA and give them the same chances of survival observed in the general population.

Several large clinical series [13, 23, 26] demonstrated that patients with HIV and NHL or HL receiving the same treatment, or included in the same protocols, may have a similar outcome of HIV-negative patients.

Clinicians should be encouraged to improve prognosis of PWA by strongly considering treating patients with HIV and lymphomas with the same protocols used for HIV-negative patients [26], thus balancing risks and benefits of using potentially immunosuppressive treatments (see following chapters).

## References

1. Antiretroviral Therapy Cohort Collaboration. Causes of death in HIV-1-infected patients treated with antiretroviral therapy, 1996–2006: collaborative analysis of 13 HIV cohort studies. Clin Infect Dis. 2010;50:1387–96.
2. Bhaskaran K, Hamouda O, Sannes M, Boufassa F, Johnson AM, Lambert PC, et al. Changes in the risk of death after HIV seroconversion compared with mortality in the general population. JAMA. 2008;300:51–9.
3. Biggar RJ, Engels E, Ly S, Kahn A, Schymura MJ, Sackoff J, et al. Survival after cancer diagnosis in persons with AIDS. J Acquir Immune Defic Syndr. 2005;39:293–9.
4. Carrieri MP, Pradier C, Piselli P, Piche M, Rosenthal E, Heudier P, et al. Reduced incidence of Kaposi's sarcoma and of systemic non-Hodgkin's lymphoma in HIV-infected individuals treated with highly active antiretroviral therapy. Int J Cancer. 2003;103:142–4.
5. Chao C, Xu L, Abrams D, Leyden W, Horberg M, Towner W, et al. Survival of non-Hodgkin lymphoma patients with and without HIV infection in the era of combined antiretroviral therapy. AIDS. 2010;24:1765–70.
6. Clifford GM, Rickenbach M, Lise M, Dal Maso L, Battegay M, Bohlius J, et al. Hodgkin lymphoma in the Swiss HIV Cohort Study. Blood. 2009;113:5737–42.
7. Coghill AE, Shiels MS, Suneja G, Engels EA. Elevated cancer-specific mortality among HIV-infected patients in the United States. J Clin Oncol. 2015;33:2376–83.
8. Dal Maso L, Rezza G, Zambon P, Tagliabue G, Crocetti E, Vercelli M, et al. Non-Hodgkin lymphoma among young adults with and without AIDS in Italy. Int J Cancer. 2001;93:430–5.
9. Dal Maso L, Franceschi S. Epidemiology of non-Hodgkin lymphoma and other haemolymphopoietic neoplasms in people with AIDS. Lancet Oncol. 2003;4:110–9.
10. Dal Maso L, Polesel J, Serraino D, Lise M, Piselli P, Falcini F, et al. Pattern of cancer risk in persons with AIDS in Italy in the HAART era. Br J Cancer. 2009;100:840–7.
11. Dal Maso L, Suligoi B, Franceschi S, Braga C, Buzzoni C, Polesel J, et al. Survival after cancer in Italian persons with AIDS, 1986–2005: a population-based estimation. J Acquir Immune Defic Syndr. 2014;66:428–35.
12. Data Collection on Adverse Events of Anti-HIV drugs (D:A:D) Study Group. Factors associated with specific causes of death amongst HIV-positive individuals in the D:A:D study. AIDS. 2010;24:1537–48.
13. Díez-Martín JL, Balsalobre P, Re A, Michieli M, Ribera JM, Canals C, et al. Comparable survival between HIV+ and HIV- non-Hodgkin and Hodgkin lymphoma patients undergoing autologous peripheral blood stem cell transplantation. Blood. 2009;113:6011–4.
14. Engels EA, Biggar RJ, Hall HI, Cross H, Crutchfield A, Finch JL, et al. Cancer risk in people infected with human immunodeficiency virus in the United States. Int J Cancer. 2008;123:187–94.
15. Franceschi S, Lise M, Clifford GM, Rickenbach M, Levi F, Maspoli M, et al. Changing patterns of cancer incidence in the early-and late-HAART periods: the Swiss HIV Cohort Study. Br J Cancer. 2010;103:416–22.

16. Frisch M, Biggar RJ, Engels EA, Goedert JJ, for the AIDS Cancer Match Registry Study Group. Association of cancer with AIDS-related immunosuppression in adults. JAMA. 2001;285:1736–45.
17. Gibson TM, Morton LM, Shiels MS, Clarke CA, Engels EA. Risk of non-Hodgkin lymphoma subtypes in HIV-infected people during the HAART era: a population-based study. AIDS. 2014;28:2313–8.
18. Gopal S, Patel MR, Yanik EL, Cole SR, Achenbach CJ, Napravnik S, et al. Temporal Trends in presentation and survival for HIV-associated lymphoma in the antiretroviral therapy era. J Natl Cancer Inst. 2013;105:1221–9.
19. Grulich AE, van Leeuwen MT, Falster MO, Vajdic CM. Incidence of cancers in people with HIV/AIDS compared with immunosuppressed transplant recipients a meta-analysis. Lancet. 2007;370:59–67.
20. Harrison KMD, Song R, Zhang X. Life expectancy after HIV diagnosis based on national HIV surveillance data from 25 States, United States. J Acquir Immune Defic Syndr. 2010;53:124–30.
21. Helleberg M, Kronborg G, Larsen CS, Pedersen G, Pedersen C, Gerstoft J, et al. Causes of death among Danish HIV patients compared with population controls in the period 1995–2008. Infection. 2012;40:627–34.
22. IARC Working Group on the Evaluation of Carcinogenic Risks to Humans. Biological agents. Volume 100B. A Review of human carcinogenesis. IARC Monogr Eval Carcinog Risks Hum. 2012;100(pt B):1–441.
23. Krishnan A, Palmer JM, Zaia JA, Tsai NC, Alvarnas J, Forman SJ. HIV status does not affect the outcome of autologous stem cell transplantation (ASCT) for non-Hodgkin lymphoma (NHL). Biol Blood Marrow Transplant. 2010;16:1302–8.
24. Lewden C, May T, Rosenthal E, Burty C, Bonnet F, Costagliola D, et al. Changes in causes of death among adults infected by HIV between 2000 and 2005: the "Mortalité 2000 and 2005" survey (ANRS EN19 and Mortavic). J Acquir Immune Defic Syndr. 2008;48:590–8.
25. Marin B, Thiébaut R, Bucher HC, Rondeau V, Costagliola D, Dorrucci M, et al. Non-AIDS-defining deaths and immunodeficiency in the era of combination antiretroviral therapy. AIDS. 2009;23:1743–53.
26. Montoto S, Shaw K, Okosun J, Gandhi S, Fields P, Wilson A, et al. HIV status does not influence outcome in patients with classical Hodgkin lymphoma treated with chemotherapy using doxorubicin, bleomycin, vinblastine, and dacarbazine in the highly active antiretroviral therapy era. J Clin Oncol. 2012;30:4111–6.
27. Norden AD, Drappatz J, Wen PY, Claus EB. Survival among patients with primary central nervous system lymphoma, 1973–2004. J Neurooncol. 2011;101:487–93.
28. Piselli P, Serraino D, Segoloni GP, Sandrini S, Piredda GB, Scolari MP, et al. Risk of de novo cancers after transplantation: results from a cohort of 7217 kidney transplant recipients, Italy 1997–2009. Eur J Cancer. 2013;49:336–44.
29. Polesel J, Clifford GM, Rickenbach M, Dal Maso L, Battegay M, Bouchardy C, et al. Non-Hodgkin's lymphoma incidence in the Swiss HIV Cohort Study before and after highly active antiretroviral therapy. AIDS. 2008;22:301–6.
30. Polesel J, Franceschi S, Suligoi B, Crocetti E, Falcini F, Guzzinati S, et al. Cancer incidence in people with AIDS. Int J Cancer. 2010;127:1437–45.
31. Puhan MA, Van Natta ML, Palella FJ, Addessi A, Meinert C, Ocular Complications of AIDS Research Group. Excess mortality in patients with AIDS in the era of highly active antiretroviral therapy: temporal changes and risk factors. Clin Infect Dis. 2010;51:947–56.
32. Robbins HA, Pfeiffer RM, Shiels MS, Li J, Hall HI, Engels EA. Excess cancers among HIV-infected people in the United States. J Natl Cancer Inst. 2015;107(4):dju503.
33. Serraino D, Carbone A, Franceschi S, Tirelli U. Increased frequency of lymphocyte depletion and mixed cellularity subtypes of Hodgkin's disease in HIV-infected patients. Italian Cooperative Group on AIDS and Tumours. Eur J Cancer. 1993;29A:1948–50.
34. Serraino D, Piselli P, Busnach G, Burra P, Citterio F, Arbustini E, et al. Risk of cancer following immunosuppression in organ transplant recipients and in HIV-positive individuals in southern Europe. Eur J Cancer. 2007;43:2117–23.

35. Serraino D, De Paoli A, Zucchetto A, Pennazza S, Bruzzone S, Spina M, et al. The impact of Kaposi sarcoma and non-Hodgkin lymphoma on mortality of people with AIDS in the highly active antiretroviral therapies era. Cancer Epidemiol. 2010;34:257–61.
36. Serraino D, Pezzotti P, Dorrucci M, Alliegro MB, Sinicco A, Rezza G. Cancer incidence in a cohort of human immunodeficiency virus seroconverters. HIV Italian Seroconversion Study Group. Cancer. 1997;79:1004–8.
37. Serraino D, Zucchetto A, Suligoi B, Bruzzone S, Camoni L, Boros S, et al. Survival after AIDS diagnosis in Italy, 1999–2006: a population-based study. J Acquir Immune Defic Syndr. 2009;52:99–105.
38. Shiels MS, Engels EA, Linet MS, Clarke CA, Li J, Hall HI, et al. The epidemic of non-Hodgkin lymphoma in the United States: disentangling the effect of HIV, 1992–2009. Cancer Epidemiol Biomarkers Prev. 2013;22:1069–78.
39. Shiels MS, Koritzinsky EH, Clarke CA, Suneja G, Morton LM, Engels EA. Prevalence of HIV infection among U.S. Hodgkin lymphoma cases. Cancer Epidemiol Biomarkers Prev. 2014;23:274–81.
40. Shiels MS, Pfeiffer RM, Gail MH, Hall HI, Li J, Chaturvedi AK, et al. Cancer burden in the HIV-infected population in the United States. J Natl Cancer Inst. 2011;103:753–62.
41. Simard EP, Engels EA. Cancer as a cause of death among people with AIDS in the United States. Clin Infect Dis. 2010;51:957–62.
42. Spagnuolo V, Travi G, Galli L, Cossarini F, Guffanti M, Gianotti N, et al. Clinical, virologic, and immunologic outcomes in lymphoma survivors and in cancer-free, HIV-1-infected patients: a matched cohort study. Cancer. 2013;119:2710–9.
43. Van Leeuwen MT, Vajdic CM, Middleton MG, McDonald AM, Law M, Kaldor JM, et al. Continuing declines in some but not all HIV-associated cancers in Australia after widespread use of antiretroviral therapy. AIDS. 2009;23:2183–90.
44. Zucchetto A, Suligoi B, De Paoli A, et al. Excess mortality for non- AIDS-defining cancers among people with AIDS. Clin Infect Dis. 2010;51:1099–101.

# Diffuse Large B-Cell Lymphoma 3

Stefan K. Barta, Kieron Dunleavy, and Nicolas Mounier

## Contents



S.K. Barta, MD, MS, MRCP (UK) (✉)
Fox Chase Cancer Center, Temple BMT Program, Temple University Health System,
333 Cottman Ave., Philadelphia, PA 19111-2497, USA
e-mail: Stefan.Barta@fccc.edu

K. Dunleavy, MD
Center for Cancer Research, National Cancer Institute,
National Institutes of Health, Bethesda, MD, USA
e-mail: dunleavk@mail.nih.gov

N. Mounier, MD
Department of Onco-Hematology, Archet Hospital,
151 Rte Saint Antoine Ginestiere BP 79, Nice 06202, France
e-mail: mounier.n@chu-nice.fr



M. Hentrich, S.K. Barta (eds.), *HIV-associated Hematological Malignancies*,
DOI 10.1007/978-3-319-26857-6_3

## 3.1 Epidemiology and Etiology

Systemic (or "non-CNS") diffuse large B-cell lymphoma (DLBCL) is the most common lymphoma accounting for approximately 30–40 % of all new lymphoma diagnoses in HIV-negative patients and 30–80 % in HIV-infected patients [1–4]. Both plasmablastic lymphoma and primary CNS lymphoma are considered variants of DLBCL, but will be discussed in detail in separate chapters (Chap. 5, Plasmablastic Lymphoma; and Chap. 7, Primary CNS Lymphoma). While in the era before 1996, when no combination antiretroviral therapy (cART) was available, the risk of developing an aggressive non-Hodgkin lymphoma (NHL) was up to 600-fold increased compared to immunocompetent patients; this risk has declined to <20-fold in the era of cART [5–9]. In DLBCL in HIV-infected patients the severity of immunosuppression is the most important risk factor for developing disease. The HIV/AIDS Cancer Match study that analyzed data of 325,516 patients diagnosed between January 1, 1996, and December 31, 2002, found that the risk of developing non-CNS DLBCL was 390.7 and 157.6 per 100,000 person years in 1990–1995 and 1996–2002, respectively. Additionally, for every decrease of the CD4 count by 50 cells/ml at the time of HIV diagnosis, the risk of developing DLBCL increased by approximately 12 % (hazard ratio [HR] 1.12; 95 % confidence interval 1.02–1.20) [10]. Many other studies report similar observations, with the risk of developing DLBCL being highest in patients with low CD4 counts, especially if <100 cells/ml, and less risk with higher CD4 counts. Both the CD4 nadir and the length of impaired immune function secondary to low CD4 counts appear to be important [11–13]. The median CD4 count at DLBCL diagnosis is typically around 200 cells/ml [14, 15]. Additionally, length of time of HIV viremia, even at low levels, has been established as risk factor for developing DLBCL [12, 13, 16, 17].

Considering that both HIV viremia and low CD4 counts increase the risk of DLBCL, it is not surprising that use of cART substantially decreases the risk of developing DLBCL [18, 19]. It should also be noted that the biology and presentation of DLBCL in patients with poorly controlled HIV are shifted toward more aggressive and often virally associated subtypes. Nevertheless, while the absolute incidence of HIV-related DLBCL has decreased over the years, patients with uncontrolled or advanced HIV now in the cART era have a similar risk for developing DLBCL when compared to patients in the early days of the HIV epidemic [20].

Although HIV itself appears not directly implicated in lymphomagenesis, the virus indirectly creates an environment in which chronic antigen stimulation, cytokine dysregulation, and coinfection with oncogenic viruses, such as the Epstein-Barr virus (EBV), in the background of genetic abnormalities and impaired immunity, can lead to the emergence of monoclonal B cells (Fig. 3.1) [2, 21]. Particularly impaired T-cell immunity toward EBV, a ubiquitous gamma herpes virus, is strongly implicated in lymphomagenesis of the immunoblastic variant of DLBCL, which occurs generally in the more immunosuppressed host compared to the centroblastic variant of DLBCL [22, 23]. While EBV is identified in neoplastic

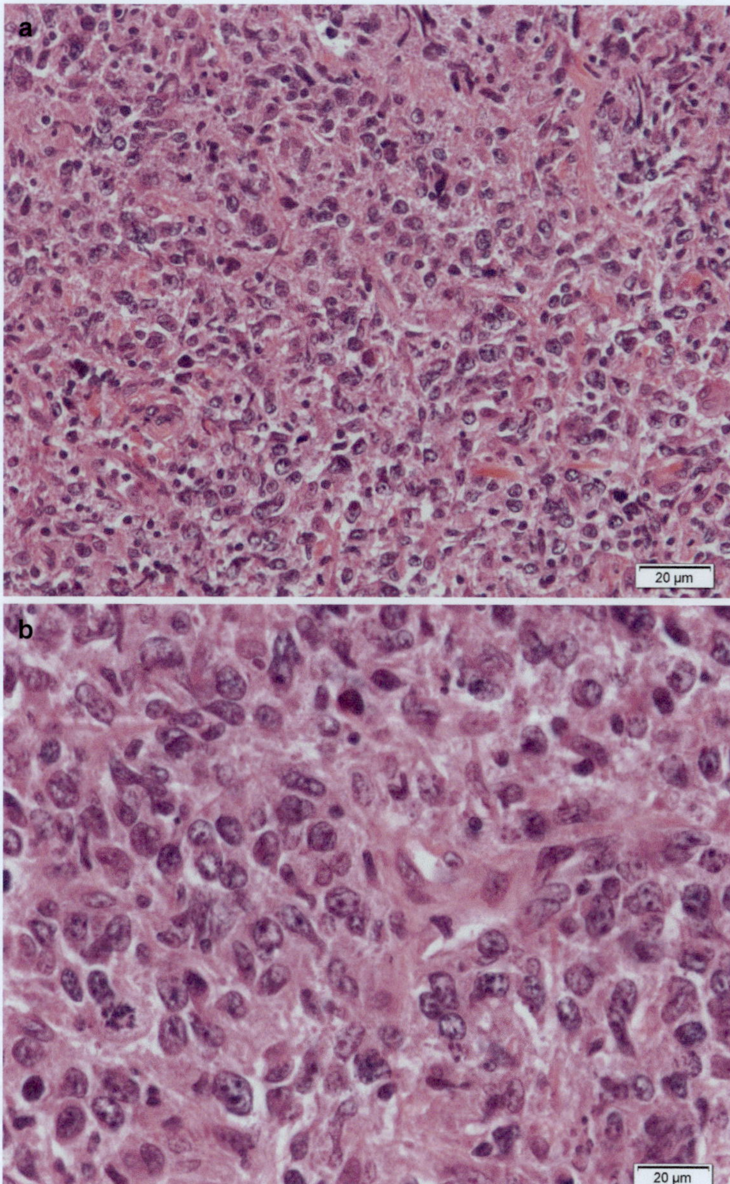


**Fig. 3.1** Diffuse large B-cell lymphoma is characterized by effacement of normal architecture by diffuse infiltration with large uniform lymphoid cells ((**a**) Hematoxylin-eosin (H&E) stain, 20× magnified view; (**b**) H&E stain, 40× magnified view). The malignant cells are uniformly positive for CD20 on immunohistochemistry (**c**). The proliferation fraction is high as determined by Ki67 staining, which is usually >40 % (**d**) (Slides are courtesy of Dr. Josette Briere)

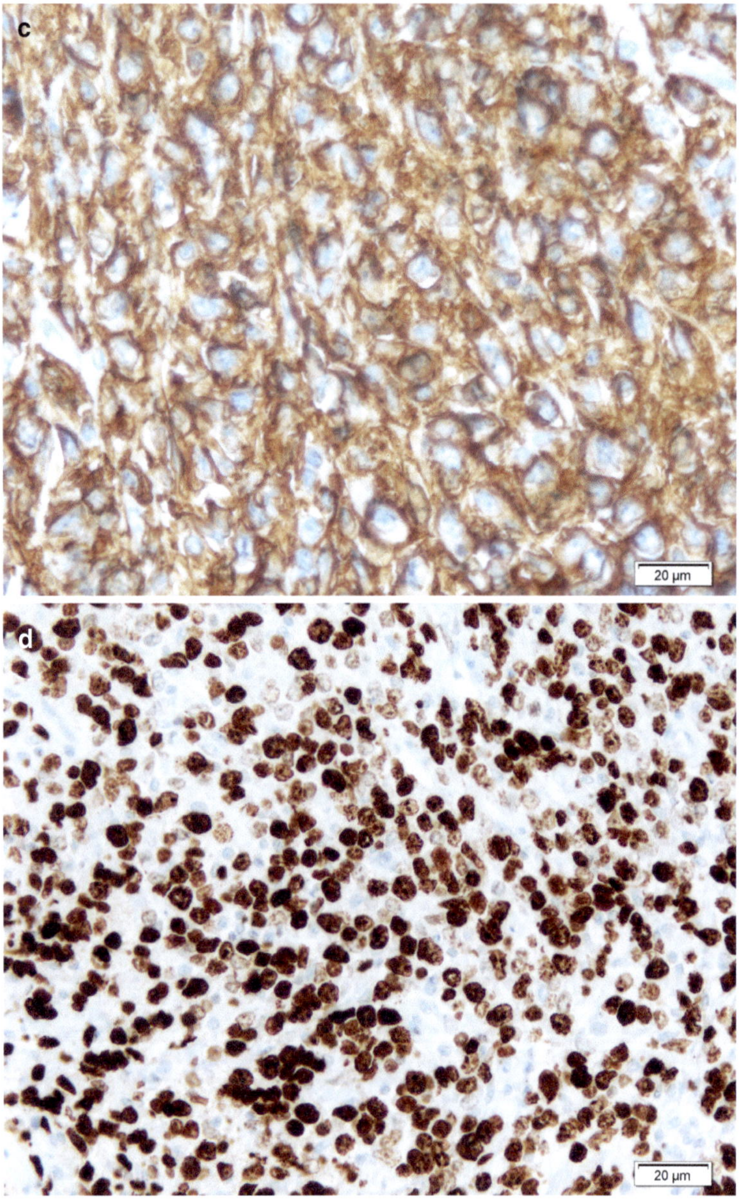


**Fig. 3.1** (continued)

lymphoma cells in 30–60 % of HIV-associated DLBCL, the incidence is much higher in the immunoblastic variant of DLBCL (80–100 %) [2, 20, 24, 25]. The immunoblastic immunophenotype is furthermore characterized by plasmacytoid features with upregulation of plasma cell markers and downregulation of mature B-cell markers [26, 27]. Generally it is thought that immunoblastic DLBCL carries a poorer prognosis, but whether this is related to the more immunosuppressed host or lymphoma-specific features remains unclear [28].

Similarly to DLBCL in immunocompetent patients, gene expression profiling in HIV-associated DLBCL can differentiate between a germinal center (GCB) and activated B-cell (ABC) subtype based on the presumed cell of origin. However, there is conflicting evidence regarding the prognostic significance of the molecular subtype when determined by immunohistochemical algorithms in HIV-associated DLBCL [29–33]. Nevertheless, most studies suggest that the non-GCB phenotype is similarly associated with a worse prognosis in HIV-positive patients. While the ABC subtype dominated in the pre-cART era (>80 %), in the current era, there has been a pathobiological shift to more favorable subtypes [20, 30, 31, 34, 35].

Recently, a subgroup within the heterogeneous entity of DLBCL termed "double-hit lymphoma" has been identified, which is characterized by rearrangement of c-myc and either BCL2 or BCL6 and is associated with a very poor prognosis [36, 37]. Additionally, overexpression of c-myc and bcl-2 and/or bcl6 protein without gene rearrangement appears to lead to worse than expected outcomes [38, 39]. In the setting of HIV, the proportion of DLBCL cases that are "double hit" and/or "double-expresser" has not been well studied [20, 33, 40].

The microenvironment in HIV-related DLBCL appears to differ from that observed in sporadic DLBCL. Liapis and colleagues described increased angiogenesis, which is in turn associated with EBV positivity, and also within the immunoblastic phenotype, reduced numbers of infiltrating T helper and regulatory T cells, but higher numbers of CD8-positive T cells [33]. These findings support the relevance of the tumor microenvironment and the important role of oncogenic viruses and dysregulated T-cell immunity in HIV-related lymphomagenesis.

## 3.2 Presentation, Evaluation, and Prognostication

DLBCL in HIV-positive patients often presents at a more advanced stage, with B symptoms (>10 % weight loss, unexplained persistent fever, drenching night sweats), and more often involves extranodal tissue in severely immunosuppressed patients [3, 28, 41–45]. Most frequently involved is the GI tract; in the pre-cART era, GI involvement as the presenting site was seen in up to 50 % of cases [46, 47], but is much less common today (<15 %) [48]. Multifocal GI involvement is not infrequent (≤23 %) [49]. Other commonly involved extranodal sites are bone marrow (13–22 %), CNS (5–15 %), liver, and lung (each ≤5 %). Therefore, thorough clinical evaluation and staging is especially important in HIV-positive patients. However, many of these observations were reported in the pre-cART era and might no longer be accurate.

Once the diagnosis of DLBCL has been established by an expert hematopathologist's careful evaluation of an excisional lymph node or tissue biopsy (core biopsies are generally considered to be inadequate), patients should undergo immediate careful clinical evaluation. The initial evaluation should focus on obtaining a comprehensive medical history to assess the symptoms related to lymphoma, performance status, B symptoms, and other comorbidities that might impact treatment decisions as well as a detailed HIV history. The latter should include assessment of prior opportunistic infections, general immune function, antiretroviral treatment history, and HIV control. Physical examination requires attention to node-bearing areas, including the Waldeyer's ring, as well as the liver and spleen size. Laboratory evaluation must include at least a complete blood count, a comprehensive metabolic panel to assess electrolytes, blood glucose, renal and liver function, uric acid, lactate dehydrogenase (LDH), hepatitis B and C serology, CD4 count, and HIV viral load. Staging examinations include at least a diagnostic X-ray computed tomography (CT) scan of the chest, abdomen, and pelvis (plus neck if cervical lymphadenopathy is present on physical examination) or a fluorodeoxyglucose (FDG) positron emission tomography (PET)-CT scan. However, because of certain confounding factors such as HIV-related reactive adenopathy, increased incidence of infections, and lipodystrophy, interpretation of FDG-PET scans can be more difficult than in the HIV-negative population, especially in patients with detectable HIV viral loads [31, 50, 51].

Given the increased incidence of bone marrow and CNS involvement in this population, we also strongly advise performing a unilateral bone marrow biopsy; imaging of the brain, preferably with gadolinium-enhanced magnetic resonance imaging (MRI); as well as a lumbar puncture for cytology and flow cytometry to rule out lymphomatous involvement. Additionally, cardiac function should be assessed in selected cases with either a cardiac MUGA (multigated acquisition) scan or an echocardiogram before treatment planning.

Prognosis for HIV-infected individuals newly diagnosed with DLBCL is determined by patient-, lymphoma- and HIV-specific factors. The significance for each of the factors has waxed and waned over the last three decades owing to changes in antiretroviral and lymphoma-directed therapy, supportive care, and a shift in lymphoma biology. The International Prognostic Index (IPI) and age-adjusted IPI (aaIPI), which were established in 1993 as prognostic scores predicting long-term survival in patients with aggressive non-Hodgkin lymphomas (NHL), have been extensively validated and remain reliable predictors of outcomes in HIV-related aggressive NHL [52–58]. HIV infection and its ensuing immunosuppression are competing risk factors that can impact outcome in this patient population. In the era before effective antiretroviral therapy became available, HIV-infected patients diagnosed with lymphoma were unable to tolerate aggressive chemotherapy, and outcomes were universally poor. However, since effective HIV control has become achievable, adequate lymphoma-directed therapy is possible in the contemporary cART era, and survival now mirrors outcomes in immunocompetent patients [14, 58] (Fig. 3.2). With regard to the impact of HIV-related factors on survival, the literature is divided. Low CD4 counts have been implicated as predictors of poor survival in several studies [57, 59–61], while others have not found such an association, especially in the cART era [54, 55, 62]. Similarly, high HIV viral load was associated with poor outcomes in some studies [63–65], while not in others [61, 64].

One explanation might be that to capture the immune deficit caused by HIV infection, a single measure alone might not be adequate. Composite scores have been developed to provide a more comprehensive measure of immune function. The

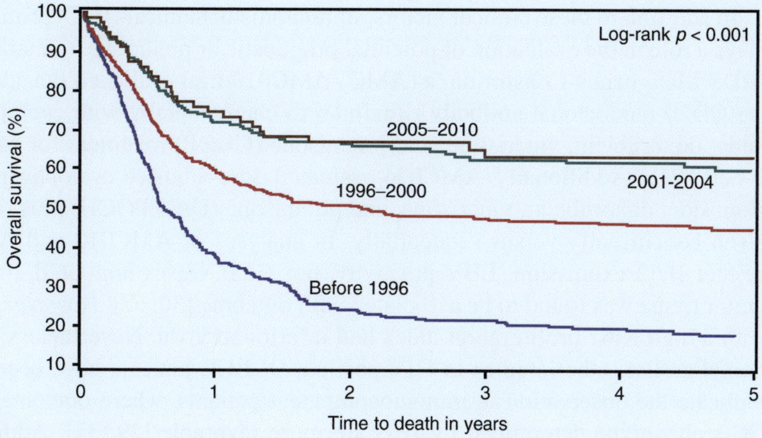


Number at risk:

| | 0 | 1 | 2 | 3 | 4 | 5 |
|---|---|---|---|---|---|---|
| 2005–2010 | 80 | 59 | 50 | 33 | 24 | 13 |
| 2001–2004 | 220 | 135 | 114 | 88 | 80 | 63 |
| 1996–2000 | 443 | 248 | 200 | 175 | 125 | 80 |
| Before 1996 | 281 | 104 | 64 | 57 | 49 | 43 |

**Fig. 3.2** Overall survival for HIV-positive patients with DLBCL during different eras of antiretroviral therapy (Adapted from Barta et al. [58])

largest prospectively performed therapeutic trial for patients with AIDS-related NHL used an HIV score to stratify intensity of treatment in a prospective trial performed in the pre-rituximab era. One point each was assigned to a history of prior AIDS, ECOG performance status (PS) >1, and a CD4 count of <100 cells/ml; patients with zero points were classified as good risk, one point was deemed intermediate risk, and two or more points were deemed high risk. This score – irrespective of intensity of lymphoma-directed therapy – was able to predict survival with 5-year overall survival ranging from 47 to 51 % for the low-risk patients, 24–28 for intermediate-risk patients, and 3–11 % for poor-risk patients [56]. A different composite HIV score, assigning points to presence of a prior history of AIDS, baseline CD4 count, and viral load, was also found to be associated with survival in patients with AIDS-related NHL treated in the rituximab era [66]. Further refinement in prognostication can potentially be achieved by combining different established patient-, lymphoma-, and HIV-related prognostic markers relevant for this specific patient into one score, such as proposed by Bower and colleagues in the pre-rituximab era (combining CD4 count and IPI) or the AIDS-related lymphoma IPI (ARL-IPI) [57, 66]. In a retrospective analysis of 487 patients treated on clinical trials for AIDS-related aggressive lymphomas, the ARL-IPI, which combines an abovementioned HIV score consisting of prior history of AIDS, baseline CD4 count, and viral load, with the age-adjusted IPI, the combined ARL-IPI was able to better predict survival than the age-adjusted IPI alone. Of note, in this analysis, 5-year overall survival was 78 % for the low-risk group, which approximates outcomes seen in HIV-negative patients with DLBCL.

In addition to these clinical factors, immunohistochemical (IHC) profiling also plays a role in the evaluation of potential prognostic or predictive biomarkers. The AIDS Malignancy Consortium's (AMC) AMC010 trial evaluated the addition of the CD20 monoclonal antibody rituximab to chemotherapy with cyclophosphamide, doxorubicin, vincristine, and prednisone (CHOP) treatment for aggressive B-cell NHL. Additionally, AMC034 evaluated dose-adjusted cyclophosphamide, etoposide, doxorubicin, vincristine, and prednisone (DA-EPOCH) plus rituximab given concurrently versus sequentially. In analyses of AMC010 and AMC034, neither Bcl2 expression, EBV positivity, nor GCB versus non-GCB subtype in tumor tissue was found to be associated with outcome [30, 67]. However, patients with a high Ki67 proliferation index had inferior survival. Nevertheless, as mentioned earlier, other studies in HIV-positive DLBCL patients have been able to replicate the observation in immunocompetent patients, where outcomes for the GCB phenotype determined by IHC are more favorable [29, 32]. Additionally, Chao and colleagues found in an analysis of 70 HIV-related DLBCL cases that EBER positivity as defined by ≥75 % EBV-encoded RNA by in situ hybridization (EBER-ish) was associated with increased mortality. The presumed mechanism of treatment resistance is EBV-related upregulation of NF-κ B leading to activation of the antiapoptotic protein BCL2 [68]. Reasons for these contradicting results may lie in different thresholds and methods of determining EBV positivity, heterogeneous treatment of patients, and lack of statistical power secondary to small patient numbers.

## 3.3 Treatment

At present there is no standard treatment for HIV-associated DLBCL. Optimal management has not been established secondary to a lack of prospective phase three trials in this patient population. Treatment recommendations are mostly based on evidence from phase two trials, retrospective series, or expert opinion. To complicate matters further, three large randomized phase three trials performed in HIV-associated DLBCL arrived at conclusions which are no longer necessarily deemed representative in regard to their findings concerning dose intensity and benefit of the CD20 monoclonal antibody rituximab. First, in a trial led by the AIDS Clinical Trials Group (ACTG), the regimen low-dose methotrexate, bleomycin, doxorubicin, cyclophosphamide, vincristine, and dexamethasone (low-dose m-BACOD) was compared with standard-dose m-BACOD; the conclusion was that the more intense regimen resulted in similar efficacy, but more toxicities [32]. Second, the French-Italian Cooperative Group (GELA and GICAT) also observed similar outcomes in patients assigned to more or less intense regimens after stratification by an HIV score irrespective of dose-intensity within each group [55]. Third, in AMC010, which assessed the addition of rituximab (R) to cyclophosphamide, doxorubicin, vincristine, and prednisone (CHOP) chemotherapy, there was no improvement in overall survival when rituximab (R) was added to chemotherapy with CHOP (cyclophosphamide, doxorubicin, vincristine, and prednisone) [67].

Interpretation of the literature is further complicated by the fact that in many early studies, patients with different subtypes of aggressive NHL, such as DLBCL, Burkitt lymphoma (BL), plasmablastic lymphoma (PBL), and primary effusion lymphoma (PEL), were all treated with the same regimens, and, frequently, only composite outcomes were reported. Similarly, patients with early stage (stage 1 and non-bulky 2) and advanced-stage disease (stages bulky 2, 3, and 4) were grouped together and mostly treated with the same protocols. These features have led to some uncertainty about how to interpret the available literature on treatment for HIV-associated DLBCL. However, despite various controversies and nonuniform approaches to treatment, the outcome of HIV-positive patients with DLBCL has steadily improved over the last three decades and today approaches the outcomes seen in HIV-negative patients (Fig. 3.2) [54, 58, 69].

## 3.4 Pre-cART Era

In the era before effective cART was available, the ability to administer lymphoma-directed therapy with curative intent to patients with AIDS was severely hampered mainly by patients' poor bone marrow reserve and the increased incidence of infectious complications. Table 3.1 summarizes the available relevant prospective phase II and III studies for the treatment of HIV-associated DLBCL in the pre-cART era. CHOP and CHOP-like regimens were used for all intermediate- and high-grade AIDS-related lymphomas. These anthracycline-based combination regimens resulted in overall response rates and complete response rates ranging from 43–85 % and 36–67 %, respectively, with a median overall ranging from 5 to 11 months [70–74]. However, less intense regimens resulted in similar survival despite achieving somewhat lower response rates [75–79]. Similarly, higher intensity regimens resulted in comparable outcomes as seen with CHOP, but with significantly more toxicities [80, 81]. As mentioned above, two trials directly compared more and less intensive regimens for patients with AIDS-related lymphomas stratified by HIV risk factors, and in both trials no significant difference in survival could be detected [56, 72]. Nevertheless, survival had remarkably improved for patients treated with chemotherapy and receiving cART compared to those treated in the pre-cART era, which was further confirmed in a study performed by investigators from the Italian National Cancer Institute [74].

## 3.5 CART Era

The arrival of effective antiretroviral therapy has had a significant positive impact on outcomes for patients with HIV-associated lymphomas. Several studies confirmed the improved outcomes and tolerability seen with CHOP therapy in patients with intermediate- and high-grade NHL in the cART era (Table 3.2). North American and European cooperative group trials demonstrated complete response rates of 48–63 % and 1-year overall survival of 60–80 % for patients with HIV-associated

**Table 3.1** Interventional trials for AIDS-related lymphomas enrolling patients in the era prior to routine use of combination antiretroviral therapy

| Study | Phase | Number of patients | Histology | Intervention | Result |
|---|---|---|---|---|---|
| Kaplan et al. [70] | III | 30 | Intermediate- and high-grade NHL | CHOP ± rGM-CSF | CRR: 67 %;<br>Median OS: 9.0 months |
| Levine et al. [78] | II | 42 | Intermediate- and high-grade NHL | Low-dose m-BACOD | ORR 51 %<br>CRR: 46 %<br>Median OS 5.6 months |
| Tirelli et al. [75] | II | 37 | "Poor-risk" (ECOG PS>2 and/or OI) aggressive NHL | Dose-reduced CHVmP-vincristine-bleomycin | ORR: 52 %;<br>CRR: 14 %;<br>Median OS: 3.5 months |
| Sawka et al. [76] | II | 30 | Aggressive NHL | Weekly etoposide, doxorubicin, cyclophosphamide, bleomycin, vincristine MTX, pred ×12 | ORR:73 %;<br>CR rate: 33 %;<br>Median OS: 8.1 months |
| Gisselbrecht et al. [80] | II | 141 | Intermediate and high grade; no active OI and PS<3 | LNH-84 | ORR: 76 %;<br>CR: 63 %;<br>Median OS: 9 months |
| Remick et al. [77] | II | 18 | Intermediate- and high-grade NHL | Low-dose oral regimen[a] | ORR: 61 %;<br>CRR: 39 %;<br>Median OS: 7 months |
| Gabarre et al. [81] | II | 32 | Intermediate and high grade; no active OI and PS<3 | LNH-84 + AZT and GCSF | ORR: 56 %<br>Median OS: 6.7 months |
| Sparano et al. [82] | II | 25 | Intermediate- and high-grade NHL | Infusional CDE + ddI and GCSF | CRR: 58 %;<br>Median OS: 18.4 months |
| Levine et al. [79] | II | 25 | Intermediate- and high-grade NHL | Low-dose m-BACOD + ddC | ORR: 76 %;<br>CRR: 56 %;<br>Median OS: 8.1 months |
| Newell et al. [71] | I/II | 14 | NHL | CEOP + GCSF | ORR: 57 %;<br>CRR: 50 %;<br>Median OS: 17 months |

| | | | | | |
|---|---|---|---|---|---|
| Tosi et al. [83] | II | 29 | High-grade NHL (included relapsed patients) | AZT + HD MTX | ORR: 79 % (untreated pts); CR rate: 44 % (untreated pts) Median OS: 12 months (all) |
| Kaplan et al. [72] | III | 192 | Intermediate- and high-grade NHL | Low-dose (LD) vs. standard-dose (SD) m-BACOD | ORR: LD: 69 %, SD 78 %; CRR: LD 41 %, SD 52 %; Median OS: LD 35 weeks, SD 31 weeks |
| Weiss et al. [84] | II | 68 | High-grade NHL | Risk-adapted therapy: CHOP for low-risk pts (no risk factors: CD4>50; ECOG PS<3; no h/o AIDS) vs. LD-CHOP or VP (2 out of 3 risk factors); followed by AZT and INF maintenance if in CR | Normal risk: CRR: 68 %; median OS 21 month High risk: VP: CRR: 28 %; median OS 2.4 months LD-CHOP: CRR: 68 %; median OS: 5.2 months |
| Kersten et al. [73] | II | 21 | NHL | CNOP + GCSF followed by AZT | ORR: 43 %; CRR: 19 %; Median OS: 5 months |
| Oksenhendler et al. [85] | II | 52 | Intermediate- and high-grade NHL | LNH84 | ORR: 85 %; CRR:71 %; Median OS: 15 months |

*NHL* non-Hodgkin Lymphoma, *rGM-CSF* recombinant granulocyte-macrophage-colony stimulating factor, *CHOP* cyclophosphamide, vincristine, doxorubicin, and prednisone, *CRR* complete response rate, *OS* overall survival, *ECOG* Eastern Cooperative Oncology Group, *PS* performance status, *OI* opportunistic infection, *CHVmP* cyclophosphamide, doxorubicin, vincristine, methotrexate, prednisone, *ORR* overall response rate, *mtx* methotrexate, *pred* prednisone, *LNH84* ACVBP×3 followed by cyclophosphamide, etoposide, methotrexate (CVM) ×3, *ACVBP* doxorubicin, cyclophosphamide, vindesine, bleomycin, and prednisolone, *AZT* azidothymidine, *GCSF* granulocyte-colony stimulating factor, *CDE* cyclophosphamide, doxorubicin and etoposide, *ddI* didanosine, *m-BACOD* methotrexate, bleomycin, doxorubicin, cyclophosphamide, vincristine, and dexamethasone, *ddC* zalcitabine, *CEOP* cyclophosphamide, epirubicin, vincristine, and prednisolone, *HD MTX* high-dose methotrexate, *pts* patients, *LD-CHOP* low-dose CHOP, *h/o* history of, *VP* vincristine and prednisone, *INF* interferon, *CNOP* cyclophosphamide, mitoxantrone, vincristine, and prednisolone.

[a] Combination of oral lomustine, etoposide, cyclophosphamide, and procarbazine

**Table 3.2** Interventional trials for AIDS-related lymphomas enrolling patients mainly in the era of combination antiretroviral therapy

| Study | Phase | Number of patients | Histology | Intervention | Result |
|---|---|---|---|---|---|
| Vaccher et al.[a] [74] | Two consecutive phase II trials | 104 | Intermediate- and high-grade NHL | CHOP or CHOP + cART | CHOP: ORR: 85 %;<br>CRR: 36 %;<br>Median OS: 7 months<br>CHOP + cART: ORR: 85 %;<br>CRR: 50 %;<br>Median OS: NR |
| Remick et al.[a] [86] | II | 20 | DLBCL, BL, BLL | Low-dose oral regimen[b] | ORR: 70 %;<br>CRR:30 %;<br>Median OS: 7.3 months |
| Ratner et al. [87] | II | 65 | Intermediate- and high-grade NHL | Modified (m) CHOP ($n=40$) and CHOP ($n=25$) | mCHOP: ORR: 60 %;<br>CRR:30 %;<br>Median DFS: 16 months<br>CHOP: ORR: 57 %;<br>CRR: 48 %;<br>Median DFS: NR |
| Gastaldi et al.[a] [88] | II | 14 | DLCL | CIOD | ORR and CRR: 93 %<br>5-year OS: 44 % |
| Little et al.[a] [35] | II | 39 | Aggressive NHL | Dose-adjusted (DA) EPOCH | ORR: 87 %;<br>CRR: 74 %;<br>OS at 53 months: 60 % |
| Tulpule et al.[a] [89] | II | 18 | Intermediate- and high-grade NHL | Low-dose CHOP + mitoguazone | ORR: 79 %;<br>CR rate 43 %;<br>Median OS: 9.9 months |

| | | | | | |
|---|---|---|---|---|---|
| Levine et al.[a] [90] | II | 24 | Intermediate- and high-grade NHL | Liposomal doxorubicin + COP | ORR: 88 %;<br>CRR: 75 %;<br>Median OS: NR (>13.4 months) |
| Sparano et al.[a] [91] | II | 98 | Intermediate- and high-grade NHL | Infusional CDE | CDE: ORR: 56 %;<br>CRR: 47 %;<br>Median OS: 6.8 months<br>CDE+cART: ORR: 58 %;<br>CRR: 44 %;<br>Median OS: 13.7 months |
| Costello et al.[a] [92] | II | 38 | Intermediate- and high-grade NHL | Intensive chemoradiation (COPx1->CHOPx3->HD MTX->HD cytarabine->radiation) | ORR: 79 %;<br>CRR: 61 %;<br>40 months OS: 43 % (30 % for non-BL) |
| Sawka et al.[a] [93] | I/II | 47 | Intermediate- and high-grade NHL | VACOP-B | ORR: 30 %;<br>CRR: 39 %;<br>Median OS: 7.2 months |
| Kaplan et al.[a] [67] | III | 150 (CHOP $n=51$; R-CHOP $n=99$) | Intermediate- and high-grade NHL | CHOP vs. R-CHOP | CHOP: ORR: 55 %;<br>CRR: 47 %;<br>Median OS: 28 months<br>R-CHOP: ORR: 66 %;<br>CRR: 58 %;<br>Median OS: 35 months |
| Spina et al.[a] [94] | Pooled results (3 Ph II) | 74 | CD20+ NHL | R-CDE | ORR: 75 %<br>CR R: 70 % (DLBCL 77 % vs. 52 % for BL)<br>2-year OS: 64 % (median OS DLBCL NR @24 months vs. 14 months for BL) |
| Navarro et al.[a] [95] | II | 23 | DLBCL | CHOP | CR R: 74 %<br>5-year OS: 63 % |

(continued)

**Table 3.2** (continued)

| Study | Phase | Number of patients | Histology | Intervention | Result |
|---|---|---|---|---|---|
| Weiss et al. [96] | II | 72 | Intermediate- and high-grade NHL | CHOP | ORR: 84 %<br>CRR: 63 % (DLBCL 66 %)<br>Median OS: 26.1 months (DLBCL 64.7 months) |
| Mounier et al.[a] [56] | III | 485 | High-grade NHL | Assignment as per HIV score:[c]<br>Good: ACVBP vs. CHOP;<br>Intermediate: CHOP vs. LD-CHOP;<br>Poor: LD-CHOP vs. VS | ORR: ACVBP: 77 %; CHOP: 58–66 %; LD-CHOP 32–48 %; VS 20 %<br>CRR: ACVBP: 61 %; CHOP: 49–51 %; LD-CHOP 20–32 %; VS 5 %<br>5-year OS: ACVBP: 51 %; CHOP: 28–47 %; LD-CHOP 11–24 %; VS 3 % |
| Boue et al. [97] | II | 52 | High-grade B-cell NHL | R-CHOP | ORR: 87 %<br>CR/Cru rate: 77 % (DLBCL 81 %)<br>2-year OS: 75 % |
| Combs et al. [98] | I/II | 12 | Intermediate- and high-grade NHL | LACE | ORR: 83 %<br>CRR: 75 %<br>Median OS: >107 months |
| Ribera et al.[a] [99] | II | 80 | DLBCL | R-CHOP | ORR: 69 %<br>CRR: 69 %<br>3-year OS: 56 % |
| Dunleavy et al. [31] | II | 33 | DLBCL | SC-EPOCH-RR | ORR: 93 %<br>CRR:91 %<br>5-year OS: 68 % |

| | | | | | |
|---|---|---|---|---|---|
| Sparano et al. [100] | II | 106 | DLBCL, BL, BLL, aggressive CD20+ NHL | R-EPOCH ($n=51$) or EPOCH->R ($n=55$) | R-EPOCH:<br>ORR: 88 %<br>CR/CRu rate:73 % (DLBCL 71 %)<br>2-year OS: 70 %<br>EPOCH->R:<br>ORR: 77 %<br>CRR: 55 % (DLBCL 46 %)<br>5-year OS: 67 % |
| Levine et al. [65] | II | 40 | CD20+ aggressive NHL | DR-COP | ORR: 68 %<br>CRR: 48 %<br>1-year OS: 70 % (DLBCL 71 %); 2-year OS: 62 % (DLBCL 56 %) |

*NHL* non-Hodgkin Lymphoma, *CHOP* cyclophosphamide, vincristine, doxorubicin, and prednisone, *cART* combination antiretroviral therapy, *ORR* overall response rate, *CRR* complete response rate, *OS* overall survival, *NR* not reached, *DLBCL* diffuse large B-cell lymphoma, *BL* Burkitt lymphoma, *BLL* Burkitt-like lymphoma, *DFS* disease-free survival, *DLCL* diffuse large cell lymphoma, *CIOD* cyclophosphamide, idarubicin, vincristine, dexamethasone, *EPOCH* infusional etoposide, oral prednisone, infusional doxorubicin, bolus cyclophosphamide, and infusional vincristine, *COP* cyclophosphamide, vincristine, and prednisone, *CDE* cyclophosphamide, doxorubicin, and etoposide, *HD MTX* high-dose methotrexate, *HD* high dose, *VACOP-B* methotrexate, doxorubicin, cyclophosphamide, vincristine, prednisone, and bleomycin, *R-CHOP* rituximab, cyclophosphamide, vincristine, doxorubicin, and prednisone, *LACE* liposomal doxorubicin, cyclophosphamide, etoposide, *SC-EPOCH-RR* short-course EPOCH with dose-dense rituximab, *R-EPOCH* rituximab concurrent with EPOCH, *EPOCH- > R* rituximab sequential after EPOCH, *DR-COP* pegylated doxorubicin, cyclophosphamide, vincristine, prednisone

[a]Not all patients were enrolled in the cART era

[b]Combination of oral lomustine, etoposide, cyclophosphamide and procarbazine

[c]HIV score: Risk factors: Eastern Cooperative Oncology Group (ECOG) performance status >1, prior AIDS, baseline CD4 count <100 cells/μL. Classification based on number of risk factors present: 0 factors = good risk, 1 factor = intermediate risk, ≥2 factors = poor risk

NHL treated with CHOP in the cART era [87, 96]. Notably, for patients with DLBCL on the German AIDS-Related Lymphoma Study Group trial, the reported CR rate was a remarkable 66 % and median overall survival 64.7 months. Results by the Spanish PETHEMA group suggested that outcomes for patient with DLBCL treated with CHOP were now similar between HIV-negative and HIV-positive patients [95].

Based on encouraging results seen in the pre-cART era with the infusional regimen CDE (cyclophosphamide, doxorubicin, and etoposide) [82], CDE and another infusional regimen, EPOCH (oral prednisone with infusional etoposide, doxorubicin, and vincristine given as a continuous infusion over 96 h followed by bolus cyclophosphamide) were further explored in the cART era. The theoretical background for the potential superiority of infusional versus bolus regimens is based on the hypothetical principle that low-dose continuous exposure of highly proliferative tumors to doxorubicin and other chemotherapy agents can overcome kinetic resistance. In addition, dynamically dose-adjusted approaches (such as dose-adjusted EPOCH) attempt to control for inter-patient variability in pharmacokinetics by using the neutrophil nadir as a surrogate marker of drug levels [101]. Between 1995 and 2000, 39 patients with AIDS-related lymphoma were treated with dose-adjusted EPOCH at the US National Cancer Institute (NCI). Twenty-five of these patients had DLBCL histology. Eighty-seven percent of all patients achieved a response and 74 % a complete response, resulting in a median overall survival of 60 % after 53 months of follow-up [35]. When progression-free survival (PFS) of the 25 patients with HIV-associated DLBCL was compared with 33 HIV-negative DLBCL patients treated at the same time at the NCI, no difference could be found (PFS 94 % for HIV positive patients after 53-month median follow-up versus 82 % in HIV-negative patients after 69-month median follow-up). Outcomes with infusional CDE in the cART era were more in line with what had been seen with the bolus regimen CHOP in a trial performed by ECOG (E3493): 44 % achieved a complete response, and median survival was 13.7 months [91].

The improved outcomes seen with the addition of the CD20-directed monoclonal antibody rituximab to CHOP therapy in immunocompetent patients with DLBCL led to a direct comparison of CHOP versus R-CHOP in HIV-associated NHL. In AMC010, 150 HIV-positive patients with intermediate- and high-grade CD20-positive NHL were randomized in a 1:2 fashion to receive either CHOP alone ($n=51$) or R-CHOP ($n=99$) followed by 3-monthly rituximab maintenance for responders. Treatment consisted of six cycles for advanced disease or three cycles followed by involved field radiation therapy (IFRT) for stage I and non-bulky stage II disease. The majority of the patients had DLBCL (80 %), but patients with BL were also included in this trial (9 %). Unexpectedly, despite higher response rates and less lymphoma-related deaths in the R-CHOP arm compared to CHOP (CR rate 58 % vs. 47 %; $p=0.15$; death due to lymphoma 14 % vs. 29 %), the overall and progression-free survivals were not statistically different between both arms (OS 139 weeks vs. 110 weeks, $p=67$; PFS 45 weeks vs. 38 weeks, $p=0.76$) [67]. Of note, 40 % of the infectious deaths in the R-CHOP arm occurred during the maintenance rituximab phase. A possible explanation for the observed lack of benefit from the addition of rituximab to CHOP in AMC010 might be the high treatment-related mortality of 36 % for patients with a CD4 count <50 cells/ml in the R-CHOP group and the lower than expected response rate in the whole group. Additionally, 9 % of the included patients had BL, a disease for which R-CHOP is deemed as an insufficient therapy (see Chap. 4, Burkitt Lymphoma). These factors might have resulted in a lower than expected effect size and a lack of statistical power to detect a significant survival benefit. However, since then other trials have explored the addition of rituximab to CHOP in HIV-related NHL (without rituximab maintenance) and found R-CHOP to be both safe and efficacious [97, 99]. Similarly, the addition of rituximab to infusional CDE also resulted in high response rates and improved survival for HIV-positive patients with DLBCL compared to historical controls [94].

Therefore, and in spite of the findings in AMC010, all future trials in CD20+ HIV-related lymphomas included rituximab as part of the initial treatment regimen. Nevertheless, following the high treatment-related mortality in patients with low CD4 counts seen in AMC010, some trials excluded patients with CD4 counts <50 cells/ml.

Given the high response rates seen in the initial NCI trial of dose-adjusted EPOCH, other trials combined rituximab with EPOCH. In AMC034, rituximab was given either consecutively with EPOCH or sequentially (weekly for six doses after completion of chemotherapy). In this "pick-the-winner" phase II trial, only the concurrent arm reached the predefined endpoint, with a CR rate of 73 % (71 % for DLBCL) versus only 55 % in the sequential arm. With concurrent R-EPOCH, 2-year overall survival reached 70 %. The NCI explored short-course EPOCH with dose-dense rituximab (SC-EPOCH-RR; EPOCH with rituximab on days 1 and 5 of each cycle) in 33 patients with HIV-associated DLBCL. Patients were treated with two cycles of EPOCH-RR, after which a CT and PET scan were performed. If CT and PET scan results were deemed negative after two cycles, one additional cycle was given; patients with positive scan results received additional cycles until their scans became negative to a maximum of six cycles (minimum number of cycles = 3). Ninety-one percent of patients achieved a complete response after a median of three cycles; PFS and OS at 5 years were 84 % and 68 %, respectively. Patients with the GCB subtype particularly benefited (non-GCB vs. GCB HR for death: 7.2; $p=0.028$) [31].

## 3.6 Treatment Recommendations

Based on the available evidence from clinical trials, many experts and cooperative groups, especially in North America, have adapted six to eight cycles of chemoimmunotherapy with rituximab and EPOCH as their standard initial regimen for the treatment of HIV-positive patients with DLBCL [20, 100, 102, 103]. While indirect evidence from retrospective analyses suggests that EPOCH might be a more efficacious chemotherapy backbone in HIV-related DLBCL than CHOP, no direct comparison of R-CHOP and R-EPOCH has been performed (Fig. 3.3) [14, 104]. Results on the completed CALGB50303 trial, which randomized immunocompetent patients with DLBCL to either R-HOP or R-EPOCH, are eagerly awaited to provide

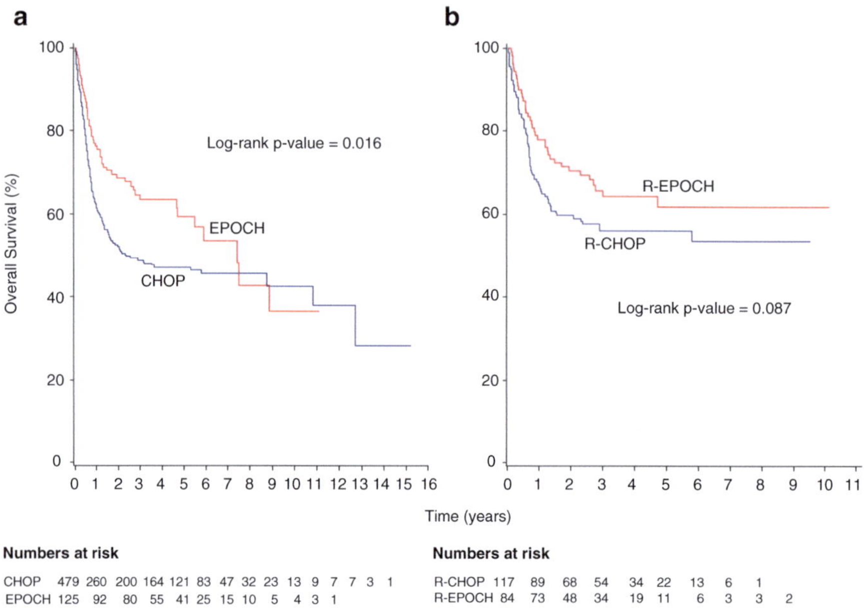


**Fig. 3.3** In a pooled retrospective analysis, HIV-positive patients with newly diagnosed diffuse large B-cell lymphoma (DLBCL) treated with infusional EPOCH achieved significantly longer overall survival than patients treated with CHOP (**a**). This was also seen when the analysis was limited to patients with DLBCL treated in the rituximab era, where treatment with R-EPOCH compared favorably to treatment with R-CHOP (**b**). This research and graph were originally published in Blood (Barta et al. [14]. © the American Society of Hematology)

further guidance. At present, both regimens [CHOP and EPOCH] are considered a valid first choice of chemotherapy for patients with advanced disease [105]. Encouragingly, outcomes with these initial regimens approach those for HIV-negative patients in the current era [45, 58, 95].

## 3.7 Areas of Uncertainty

### 3.7.1 Early-Stage Disease

Most HIV-positive patients present with advanced lymphoma, and only 10–30 % present with early-stage DLBCL (stages I and non-bulky stage II) [67, 97, 99]. Often these patients are excluded from clinical trials, and therefore, recommendations must rely on extrapolation of data from HIV-negative patients. We favor treating patients with early-stage DLBCL with chemoimmunotherapy alone (e.g., six cycles of R-CHOP) and avoid abbreviated chemotherapy followed by radiation therapy, as HIV-associated DLBCL tends to be associated with higher stages, more advanced and aggressive disease, as well as higher rates of bone marrow and extranodal involvement.

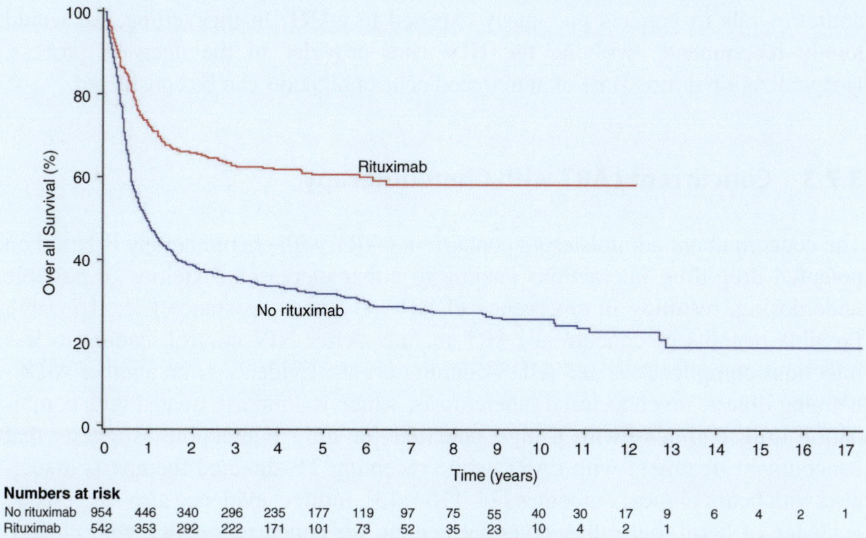


**Fig. 3.4** Overall survival has improved significantly for HIV-positive patients treated with rituximab-containing regimens when compared to patients who did not receive rituximab (Kaplan-Meier curve: log-rank $p<0.001$; HR for overall survival in multivariate analysis: 0.51, [95 % CI 0.38–0.71; $p<0.0001$]). This research and graph were originally published in Blood (Barta et al. [14]. © the American Society of Hematology)

## 3.7.2 Rituximab for Patients with Low CD4 Counts

A high treatment-related mortality, especially secondary to infectious deaths, has been observed in patients with CD4 counts <50 cells/ml in AMC010 and AMC034 (36 % and 38 %, respectively) versus only 5–6 % in patients with CD4 counts ≥50 cells/ml [104]. However, other studies that included rituximab as part of the initial treatment regimen did not observe such a high treatment-related mortality rate, even in patients with low CD4 counts [31, 94, 97, 99]. While the addition of rituximab has clearly resulted in improved survival for HIV-positive patients with newly diagnosed DLBCL (Fig. 3.4) [106], the benefit of rituximab in patients with low CD4 counts (<50 cells/ml) has not been fully established. In a large retrospective database analysis, the addition of rituximab to chemotherapy resulted in significantly higher complete response rates and overall survival for patients with CD4 counts ≥50 cells/ml (OR 2.84 for CR rate and HR for OS 0.55; $p<0.001$ for both), but no significant benefit was seen in those patients with lower CD4 counts (OR 1.36 for CR, $p=0.44$; HR for OS 1.08, $p=0.76$) [14]. However, in many other studies, rituximab has been used safely in patients with CD4 counts <50 cells/ml. Therefore, we recommend adding rituximab to chemotherapy for most patients irrespective of their CD4 count. Nevertheless, factors that might indicate a higher risk of mainly infectious complications in these patients with very low CD4 counts are a history of prior or ongoing opportunistic infection and a low likelihood of adequate HIV control with antiretrovirals in patients previously exposed to cART. In this setting, we would highly recommend involving the HIV care provider in the decision process. Hospitalization during time of anticipated neutrophil nadir can be considered.

### 3.7.3 Concurrent cART with Chemotherapy

The concern about administering concurrent cART with chemotherapy is based on potential drug-drug interactions leading to either increased toxicities or possible underdosing, resulting in emergence of HIV or cancer resistance [87, 107–109]. Possible benefits of concurrent cART include better HIV control leading to less infectious complications and AIDS-defining events. Evidence from another AIDS-defining illness, mycobacterial tuberculosis, which is similarly treated with combination drug regimens with a high potential for drug interactions, suggests that concomitant treatment with cART while receiving TB-directed therapy is associated with better clinical outcomes [74, 110–113]. Indirect evidence also suggests no evidence of harm, but rather potential benefit, for concurrent cART with chemotherapy [14]. While the authors recommend concurrent cART with chemotherapy, they recognize that it is reasonable to suspend cART therapy during treatment, especially if treatment duration is brief, such as with SC-EPOCH-RR or for early disease. Unstructured interruption of cART administration can lead to antiretroviral resistance and must be avoided at all cost. For a more detailed discussion of this topic, we refer the reader to Chap. 17, Chemotherapy and Interactions with cART.

### 3.7.4 Relapsed Disease

The only prospective trials for relapsed HIV-associated NHL not involving hematopoietic stem cell transplantation have been published in the pre-rituximab era and add little to inform current treatment strategies [114–117]. In a retrospective series of patients treated by AMC institutions, the 1-year survival of patients with relapsed or refractory AIDS-related lymphomas who did not undergo autologous stem cell transplantation was only 37 %. Complete responses with different second-line salvage regimens ranged from 5 to 39 %. Patients with primary refractory disease did worse than patients who experienced a relapse after having achieved a response (1-year OS 31 % vs. 59 %; $p=0.02$), and patients who underwent autologous stem cell transplantation (ASCT) as part of their salvage therapy lived longer than patients who did not (1-year OS: 63.2 % vs. 37.2 %). However, in this series, patients who achieved either a partial or complete response to first-line salvage therapy had similar 1-year survival to patients who underwent ASCT (87.5 % for ASCT vs. 81.8 % for non-ASCT) [118].

Given the convincing evidence that most HIV-positive patients in the current era can tolerate dose-intense multiagent regimens such as those used for BL or as preparative regimes for ASCT, we would recommend approaching HIV-positive patients with relapsed or refractory DLBCL in a manner similar to immunocompetent patients. High-dose salvage regimens such as ICE (ifosfamide, carboplatin, etoposide), DHAP (dexamethasone, cytarabine, cisplatin), or GDP (gemcitabine, dexamethasone, cisplatin) in combination with rituximab appear to have similar efficacy and should be used for appropriate patients based on data in HIV-negative patients with relapsed or refractory aggressive NHL [119, 120]. Patients with chemosensitive disease, who are transplant eligible, should proceed to hematopoietic stem cell transplantation (HCT), which is discussed in detail in Chap. 12, Autologous Stem Cell Transplantation; and Chap. 13, Allogeneic Stem Cell Transplantation. In HIV-negative DLBCL, many new agents are in development, particularly inhibitors of the NF-kappa B pathway and B-cell receptor signaling. Ibrutinib has demonstrated good efficacy in relapsed HIV-negative ABC DLBCL; therefore, such agents should be considered in patients with relapsed ABC tumors [121]. Ultimately, advances in understanding tumor biology and developing rational agents to target new pathways should not be different in the HIV-positive setting.

Improvements in supportive care, such as CNS and antimicrobial prophylaxis, have significantly contributed to the improved outcomes for HIV-positive patients with cancer and will be discussed in detail separately in Chap. 18, Special Considerations.

## References


1. Beral V, Peterman T, Berkelman R, et al. AIDS-associated non-Hodgkin lymphoma. Lancet. 1991;337:805–9.
2. Swerdlow SH, Campo E, Harris NL, et al. WHO classification of tumours of haematopoietic and lymphoid tissues. 4th ed. Lyon: International Agency for Research on Cancer; 2008.
3. Besson C, Goubar A, Gabarre J, et al. Changes in AIDS-related lymphoma since the era of highly active antiretroviral therapy. Blood. 2001;98:2339–44.
4. Raphael M, Gentilhomme O, Tulliez M, et al. Histopathologic features of high-grade non-Hodgkin's lymphomas in acquired immunodeficiency syndrome. The French Study Group of Pathology for Human Immunodeficiency Virus-Associated Tumors. Arch Pathol Lab Med. 1991;115:15–20.
5. Coté TR, Biggar RJ, Rosenberg PS, et al. Non-Hodgkin's lymphoma among people with AIDS: incidence, presentation and public health burden. Int J Cancer. 1997;73:645–50.
6. Bohlius J, Schmidlin K, Costagliola D, et al. Incidence and risk factors of HIV-related non-Hodgkin's lymphoma in the era of combination antiretroviral therapy: a European multicohort study. Antivir Ther. 2009;14:1065–74.
7. The Antiretroviral Therapy Cohort Collaboration. The changing incidence of AIDS events in patients receiving highly active antiretroviral therapy. Arch Intern Med. 2005;165:416–23.
8. Gibson TM, Morton LM, Shiels MS, et al. Risk of non-Hodgkin lymphoma subtypes in HIV-infected people during the HAART era: a population-based study. AIDS. 2014;28:2313–8.
9. Silverberg MJ, Chao C, Leyden WA, et al. HIV infection, immunodeficiency, viral replication, and the risk of cancer. Cancer Epidemiol Biomarkers Prev. 2011;20:2551–9.
10. Biggar RJ, Chaturvedi AK, Goedert JJ, et al. AIDS-related cancer and severity of immunosuppression in persons with AIDS. J Natl Cancer Inst. 2007;99:962–72.
11. Pluda JM, Yarchoan R, Jaffe ES, et al. Development of non-Hodgkin lymphoma in a cohort of patients with severe human immunodeficiency virus (HIV) infection on long-term antiretroviral therapy. Ann Intern Med. 1990;113:276–82.

12. Engels EA, Pfeiffer RM, Landgren O, et al. Immunologic and virologic predictors of AIDS-related non-hodgkin lymphoma in the highly active antiretroviral therapy era. J Acquir Immune Defic Syndr. 2010;54:78–84.
13. Guiguet M, Boué F, Cadranel J, et al. Effect of immunodeficiency, HIV viral load, and antiretroviral therapy on the risk of individual malignancies (FHDH-ANRS CO4): a prospective cohort study. Lancet Oncol. 2009;10:1152–9.
14. Barta SK, Xue X, Wang D, et al. Treatment factors affecting outcomes in HIV-associated non-Hodgkin lymphomas: a pooled analysis of 1546 patients. Blood. 2013;122:3251–62.
15. Bower M, Fisher M, Hill T, et al. CD4 counts and the risk of systemic non-Hodgkin's lymphoma in individuals with HIV in the UK. Haematologica. 2009;94:875–80.
16. Achenbach CJ, Buchanan AL, Cole SR, et al. HIV viremia and incidence of non-Hodgkin lymphoma in patients successfully treated with antiretroviral therapy. Clin Infect Dis. 2014;58(11):1599–606.
17. Zoufaly A, Stellbrink HJ, Heiden MA, et al. Cumulative HIV viremia during highly active antiretroviral therapy is a strong predictor of AIDS-related lymphoma. J Infect Dis. 2009;200:79–87.
18. Clifford GM, Polesel J, Rickenbach M, et al. Cancer risk in the Swiss HIV cohort study: associations with immunodeficiency, smoking, and highly active antiretroviral therapy. J Natl Cancer Inst. 2005;97:425–32.
19. Franceschi S, Lise M, Clifford GM, et al. Changing patterns of cancer incidence in the early- and late-HAART periods: the Swiss HIV cohort study. Br J Cancer. 2010;103:416–22.
20. Little RF, Dunleavy K. Update on the treatment of HIV-associated hematologic malignancies. ASH Educ Prog Book. 2013;2013:382–8.
21. Carbone A, Vaccher E, Gloghini A, et al. Diagnosis and management of lymphomas and other cancers in HIV-infected patients. Nat Rev Clin Oncol. 2014;11:223–38.
22. Ometto L, Menin C, Masiero S, et al. Molecular profile of Epstein-Barr virus in human immunodeficiency virus type 1-related lymphadenopathies and lymphomas. Blood. 1997;90:313–22.
23. Hamilton-Dutoit SJ, Pallesen G, Karkov J, et al. Identification of EBV-DNA in tumour cells of AIDS-related lymphomas by in-situ hybridisation. Lancet. 1989;1:554–2.
24. Carbone A, Tirelli U, Gloghini A, et al. Human immunodeficiency virus-associated systemic lymphomas may be subdivided into two main groups according to Epstein-Barr viral latent gene expression. J Clin Oncol. 1993;11:1674–81.
25. Ambinder RF. Epstein-Barr virus associated lymphoproliferations in the AIDS setting. Eur J Cancer. 2001;37:1209–16.
26. Cesarman E. Pathology of lymphoma in HIV. Curr Opin Oncol. 2013;25:487–94.
27. Chadburn A, Abdul-Nabi AM, Teruya BS, et al. Lymphoid proliferations associated with human immunodeficiency virus infection. Arch Pathol Lab Med. 2013;137:360–70.
28. Gabarre J, Raphael M, Lepage E, et al. Human immunodeficiency virus-related lymphoma: relation between clinical features and histologic subtypes. Am J Med. 2001;111:704–11.
29. Hoffmann C, Tiemann M, Schrader C, et al. AIDS-related B-cell lymphoma (ARL): correlation of prognosis with differentiation profiles assessed by immunophenotyping. Blood. 2005;106:1762–9.
30. Chadburn A, Chiu A, Lee JY, et al. Immunophenotypic analysis of AIDS-related diffuse large B-cell lymphoma and clinical implications in patients from AIDS malignancies consortium clinical trials 010 and 034. J Clin Oncol. 2009;27:5039–48.
31. Dunleavy K, Little RF, Pittaluga S, et al. The role of tumor histogenesis, FDG-PET, and short-course EPOCH with dose-dense rituximab (SC-EPOCH-RR) in HIV-associated diffuse large B-cell lymphoma. Blood. 2010;115:3017–24.
32. Xicoy B, Ribera J-M, Mate J-l, et al. Immunohistochemical expression profile and prognosis in patients with diffuse large B-cell lymphoma with or without human immunodeficiency virus infection. Leuk Lymphoma. 2010;51:2063–9.
33. Liapis K, Clear A, Owen A, et al. The microenvironment of AIDS-related diffuse large B-cell lymphoma provides insight into the pathophysiology and indicates possible therapeutic strategies. Blood. 2013;122:424–33.

34. Morton LM, Kim CJ, Weiss LM, et al. Molecular characteristics of diffuse large B-cell lymphoma in human immunodeficiency virus-infected and -uninfected patients in the pre-highly active antiretroviral therapy and pre-rituximab era. Leuk Lymphoma. 2014;55:551–7.
35. Little RF, Pittaluga S, Grant N, et al. Highly effective treatment of acquired immunodeficiency syndrome-related lymphoma with dose-adjusted EPOCH: impact of antiretroviral therapy suspension and tumor biology. Blood. 2003;101:4653–9.
36. Kanungo A, Medeiros LJ, Abruzzo LV, et al. Lymphoid neoplasms associated with concurrent t(14;18) and 8q24/c-MYC translocation generally have a poor prognosis. Mod Pathol. 2006;19:25–33.
37. van Imhoff GW, Boerma EJ, van der Holt B, et al. Prognostic impact of germinal center-associated proteins and chromosomal breakpoints in poor-risk diffuse large B-cell lymphoma. J Clin Oncol. 2006;24:4135–42.
38. Johnson NA, Slack GW, Savage KJ, et al. Concurrent expression of MYC and BCL2 in diffuse large B-cell lymphoma treated with rituximab plus cyclophosphamide, doxorubicin, vincristine, and prednisone. J Clin Oncol. 2012;30:3452–9.
39. Green TM, Young KH, Visco C, et al. Immunohistochemical double-hit score is a strong predictor of outcome in patients with diffuse large B-cell lymphoma treated with rituximab plus cyclophosphamide, doxorubicin, vincristine, and prednisone. J Clin Oncol. 2012;30:3460–7.
40. Gaidano G, Pasqualucci L, Capello D, et al. Aberrant somatic hypermutation in multiple subtypes of AIDS-associated non-Hodgkin lymphoma. Blood. 2003;102:1833–41.
41. Levine AM. Acquired immunodeficiency syndrome-related lymphoma. Blood. 1992;80:8–20.
42. Matthews GV, Bower M, Mandalia S, et al. Changes in acquired immunodeficiency syndrome-related lymphoma since the introduction of highly active antiretroviral therapy. Blood. 2000;96:2730–4.
43. Little RF, Gutierrez M, Jaffe ES, et al. HIV-associated non-Hodgkin lymphoma: incidence, presentation, and prognosis. JAMA. 2001;285:1880–5.
44. Levine AM, Seneviratne L, Espina BM, et al. Evolving characteristics of AIDS-related lymphoma. Blood. 2000;96:4084–90.
45. Coutinho R, Pria AD, Gandhi S, et al. HIV status does not impair the outcome of patients diagnosed with diffuse large B-cell lymphoma treated with R-CHOP in the cART era. AIDS. 2014;28:689–97.
46. Imrie KR, Sawka CA, Kutas G, et al. HIV-associated lymphoma of the gastrointestinal tract: the university of Toronto AIDS-lymphoma study group experience. Leuk Lymphoma. 1995;16:343–9.
47. Beck PL, Gill MJ, Sutherland LR. HIV-associated non-Hodgkin's lymphoma of the gastrointestinal tract. Am J Gastroenterol. 1996;91:2377–81.
48. Diamond C, Taylor TH, Aboumrad T, et al. Changes in acquired immunodeficiency syndrome-related non-Hodgkin lymphoma in the era of highly active antiretroviral therapy: incidence, presentation, treatment, and survival. Cancer. 2006;106:128–35.
49. Heise W, Arasteh K, Mostertz P, et al. Malignant gastrointestinal lymphomas in patients with AIDS. Digestion. 1997;58:218–24.
50. Mhlanga JC, Durand D, Tsai HL, et al. Differentiation of HIV-associated lymphoma from HIV-associated reactive adenopathy using quantitative FDG PET and symmetry. Eur J Nucl Med Mol Imaging. 2014;41:596–604.
51. Sathekge M, Maes A, Van de Wiele C. FDG-PET imaging in HIV infection and tuberculosis. Semin Nucl Med. 2013;43:349–66.
52. Navarro J, Ribera J, Oriol A, et al. International prognostic index is the best prognostic factor for survival in patients with AIDS-related non-Hodgkin's lymphoma treated with CHOP. A multivariate study of 46 patients. Haematologica. 1998;83:508–13.
53. Rossi G, Donisi A, Casari S, et al. The International prognostic index can be used as a guide to treatment decisions regarding patients with human immunodeficiency virus-related systemic non-Hodgkin lymphoma. Cancer. 1999;86:2391–7.

54. Lim ST, Karim R, Tulpule A, et al. Prognostic factors in HIV-related diffuse large-cell lymphoma: before versus after highly active antiretroviral therapy. J Clin Oncol. 2005;23:8477–82.
55. Miralles P, Berenguer J, Ribera JM, et al. Prognosis of AIDS-related systemic non-Hodgkin lymphoma treated with chemotherapy and highly active antiretroviral therapy depends exclusively on tumor-related factors. J Acquir Immune Defic Syndr. 2007;44:167–73.
56. Mounier N, Spina M, Gabarre J, et al. AIDS-related non-Hodgkin lymphoma: final analysis of 485 patients treated with risk-adapted intensive chemotherapy [see comment]. Blood. 2006;107:3832–40.
57. Bower M, Gazzard B, Mandalia S, et al. A prognostic index for systemic AIDS-related non-Hodgkin lymphoma treated in the era of highly active antiretroviral therapy. Ann Intern Med. 2005;143:265–73.
58. Barta SK, Samuel MS, Xue X, et al. Changes in the influence of lymphoma- and HIV-specific factors on outcomes in AIDS-related non-Hodgkin lymphoma. Ann Oncol. 2015.
59. Bohlius J, Schmidlin K, Costagliola D, et al. Prognosis of HIV-associated non-Hodgkin lymphoma in patients starting combination antiretroviral therapy. AIDS. 2009; 23(15):2029–37.
60. Straus DJ, Huang J, Testa MA, et al. Prognostic factors in the treatment of human immunodeficiency virus-associated non-Hodgkin's lymphoma: analysis of AIDS Clinical Trials Group protocol 142–low-dose versus standard-dose m-BACOD plus granulocyte-macrophage colony-stimulating factor. National Institute of Allergy and Infectious Diseases. J Clin Oncol. 1998;16:3601–6.
61. Tedeschi R, Bortolin MT, Bidoli E, et al. Assessment of immunovirological features in HIV related non-Hodgkin lymphoma patients and their impact on outcome. J Clin Virol. 2012;53:297–301.
62. Lim ST, Karim R, Nathwani BN, et al. AIDS-related Burkitt's lymphoma versus diffuse large-cell lymphoma in the pre-highly active antiretroviral therapy (HAART) and HAART eras: significant differences in survival with standard chemotherapy. J Clin Oncol. 2005;23:4430–8.
63. Bortolin MT, Zanussi S, Talamini R, et al. Predictive value of HIV type 1 DNA levels on overall survival in HIV-related lymphoma patients treated with high-dose chemotherapy (HDC) plus autologous stem cell transplantation (ASCT). AIDS Res Hum Retroviruses. 2010;26:245–51.
64. Long JL, Engels EA, Moore RD, et al. Incidence and outcomes of malignancy in the HAART era in an urban cohort of HIV-infected individuals. AIDS. 2008;22:489–96.
65. Levine AM, Noy A, Lee JY, et al. Pegylated liposomal doxorubicin, rituximab, cyclophosphamide, vincristine, and prednisone in AIDS-related lymphoma: AIDS malignancy consortium study 047. J Clin Oncol. 2013;31:58–64.
66. Barta SK, Xue X, Wang D, et al. A new prognostic score for AIDS-related lymphomas in the rituximab-era. Haematologica. 2014;99:1731–7.
67. Kaplan LD, Lee JY, Ambinder RF, et al. Rituximab does not improve clinical outcome in a randomized phase 3 trial of CHOP with or without rituximab in patients with HIV-associated non-Hodgkin lymphoma: AIDS-malignancies consortium trial 010. Blood. 2005;106:1538–43.
68. Chao C, Silverberg MJ, Martinez-Maza O, et al. Epstein-Barr virus infection and expression of B-cell oncogenic markers in HIV-related diffuse large B-cell Lymphoma. Clin Cancer Res. 2012;18:4702–12.
69. Gopal S, Patel MR, Yanik EL, et al. Temporal trends in presentation and survival for HIV-associated lymphoma in the antiretroviral therapy era. J Natl Cancer Inst. 2013;105:1221–9.
70. Kaplan L, Kahn J, Crowe S, et al. Clinical and virologic effects of recombinant human granulocyte- macrophage colony-stimulating factor in patients receiving chemotherapy for human immunodeficiency virus-associated non-Hodgkin's lymphoma: results of a randomized trial. J Clin Oncol. 1991;9:929–40.
71. Newell M, Goldstein D, Milliken S, et al. Phase I/II trial of filgrastim (r-metHuG-CSF), CEOP chemotherapy and antiretroviral therapy in HIV-related non-Hodgkin's lymphoma. Ann Oncol. 1996;7:1029–36.

72. Kaplan LD, Straus DJ, Testa MA, et al. Low-dose compared with standard-dose m-BACOD chemotherapy for non-Hodgkin's lymphoma associated with human immunodeficiency virus infection. National Institute of Allergy and Infectious Diseases AIDS Clinical Trials Group. N Engl J Med. 1997;336:1641–8.
73. Kersten MJ, Verduyn TJ, Reiss P, et al. Treatment of AIDS-related non-Hodgkin's lymphoma with chemotherapy (CNOP) and r-hu-G-CSF: clinical outcome and effect on HIV-1 viral load. Ann Oncol. 1998;9:1135–8.
74. Vaccher E, Spina M, di Gennaro G, et al. Concomitant cyclophosphamide, doxorubicin, vincristine, and prednisone chemotherapy plus highly active antiretroviral therapy in patients with human immunodeficiency virus-related, non-Hodgkin lymphoma. Cancer. 2001;91:155–63.
75. Tirelli U, Errante D, Oksenhendler E, et al. Prospective study with combined low-dose chemotherapy and zidovudine in 37 patients with poor-prognosis AIDS-related non-Hodgkin lymphoma. Ann Oncol. 1992;3:843–7.
76. Sawka CA, Shepherd FA, Brandwein J, et al. Treatment of AIDS-related non-Hodgkin's lymphoma with a twelve week chemotherapy program. Leuk Lymphoma. 1992;8:213–20.
77. Remick S, McSharry J, Wolf B, et al. Novel oral combination chemotherapy in the treatment of intermediate- grade and high-grade AIDS-related non-Hodgkin's lymphoma. J Clin Oncol. 1993;11:1691–702.
78. Levine AM, Wernz JC, Kaplan L, et al. Low-dose chemotherapy with central nervous system prophylaxis and zidovudine maintenance in AIDS-related lymphoma. A prospective multi-institutional trial. JAMA. 1991;266:84–8.
79. Levine AM, Tulpule A, Espina B, et al. Low dose methotrexate, bleomycin, doxorubicin, cyclophosphamide, vincristine, and dexamethasone with zalcitabine in patients with acquired immunodeficiency syndrome-related lymphoma. Effect on human immunodeficiency virus and serum interleukin-6 levels over time. Cancer. 1996;78:517–26.
80. Gisselbrecht C, Oksenhendler E, Tirelli U, et al. Human immunodeficiency virus-related lymphoma treatment with intensive combination chemotherapy. French-Italian Cooperative Group. Am J Med. 1993;95:188–96.
81. Gabarre J, Lepage E, Thyss A, et al. Chemotherapy combined with zidovudine and GM-CSF in human immunodeficiency virus-related non-Hodgkin's lymphoma. Ann Oncol. 1995;6:1025–32.
82. Sparano J, Wiernik P, Hu X, et al. Pilot trial of infusional cyclophosphamide, doxorubicin, and etoposide plus didanosine and filgrastim in patients with human immunodeficiency virus-associated non-Hodgkin's lymphoma. J Clin Oncol. 1996;14:3026–35.
83. Tosi P, Gherlinzoni F, Mazza P, et al. 3′-azido 3′-deoxythymidine + methotrexate as a novel antineoplastic combination in the treatment of human immunodeficiency virus-related non-Hodgkin's lymphomas. Blood. 1997;89:419–25.
84. Weiss R, Huhn D, Mitrou P, et al. HIV-related non-Hodgkin's lymphoma: CHOP induction therapy and interferon-alpha-2b/zidovudine maintenance therapy. Leuk Lymphoma. 1998;29:103–18.
85. Oksenhendler E, Gerard L, Dubreuil M-L, et al. Intensive chemotherapy (LNHIV-91 regimen) and G-CSF for HIV associated non-Hodgkin's lymphoma. Leuk Lymphoma. 2000;39:87–95.
86. Remick SC, Sedransk N, Haase RF, et al. Oral combination chemotherapy in conjunction with filgrastim (G-CSF) in the treatment of AIDS-related non-Hodgkin's lymphoma: evaluation of the role of G-CSF; quality-of-life analysis and long-term follow-up. Am J Hematol. 2001;66:178–88.
87. Ratner L, Lee J, Tang S, et al. Chemotherapy for human immunodeficiency virus-associated non-Hodgkin's lymphoma in combination with highly active antiretroviral therapy. J Clin Oncol. 2001;19:2171–8.
88. Gastaldi R, Martino P, Gentile G, et al. High dose of idarubicin-based regimen for diffuse large cell AIDS-related non-Hodgkin's lymphoma patients: a pilot study. Haematologica. 2001;86:1051–9.

89. Tulpule A, Espina BM, Pedro Santabarbara AB, et al. Treatment of AIDS related non-Hodgkin's lymphoma with combination mitoguazone dihydrochloride and low dose CHOP chemotherapy: results of a phase II study. Invest New Drugs. 2004;22:63–8.
90. Levine AM, Tulpule A, Espina B, et al. Liposome-encapsulated doxorubicin in combination with standard agents (cyclophosphamide, vincristine, prednisone) in patients with newly diagnosed AIDS-related non-Hodgkin's lymphoma: results of therapy and correlates of response. J Clin Oncol. 2004;22:2662–70.
91. Sparano JA, Lee S, Chen MG, et al. Phase II trial of infusional cyclophosphamide, doxorubicin, and etoposide in patients with HIV-associated non-Hodgkin's lymphoma: an eastern cooperative oncology group trial (E1494). J Clin Oncol. 2004;22:1491–500.
92. Costello RT, Zerazhi H, Charbonnier A, et al. Intensive sequential chemotherapy with hematopoietic growth factor support for non-Hodgkin lymphoma in patients infected with the human immunodeficiency virus. Cancer. 2004;100:667–76.
93. Sawka CA, Shepherd FA, Franssen E, et al. A prospective, non-randomised phase 1-2 trial of VACOP-B with filgrastim support for HIV-related non-Hodgkin's lymphoma. Biotechnol Annu Rev Elsevier. 2005;11:381–9.
94. Spina M, Jaeger U, Sparano JA, et al. Rituximab plus infusional cyclophosphamide, doxorubicin, and etoposide in HIV-associated non-Hodgkin lymphoma: pooled results from 3 phase 2 trials [see comment]. Blood. 2005;105:1891–7.
95. Navarro JT, Lloveras N, Ribera JM, et al. The prognosis of HIV-infected patients with diffuse large B-cell lymphoma treated with chemotherapy and highly active antiretroviral therapy is similar to that of HIV-negative patients receiving chemotherapy. Haematologica. 2005;90:704–6.
96. Weiss R, Mitrou P, Arasteh K, et al. Acquired immunodeficiency syndrome-related lymphoma. Cancer. 2006;106:1560–8.
97. Boue F, Gabarre J, Gisselbrecht C, et al. Phase II trial of CHOP plus rituximab in patients with HIV-associated non-Hodgkin's lymphoma. J Clin Oncol. 2006;24:4123–8.
98. Combs S, Neil N, Aboulafia DM. Liposomal doxorubicin, cyclophosphamide, and etoposide and antiretroviral therapy for patients with AIDS-related lymphoma: a pilot study. Oncologist. 2006;11:666–73.
99. Ribera JM, Oriol A, Morgades M, et al. Safety and efficacy of cyclophosphamide, adriamycin, vincristine, prednisone and rituximab in patients with human immunodeficiency virus-associated diffuse large B-cell lymphoma: results of a phase II trial. Br J Haematol. 2008;140:411–9.
100. Sparano JA, Lee JY, Kaplan LD, et al. Rituximab plus concurrent infusional EPOCH chemotherapy is highly effective in HIV-associated B-cell non-Hodgkin lymphoma. Blood. 2010;115:3008–16.
101. Wilson WH, Grossbard ML, Pittaluga S, et al. Dose-adjusted EPOCH chemotherapy for untreated large B-cell lymphomas: a pharmacodynamic approach with high efficacy. Blood. 2002;99:2685–93.
102. Dunleavy K, Wilson WH. How I treat HIV-associated lymphoma. Blood. 2012;119:3245–55.
103. Zelenetz AD, Gordon LI, Wierda WG, et al. Non-Hodgkin's lymphomas, version 4.2014. J Natl Compr Canc Netw. 2014;12:1282–303.
104. Barta SK, Lee JY, Kaplan LD, et al. Pooled analysis of AIDS malignancy consortium trials evaluating rituximab plus CHOP or infusional EPOCH chemotherapy in HIV-associated non-Hodgkin lymphoma. Cancer. 2012;118:3977–83.
105. Bower M, Palfreeman A, Alfa-Wali M, et al. British HIV association guidelines for HIV-associated malignancies 2014. HIV Med. 2014;15 Suppl 2:1–92.
106. Castillo JJ, Echenique IA. Rituximab in combination with chemotherapy versus chemotherapy alone in HIV-associated non-Hodgkin lymphoma: a pooled analysis of 15 prospective studies. Am J Hematol. 2012;87:330–3.
107. Cruciani M, Gatti G, Vaccher E, et al. Pharmacokinetic interaction between chemotherapy for non-Hodgkin's lymphoma and protease inhibitors in HIV-1-infected patients. J Antimicrob Chemother. 2005;55:546–9.

108. Cheung MC, Hicks LK, Leitch HA. Excessive neurotoxicity with ABVD when combined with protease inhibitor, ÄìBased antiretroviral therapy in the treatment of AIDS-related Hodgkin lymphoma. Clin Lymphoma Myeloma Leuk. 2010;10:E22–5.
109. Bower M, McCall-Peat N, Ryan N, et al. Protease inhibitors potentiate chemotherapy-induced neutropenia. Blood. 2004;104:2943–6.
110. Miro JM, Manzardo C, Mussini C, et al. Survival outcomes and effect of early vs. deferred cART among HIV-infected patients diagnosed at the time of an AIDS-defining event: a cohort analysis. PLoS One. 2011;6:e26009.
111. Manzardo C, Esteve A, Ortega N, et al. Optimal timing for initiation of highly active antiretroviral therapy in treatment-naive human immunodeficiency virus-1-infected individuals presenting with AIDS-defining diseases: the experience of the PISCIS Cohort. Clin Microbiol Infect. 2012;25:1469–0691. doi:10.1111/j.1469-0691.2012.03991.x.
112. Shao H, Crump JA, Ramadhani HO, et al. Early versus delayed fixed dose combination abacavir/lamivudine/zidovudine in patients with HIV and tuberculosis in Tanzania. AIDS Res Hum Retroviruses. 2009;25:1277–85.
113. Sinha S, Shekhar R, Singh G, et al. Early versus delayed initiation of antiretroviral therapy for Indian HIV-infected individuals with tuberculosis on antituberculosis treatment. BMC Infect Dis. 2012;12:168.
114. Tirelli U, Errante D, Spina M, et al. Second-line chemotherapy in human immunodeficiency virus-related non-Hodgkin's lymphoma: evidence of activity of a combination of etoposide, mitoxantrone, and prednimustine in relapsed patients. Cancer. 1996;77:2127–31.
115. Levine AM, Tulpule A, Tessman D, et al. Mitoguazone therapy in patients with refractory or relapsed AIDS-related lymphoma: results from a multicenter phase II trial. J Clin Oncol. 1997;15:1094–103.
116. Bi J, Espina BM, Tulpule A, et al. High-dose cytosine-arabinoside and cisplatin regimens as salvage therapy for refractory or relapsed AIDS-related non-Hodgkin's lymphoma. J Acquir Immune Defic Syndr. 2001;28:416–21.
117. Spina M, Vaccher E, Juzbasic S, et al. Human immunodeficiency virus-related non-Hodgkin lymphoma: activity of infusional cyclophosphamide, doxorubicin, and etoposide as second-line chemotherapy in 40 patients. Cancer. 2001;92:200–6.
118. Bayraktar UD, Ramos JC, Petrich A, et al. Outcome of patients with relapsed/refractory acquired immune deficiency syndrome-related lymphoma diagnosed 1999–2008 and treated with curative intent in the AIDS Malignancy Consortium. Leuk Lymphoma. 2012;53:2383–9.
119. Gisselbrecht C, Glass B, Mounier N, et al. Salvage regimens with autologous transplantation for relapsed large B-cell lymphoma in the rituximab era. J Clin Oncol. 2010;28:4184–90.
120. Crump M, Kuruvilla J, Couban S, et al. Randomized comparison of gemcitabine, dexamethasone, and cisplatin versus dexamethasone, cytarabine, and cisplatin chemotherapy before autologous stem-cell transplantation for relapsed and refractory aggressive lymphomas: NCIC-CTG LY.12. J Clin Oncol. 2014;32:3490–6.
121. Wilson WH, Gerecitano JF, Goy A, et al. The Bruton's Tyrosine Kinase (BTK) inhibitor, ibrutinib (PCI-32765), has preferential activity in the ABC subtype of relapsed/refractory de novo Diffuse Large B-Cell Lymphoma (DLBCL): interim results of a multicenter, open-label, phase 2 study. ASH Annu Meet Abstr. 2012;120:686.

# Burkitt Lymphoma

**4**

Silvia Montoto, Ariela Noy, and Josep M. Ribera

## Contents



## 4.1 History, Pathogenesis and Epidemiology of Burkitt Lymphoma (BL)

Burkitt lymphoma was first described by Dennis Burkitt in 1958 in the paper entitled 'A sarcoma involving the jaws of African children' [1], following his observation of several children with multiple jaw tumours in Uganda, where he was working as a surgeon for the British government. These small round cell


S. Montoto, MD (✉)
Haemato-oncology Department, St Bartholomew's Hospital, Barts Cancer Institute, Queen Mary University of London, London, UK
e-mail: s.montoto@qmul.ac.uk

A. Noy, MD
Hematology Division, Lymphoma Service, Memorial Sloan-Kettering Cancer Center, New York, NY, USA
e-mail: noya@mskcc.org

J.M. Ribera, MD
Clinical Hematology Service, IJC-Institut de Recerca Contra la Leucèmia Josep Carreras, Universitat Autònoma de Barcelona, Badalona, Spain
e-mail: jribera@iconcologia.net




M. Hentrich, S.K. Barta (eds.), *HIV-associated Hematological Malignancies*,
DOI 10.1007/978-3-319-26857-6_4

tumours were later recognised to be lymphomas. Burkitt defined a geographic 'lymphoma belt' with a high incidence of BL [2]. The 'lymphoma belt' corresponds closely to the distribution of several insect-transmitted diseases leading to the hypothesis that BL might be driven by a virus. When MA Epstein, a pathologist with a special interest in virology, obtained tumour samples from Burkitt, he was able to demonstrate the presence of herpes-like particles in the tumours. The epidemiological and pathogenic relationship between the newly described Epstein-Barr virus (EBV) and African cases of BL was further demonstrated in several studies. In parallel, the observation that the 'lymphoma belt' mimicked the distribution of malaria and that successful malaria-eradication campaigns resulted in a decreased incidence of BL supported a role for malaria in the pathogenesis of BL, possibly by causing hyperplasia of B-lymphocytes and an increase in the circulation of EBV-infected memory B-cells. Whereas it is clear that both EBV and malaria play a significant role in the development of BL, the exact mechanism is still not well understood [3].

Subsequent to the description of the so-called 'endemic' BL, other cases categorised as 'sporadic' or 'immunodeficiency-associated' BL were described. Before the discovery of HIV, most of the 'immunodeficiency-associated' BL cases were described in patients receiving immunosuppressive drugs, i.e. in transplant recipients. Nowadays most cases of BL in immunodeficient patients are seen in the context of HIV infection. The incidence of non-Hodgkin lymphoma (NHL) is 11-fold in patients with HIV infection in comparison with the general population [4], and BL is the second commonest subtype. BL presents in individuals with HIV with relatively preserved CD4 counts and, thus, has not seen a dramatic declined in its incidence since the advent of highly active antiretroviral therapy (HAART) [5], in contrast with other types of NHL such as primary central nervous system lymphoma.

## 4.2 Pathological and Molecular Features

BL is characterised by a monotonous infiltration composed of small-medium round lymphocytes with a basophilic cytoplasm and vacuoles (the latter might be evident only on smear preparations). The proliferation fraction is typically approaching 100 %. The high proliferation rate and its counterpart, a high rate of apoptotic cell death, is responsible for the characteristic 'starry sky' pattern, composed of macrophages that phagocyte apoptotic tumour cells. The lymphocytes express B-cell markers such as CD19, CD20, CD22 and CD79a, as well as IgM, CD10 and bcl-6. They are negative for bcl-2 and TdT. The molecular hallmark of BL is the reciprocal translocation of *MYC* oncogene, located in chromosome 8, with either immunoglobulin heavy chain (*IgH*) in t(8;14) (the most frequent translocation) or light chains [*IgK* in t(2;8) or *IgL* in t(8;22)]. These translocations approximate the immunoglobulin enhancer to *MYC*, leading to the constitutive and deregulated expression of *MYC*, which plays a major role in the regulation of cell proliferation, differentiation and apoptosis.

## 4.3 Clinical Characteristics

BL is a very aggressive lymphoma. Therefore, patients typically present with a short history of rapidly growing masses. B-symptoms are present in around one third of the patients, and the majority (55–78 %) have a poor performance status at diagnosis (ECOG PS ≥2) [6–8]. In addition to peripheral lymphadenopathy, extra-nodal involvement is common. Frequent extra-nodal sites of disease include the bowel, bone marrow (BM) and central nervous system (CNS). CNS or BM infiltration is associated with a poor outcome in several studies. The incidence of CNS involvement ranges from 8 to 28 % [6, 7, 9, 10]. The presence of >20–25 % infiltration in the BM defines Burkitt leukaemia or acute lymphoblastic leukaemia 3 (ALL3). The majority of the patients have advanced stage at diagnosis (Ann Arbor III–IV) with an elevated LDH (>ULN: 78–100 %) [7, 8, 10], reflecting the high tumour burden. Although many patients present with peripheral lymphadenopathy, compression symptoms (such as bowel obstruction or acute renal failure secondary to hydronephrosis) may occur. Another characteristic feature is tumour lysis syndrome, due to the rapid cell turnover. This is a life-threatening complication that can appear not only after starting treatment but also spontaneously as the initial manifestation. In comparison with BL in immunocompetent patients, those with BL in the setting of HIV infection have been reported to have a higher incidence of poor PS and high LDH [8], although this has not been documented in other series [7].

## 4.4 Treatment of Patients with BL

The management of adult patients with BL in the general population has followed the advances seen in the childhood setting, and, in turn, the treatment of BL in patients with HIV infection has developed from the improvements achieved in the management of adult immunocompetent patients with BL. Hence, a review of how the treatment of BL has evolved, first in children and subsequently in adults, provides a better understanding of the current management of BL in patients with HIV infection.

It was evident soon after the description of BL that surgery was not a good treatment option. Following the initial observations by Burkitt et al. of durable responses to single-agent methotrexate (MTX), several combination regimens were developed [2]. In 1986, Murphy et al. published the results of an intensive chemotherapy regimen including high-dose fractionated cyclophosphamide, high-dose MTX and cytarabine (Ara-C) in children [11]. The response rate was 93 % and the 2-year disease-free survival (DFS) in patients with stage III, 81 %. The results in patients with stage IV (either CNS or BM involvement) were significantly worse. Subsequently, Magrath et al. demonstrated 2-year event-free survival of 80 % in both children and adults with the 89-C-41 protocol [12]. 89-C-41 added an alternating regimen with ifosfamide, etoposide and Ara-C and more intensive CNS prophylaxis and constitutes the backbone of the current CODOX-M/IVAC regimen.

In the pre-HAART era, the outcome of patients with NHL and HIV infection treated with the conventional regimens used in the general population was extremely poor, partly because of the significantly increased chemotherapy toxicity in patients with poor HIV control and also frequent opportunistic infections. Consequently, HIV patients were frequently offered alternative (sequential) or palliative regimens. The advent of HAART resulted in a switch in the management of patients with diffuse large B-cell lymphoma (DLBCL), who were subsequently treated with the same conventional regimens administered to immunocompetent patients. This resulted in a significant improvement in the outcome of patients with DLBCL in the HAART era. In contrast, patients with BL and HIV who continued receiving non-intensive chemotherapy regimens had outcomes in the HAART era which remained as poor as previously [10]. Infusional regimens such as CDE (cyclophosphamide, doxorubicin and etoposide) or EPOCH (etoposide, doxorubicin, vincristine, cyclophosphamide and prednisone) result in complete response (CR) rates of 44–74 % with OS at 2 years around 50 % (Table 4.1). Most of the studies analysing the role of infusional regimens in patients with HIV and lymphoma include several histological subtypes making it difficult to tease out the results in the subgroup of patients with BL, but Spina et al. demonstrated that BL histology was associated with a worse prognosis in patients treated with R-CDE [13].

The realisation that HAART provides excellent control of HIV infection led to the investigation of the intensive regimens commonly used in immunocompetent patients to treat BL in the HIV setting, and several retrospective and phase II studies showed their feasibility and efficacy with OS ranging from 47 % in patients with stage IV to 78 % at 4 years (Table 4.2). Although clearly more toxic than conventional or infusional regimens, Montoto et al. reported that it is possible to achieve an excellent immunological recovery after treatment with the intensive CODOX-M/IVAC regimen [14]. Furthermore, Ribera et al. have demonstrated comparable outcomes in BL with or without HIV infection treated with the same intensive regimens, in spite of an increased toxicity in patients with HIV [7].

The advent of rituximab has dramatically improved the outcome of patients with CD20+ B-cell lymphomas, specifically those with DLBCL. CD20 expression on BL cells makes rituximab an attractive agent. Several phase II studies have

**Table 4.1** Infusional regimens

| Series, year | Regimen | *N* patients with BL | CR | 2-year OS | 2-year EFS | Comments |
|---|---|---|---|---|---|---|
| Little [17], 2003 | DA-EPOCH | 7 | 74 % | 60 % (43 % in BL)[a] | 73 %[a] | ARL=39 |
| Sparano [18], 2004 | CDE | 22 | 44 % | 45 % | 38 % | ARL=55 |
| Spina [13], 2005 | R-CDE | 21 | 70 % | 64 % | 52 % | ARL=74 |
| Dunleavy [8], 2013 | SC-EPOCH-RR | 11 | NR | 92 %[b] | 92 %[b] | |

*CR* complete response, *OS* overall survival, *EFS* event-free survival, *DA-EPOCH* dose-adjusted EPOCH (etoposide, doxorubicin, vincristine, cyclophosphamide and prednisone), *ARL* AIDS-related lymphoma, *CDE* cyclophosphamide, doxorubicin and etoposide, *R* rituximab, *SC-EPOCH-RR* short-course EPOCH-rituximab, *NR* not reported

[a]At 53 months

[b]At 73 months

**Table 4.2** Intensive regimens

| Series, year | Regimen | *N* | CR | 2-year OS | 2-year EFS | TRM |
|---|---|---|---|---|---|---|
| Cortes [9], 2002 | HyperCVAD | 13 | 92 % | 48 % | 52 %[a] | 15 % |
| Wang [6], 2003 | CODOX-M/IVAC | 8 | 63 % | NR | 60 % | 12.5 % |
| Galicier, 2007 | LMB-86 | 63[b] | 70 | 47 % | 44 % | 11 % |
| Oriol, 2008 | B-ALL/NHL2002 | 19 | 84 % | 73 % | 87 %[a] | 16 % |
| Ribera, 2013 | Burkimab | 38 | 82 % | 78 %[c] | 80 %[ac] | 26 % |

*CR* complete response, *OS* overall survival, *EFS* event-free survival, *TRM* treatment-related mortality, *HyperCVAD* cyclophosphamide, vincristine, doxorubicin, dexamethasone, methotrexate and cytarabine, *CODOX-M/IVAC* cyclophosphamide, vincristine, doxorubicin, methotrexate, ifosfamide, etoposide and cytarabine, *LMB-86* cyclophosphamide, vincristine, prednisone, doxorubicin, methotrexate, etoposide and cytarabine, *B-ALL/NHL2002* cyclophosphamide, prednisone, rituximab, vincristine, dexamethasone, teniposide, doxorubicin, methotrexate, ifosfamide, etoposide and cytarabine, *Burkimab* cyclophosphamide, prednisone, rituximab, vincristine, dexamethasone, teniposide, doxorubicin, methotrexate, ifosfamide, etoposide and cytarabine

[a]*DFS* disease-free survival

[b]All stage IV

[c]At 4 years

demonstrated the feasibility of adding rituximab to intensive regimens, both in HIV-positive and HIV-negative patients [15, 16]. However, given the rarity of this type of lymphoma, no randomised trials have been performed. The historical comparison of rituximab-containing regimens with their rituximab-free counterparts suggests that rituximab improves the outcome, and it is now routinely incorporated into the management of patients with BL and HIV infection.

In a very different approach from the intensive regimens mentioned above, the US National Cancer Institute has developed their infusional regimen EPOCH into the 'SC-EPOCH-RR'. This involves a short course of EPOCH (without dose adjustment: all patients receive a fixed dose of 750 mg of cyclophosphamide) with a double dose of rituximab for those with low-risk disease and 6 cycles for the remainder. Dunleavy et al. treated 11 patients with HIV infection and BL (none of them presented with CNS involvement) with this regimen and reported an excellent OS at 73 months of 92 % [8].

In summary, the outcome of patients with BL and HIV infection is improved and may be equivalent to that of patients in the general population when they are treated with the same regimens. The optimal Burkitt regimen has yet to be defined. CTSU 9177 is an ongoing US national study exploring EPOCH-R irrespective of HIV status. Additional insights into BL pathogenesis may also result in targeted therapies incorporated into upfront regimens or used for those with relapsed and refractory disease.

## References

1. Burkitt D. A sarcoma involving the jaws in African children. Br J Surg. 1958;46(197):218–23.
2. Magrath I. Denis Burkitt and the African lymphoma. Ecancermedicalscience. 2009;3:159.

3. Brady G, MacArthur GJ, Farrell PJ. Epstein-Barr virus and Burkitt lymphoma. J Clin Pathol. 2007;60(12):1397–402.
4. Gibson TM, Morton LM, Shiels MS, Clarke CA, Engels EA. Risk of non-Hodgkin lymphoma subtypes in HIV-infected people during the HAART era: a population-based study. AIDS. 2014;28(15):2313–8.
5. International Collaboration on HIV and Cancer. Highly active antiretroviral therapy and incidence of cancer in human immunodeficiency virus-infected adults. J Natl Cancer Inst. 2000;92(22):1823–30.
6. Wang ES, Straus DJ, Teruya-Feldstein J, et al. Intensive chemotherapy with cyclophosphamide, doxorubicin, high-dose methotrexate/ifosfamide, etoposide, and high-dose cytarabine (CODOX-M/IVAC) for human immunodeficiency virus-associated Burkitt lymphoma. Cancer. 2003;98(6):1196–205.
7. Ribera JM, Garcia O, Grande C, et al. Dose-intensive chemotherapy including rituximab in Burkitt's leukemia or lymphoma regardless of human immunodeficiency virus infection status: final results of a phase 2 study (Burkimab). Cancer. 2013;119(9):1660–8.
8. Dunleavy K, Pittaluga S, Shovlin M, et al. Low-intensity therapy in adults with Burkitt's lymphoma. N Engl J Med. 2013;369(20):1915–25.
9. Cortes J, Thomas D, Rios A, et al. Hyperfractionated cyclophosphamide, vincristine, doxorubicin, and dexamethasone and highly active antiretroviral therapy for patients with acquired immunodeficiency syndrome-related Burkitt lymphoma/leukemia. Cancer. 2002;94(5): 1492–9.
10. Lim ST, Karim R, Nathwani BN, Tulpule A, Espina B, Levine AM. AIDS-related Burkitt's lymphoma versus diffuse large-cell lymphoma in the pre-highly active antiretroviral therapy (HAART) and HAART eras: significant differences in survival with standard chemotherapy. J Clin Oncol. 2005;23(19):4430–8.
11. Murphy SB, Bowman WP, Abromowitch M, et al. Results of treatment of advanced-stage Burkitt's lymphoma and B cell (SIg+) acute lymphoblastic leukemia with high-dose fractionated cyclophosphamide and coordinated high-dose methotrexate and cytarabine. J Clin Oncol. 1986;4(12):1732–9.
12. Magrath I, Adde M, Shad A, et al. Adults and children with small non-cleaved-cell lymphoma have a similar excellent outcome when treated with the same chemotherapy regimen. J Clin Oncol. 1996;14(3):925–34.
13. Spina M, Jaeger U, Sparano JA, et al. Rituximab plus infusional cyclophosphamide, doxorubicin, and etoposide in HIV-associated non-Hodgkin lymphoma: pooled results from 3 phase 2 trials. Blood. 2005;105(5):1891–7.
14. Montoto S, Wilson J, Shaw K, et al. Excellent immunological recovery following CODOX-M/IVAC, an effective intensive chemotherapy for HIV-associated Burkitt's lymphoma. AIDS. 2010;24(6):851–6.
15. Hoelzer D, Walewski J, Dohner H, et al. Improved outcome of adult Burkitt lymphoma/leukemia with rituximab and chemotherapy: report of a large prospective multicenter trial. Blood. 2014;124(26):3870–9.
16. Evens AM, Carson KR, Kolesar J, et al. A multicenter phase II study incorporating high-dose rituximab and liposomal doxorubicin into the CODOX-M/IVAC regimen for untreated Burkitt's lymphoma. Ann Oncol. 2013;24(12):3076–81.
17. Little RF, Pittaluga S, Grant N, et al. Highly effective treatment of acquired immunodeficiency syndrome-related lymphoma with dose-adjusted EPOCH: impact of antiretroviral therapy suspension and tumor biology. Blood. 2003;101(12):4653–9.
18. Sparano JA, Lee S, Chen MG, et al. Phase II trial of infusional cyclophosphamide, doxorubicin, and etoposide in patients with HIV-associated non-Hodgkin's lymphoma: an Eastern Cooperative Oncology Group Trial (E1494). J Clin Oncol. 2004;22(8):1491–500.

# 5 AIDS-Related Plasmablastic Lymphoma

Paul G. Rubinstein and Christoph Wyen

## Contents



## 5.1 Introduction

In 1997 a new entity was added to the World Health Organization (WHO) classification of lymphomas as a subset of diffuse large B cell lymphoma (DLBCL) called plasmablastic lymphoma (PBL) [1–4]. Its classification was prompted by its plasmacytoid appearance, with an elevated proliferation index, post-germinal

P.G. Rubinstein, MD (✉)
Section of Hematology/Oncology, Department of Medicine, John H. Stroger Jr. Hospital of Cook County (Cook County Hospital), Chicago, IL, USA

Rush University Medical Center, Chicago, IL, USA

The Ruth M. Rothstein CORE Center, Chicago, IL, USA
e-mail: prubinstein@cookcountyhhs.org

C. Wyen, MD
First Department of Internal Medicine, University of Cologne, Cologne, Germany
e-mail: christoph.wyen@uk-koeln.de

 
M. Hentrich, S.K. Barta (eds.), *HIV-associated Hematological Malignancies*,
DOI 10.1007/978-3-319-26857-6_5

phenotype with loss of the mature B cell markers, CD20, and strong expression of mature plasma cell antigens, i.e., CD138 [2–8]. The initial description was that this lymphoma affects primarily mucosal sites, particularly the oropharynx, and is characterized by poor outcome and is present predominantly in patients infected with HIV [1], though cases have also been reported in patients with advanced age or poor immune function [5]. Here we examine the epidemiology, pathogenesis, diagnosis, and treatments for PBL and future directions to gain insight on how to better understand and manage this entity in patients infected with HIV.

## 5.2 Epidemiology/Presentation

Since the start of the HIV epidemic, the incidence of AIDS-related lymphomas (ARL) has decreased dramatically. The implementation of combined antiretroviral therapy (cART) in the mid-1990s decreased the incidence of ARL from over 100 times to just about 25 times that of patients not infected with HIV [9]. In 1993, over 7000 patients were diagnosed with ARL in the United States compared to just about 2000 in 2005 [9]. The incidence of all ARL is on the decline with the exception of Burkitt lymphoma, which has remained stable [10–12]. The epidemiology of PBL, however, has not been well studied in either the HIV- or non-HIV-infected population due to the rarity of the diagnosis. Studies estimated that PBL represents 2.6–12 % of all ARL [13, 14]. In a retrospective study of 138 cases of ARL at John H. Stroger Jr. Hospital of Cook County, only 6 % of the cohort were diagnosed with PBL compared to DLBCL (49 %) and Burkitt lymphoma (22 %) [15]. Based on a literature review of 167 cases of PBL, 69 % of these patients were found to be infected with HIV [16]. There is a male predominance in patients diagnosed with AIDS-related PBL as well as all ARL though epidemiologically, more men are infected with HIV than women. In general, patients with HIV diagnosed with PBL were younger (39 vs. 58 median years of age) and had more disease presenting more in the oral cavity than those without [16]. The median CD4+ T cell count ranges from 87 to 206 cells/mm$^3$ at presentation (Table 5.2). Sixty percent of the patients present with advanced disease, and the most common areas affected are the head and neck, colon, and extranodal sites [4, 16].

## 5.3 Diagnosis

PBLs morphologically are composed of large cells, plasmacytoid in nature, that exhibit immunoblastic or plasmablastic features. It is a lymphoma of post-germinal center origin, which exhibits very little or complete absence of expression of the mature B cell antigens, CD20 and 79a, as well as the common lymphocyte antigen (CD45) [1–6, 17]. It expresses the multiple myeloma oncogene-1(MUM-1), consistent with its post-germinal center origin, and is positive for the plasma cell-associated markers CD138 (syndecan-1) and CD38 (Fig. 5.1) [1–6]. It characteristically has a high proliferation index, above 60 % [1–6]. However, in contrast to plasma cell

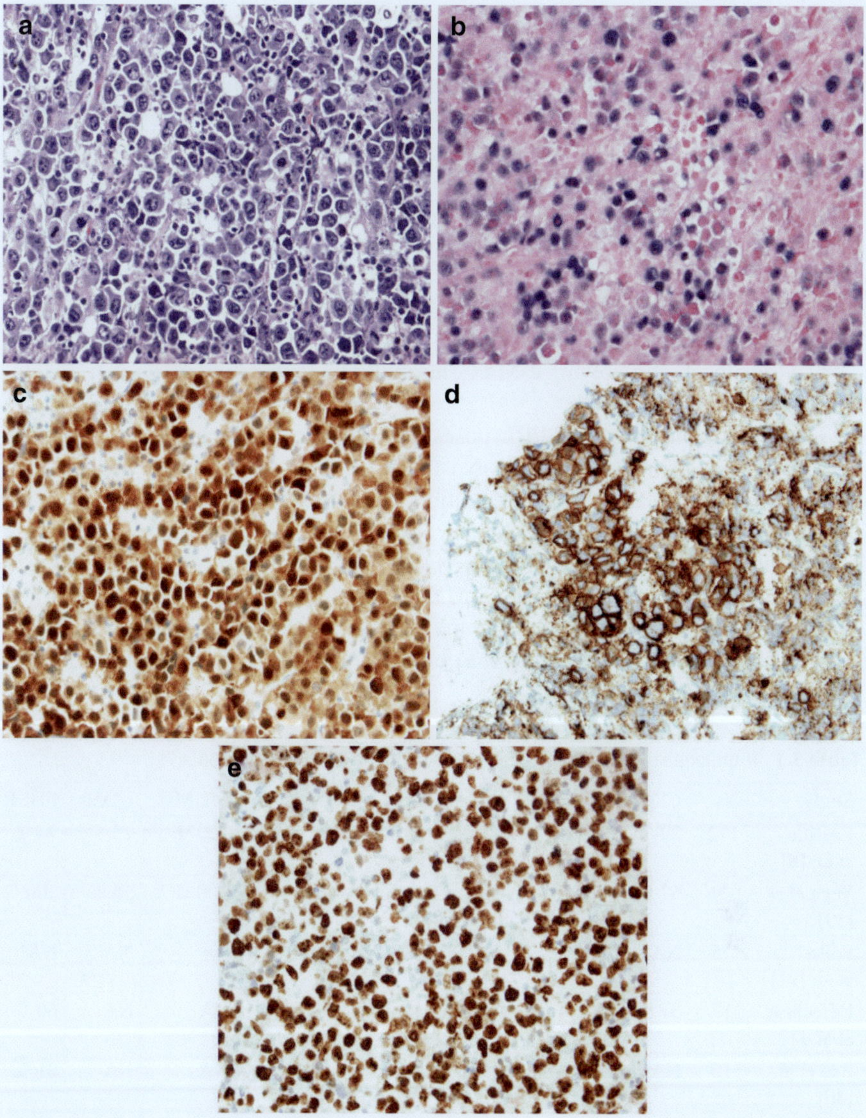


**Fig. 5.1** Phenotypic analysis of a lymph node biopsy from a HIV-positive patient with plasmablastic lymphoma. (**a**) Hematoxylin- and eosin-stained section showed large cells with eccentric nuclei and multiple mitotic figures (400×). (**b**) In situ hybridization for the Epstein-Barr virus (*EBV*)-encoded RNA (*EBER*) detected cells that contain EBV. Note that all the large plasmacytoid cells were positive for EBV, compared to the smaller non-neoplastic cells (in situ hybridization; 400×). (**c**) Immunohistochemical staining for MUM-1 (multiple myeloma oncogene-1) showed diffuse positivity in the larger plasmacytoid cells (immunoperoxidase staining; 400×). (**d**) CD138/syndecan1, a plasma cell marker, outlines the plasmacytoid neoplastic cells (immunoperoxidase staining; 400×). (**e**) Over 90 % of the large cells were positive for Ki-67, a proliferation marker, indicating that the neoplastic cells were actively undergoing division (immunoperoxidase; 400×). Note: The number of MUM-1 or Ki-67 positive cells does not match the EBER positive cells

myeloma, where CD56 is present in 70–80 % of the cases, only 30–56 % of PBLs demonstrate CD56 expression [17–19].

The oncogenic virus, Epstein-Barr virus (EBV), is commonly present in many ARL as well as in HIV-associated Hodgkin lymphoma (HIV-cHL) [19]. About 68–100 % of the cases of PBL demonstrate EBV positivity, as detected by EBER (Epstein-Barr virus-encoded RNA) in situ hybridization [1, 2, 4, 19]. Other methods of EBV detection are less reliable in PBL. For example, the EBV-associated latent membrane protein-1 (LMP-1) is rarely expressed in PBL, though present in EBV-associated HIV-cHL (Table 5.1) [1, 2, 4, 5, 8, 16, 17, 19, 21, 22]. The other major oncogenic virus associated with ARL, HHV8, has been only very rarely identified in PBL [2, 17]. In addition, recent studies have demonstrated that 50 % of the cases carry a translocation involving c-MYC, normally in conjunction with other cytogenetic abnormalities [23–25].

The immunophenotype of PBL poses a diagnostic dilemma, as it can overlap with other neoplasms with a plasmablastic morphology. For example, plasma cell myeloma with plasmablastic differentiation, in addition to its morphologic similarities, can also express CD138, CD38, and MUM-1 [19, 23]. In some instances these neoplasms are CD56 negative in addition to being negative for mature B cell markers, such as CD20 and 79a [19, 23]. C-MYC translocations have also been identified [23–25]. The clinical context, the immune deficient status, EBV positivity by EBER, and lymphadenopathy (rare in plasma cell myeloma) can help distinguish the two entities (Table 5.1).

**Table 5.1** Immunohistochemical characteristics of plasmablastic lymphoma

| Study | *N* | CD45 | CD79a | CD20 | CD38 | CD138 | MUM-1 | CD56 | EBER |
|---|---|---|---|---|---|---|---|---|---|
| Castillo et al. [8] | 112 | 29 % | 14 % | 3 % | 100 % | 84 % | 100 % | 25 % | 74 % |
| Vega et al. [19] | 9 | 67 % | 17 % | NA | 100 % | 100 % | 100 % | 56 % | 100 % |
| Folks et al. [21] | 5 | NA | 20 % | 20 % | 80 % | 100 % | NA | NA | NA[a] |
| Delecluse et al. [1] | 17 | 37 % | NA | NA | NA | NA | NA | NA | 60 % |
| Lee et al. [40] | 16 | NA | NA | 0 % | NA | 100 % | NA | NA | 81 % |
| Carbone et al. [5] | 7 | NA | NA | NA | NA | 100 % | 86 % | NA | 86 % |
| Castillo et al. [16] | 157 | 50 % | 51 % | 17 % | NA | NA | NA | 67 % | 82 % |
| Castillo et al. [17] | | 65 % | NA | 0 % | 89 % | 87 % | 100 % | 36 % | 95 % |
| Bogusz et al. [22] | 9 | NA | NA | 0 % | 40–100 %[b] | 33–80 %[b] | 100 % | 0 % | 100 % |

*NA* not assessed in the study

[a]EBER was not assessed in this study, though LMP1 was 0 % positive in this cohort

[b]The study of Bogusz et al. examined the difference in the immunohistochemical signature in patients with c-MYC-positive and c-MYC-negative translocated cases of PBL. In the cases of CD38 and 138, the difference ranged from 40 to 100 % and 33 to 80 %, respectively

**Table 5.2** Studies evaluating outcomes of AIDS-related plasmablastic lymphoma

| Study | Year | *N* | CD4+ T cell count[a] | Treatment | Median survival (months) |
|---|---|---|---|---|---|
| Castillo et al. [8] | 1997–2007 | 112 | 178 | CHOP, EPOCH, CODOX-M/IMVAC | 15 months |
| Castillo et al. [17] | 2000–2010 | 50 | 206 | CHOP/CHOP-like (63 %) | 11 months |
| | | | | Others (37 %) | |
| Castillo et al. [16] | 1997–2006 | 70 | 165 | CHOP/CHOP-like | 14 months |
| | | | | Intensive regimens, i.e., CODOX-M/IMVAC | 14 months |
| Noy et al. [38] | 2013 | 19 | 110 | DA-EPOCH, CDE, CHOP | 12 months (67 %) |
| Ibrahim et al. [39] | 2014 | 25 | 87 | DA-EPOCH ($n=14$) | 17 months |
| | | | | CHOP/CHOP-like ($n=11$) | 7 months |
| Lee et al. [40] | 2014 | 12 | 152 | DA-EPOCH (58 %) | 17 months |
| Schommers et al. [41] | 2013 | 18 | 85 | CHOP (50 %) | 5 months |

[a]Median CD4+ T cell count (cells/$mm^3$) at diagnosis. Dose-adjusted etoposide, prednisone, vincristine, cyclophosphamide, and doxorubicin (DA-EPOCH). Cyclophosphamide, doxorubicin, vincristine, and prednisone (CHOP). Cyclophosphamide, doxorubicin, methotrexate, ifosfamide, etoposide, cytarabine (CODOX-M/IVAC)

## 5.4 Pathogenesis

Like many ARL, PBL is associated with the oncogenic virus EBV [4, 20]. EBV has been shown to alter cell cycle regulation, inhibit apoptosis, and inhibit tumor suppressor genes [4, 20, 26–28]. As with many other oncogenic viruses, EBV also expresses miRNAs, which interfere with normal cellular function by destroying target RNAs, thus preventing specific protein expression. EBV, HHV8, and HPV, all oncogenic viruses, associated with cancers in HIV-infected patients, together express over 40 viral-associated miRNAs [29–31]. The EBV-associated miRNA, MiR-BHRF1-1, for example, inhibits the tumor suppressor gene p53 and miR-BART1, which activates BCL-2, an antiapoptotic protein [31–33]. In addition, via an unclear mechanism, EBV has been associated with the overexpression of c-MYC, and translocations with c-MYC have been identified more frequently in EBV-positive cancers than in those which are EBV negative [4, 21].

Terminal B cell differentiation is induced by the transcription factor, PR domain zinc finger protein 1, also known as BLIMP1. BLIMP1, highly expressed in PBL, represses mature B cell genes and helps promotes the gene transcription and ultimately plasma cell differentiation [4, 34, 35]. BLIMP1 also suppresses c-MYC, in addition to other tumor suppressors preventing uncontrolled cell division. While the mechanism of transformation is not exactly clear, and likely multifactorial, the overexpression of c-MYC is likely required to overcome the protective effect of BLIMP1 [4, 23, 25, 34–36]. It is interesting to note that c-MYC translocations are also present in plasma cell myeloma [23, 25, 34–36]. While the incidence of c-MYC translocations are low, 0–15 %, in plasma cell myeloma, in more poorly differentiated forms, i.e., plasmablastic plasma cell myeloma, the rate of c-MYC rearrangements has been reported as high as 45 %, suggesting a possible mechanistic link in the pathogenesis of plasmablastic cell myeloma and PBL [23–25, 37].

## 5.5 Treatment

Currently there is no standard of care with respect to chemotherapy in PBL in patients with HIV due to the rarity of the condition. In addition, no data regarding outcomes of therapy before cART are available as this entity became recognized in 1997 [1, 2, 4]. Few prospective studies have analyzed the effects of chemotherapy on AIDS-associated PBL; thus, most studies have been retrospective in nature (Table 5.2). All of these studies have poor median overall survival (OS) of 5–17 months (Table 5.2) [4, 8, 16, 17, 38–41]. One retrospective study demonstrated improved OS with infusional daEPOCH (dose-adjusted etoposide, prednisone, vincristine, cyclophosphamide, and doxorubicin) vs. CHOP (cyclophosphamide, doxorubicin, vincristine, and prednisone) (17 vs. 7 months, $p<0.04$) though a study by Castillo et al. demonstrated no OS benefit of CHOP or CHOP-like chemotherapy vs. more intensive regimens like CODOX-M/IVAC (cyclophosphamide, doxorubicin, methotrexate, ifosfamide, etoposide, cytarabine) [4, 8, 16, 17, 38–41]. There appears to be great variability in survival. For example, in a study of the German AIDS-related lymphoma cohort, the median survival was only 5 months, with a range of 0–76 months. Univariate analysis showed than an elevated international prognostic index was prognostic for poorer outcomes. Other studies have demonstrated that the presence of the c-MYC translocation (t8:14) correlates with decreased survival [4, 22, 38–41].

Treatment for AIDS-associated PBL should be initiated in conjunction with cART. A study by Barta et al. demonstrated that there was an increase in rates of complete remission (CR) and a trend toward improved overall survival (OS) for ARL treated with concurrent cART [42]. While this study did not look at PBL specifically, a study by Castillo et al. also demonstrated improved over OS in AIDS-related PBL when treated with concurrent antiviral therapy [43]. In these studies, the regimes utilized were heterogeneous; however, it is clear that a median survival of only 5–17 months indicates that newer therapies should be investigated to improve outcomes (Table 5.2).

## 5.6 New Approaches

New approaches are being investigated to take advantage that many ARL are co-infected with oncogenic viruses EBV and HHV8 [20]. Two agents, a histone deacetylase inhibitor, vorinostat, and the proteasome inhibitor, bortezomib, have been found to induce the lytic replication cycle of both EBV and HHV8, thus inducing cell lysis of all cells infected [44, 45]. In the case of ARL, the lytic activation of the oncogenic virus will destroy the tumor itself. The drug bortezomib is of particular interest, as it is also particularly effective against multiple myeloma, which shares many molecular and immunohistochemical features with PBL, as stated above [46]. Bortezomib in addition has activity against post-germinal center DLBCL [47]. Vorinostat also has activity against T cell lymphomas [48]. In light of these data, the AIDS Malignancy Consortium (AMC) has just completed a trial of bortezomib plus ifosfamide, etoposide, and carboplatin with or without rituximab (RICE) for relapsed or refractory ARL or relapsed/refractory HIV-associated Hodgkin lymphoma [49]. In the upfront setting for ARL, the AMC is also studying vorinostat plus daEPOCH with or without rituximab [50]. Another drug that may be effective in combination with other agents is the Bruton's tyrosine kinase inhibitor, ibrutinib. This drug is particularly effective against post-germinal center DLBCL, indolent lymphomas, and chronic lymphocytic leukemia [51].

**Conclusions**

PBL comprises about 2–12 % of all ARL. It affects HIV-infected patients more than HIV-negative patients, and it has a propensity for presenting in the oropharynx. It is almost always EBV positive and, in 50 % of the cases, has a c-MYC chromosomal alteration. It has an immunohistochemical signature close to plasma cell myeloma.

Current therapies provide only a median survival of 5 months to 1 year. More targeted therapies like bortezomib, vorinostat, or ibrutinib, in combination with chemotherapy targeting a non-germinal phenotype and the oncogenic virus, may lead to more promising and sustained survival results.

## References


1. Delecluse HJ, Anagnostopoulos I, Dallenbach F, et al. Plasmablastic lymphomas of the oral cavity: a new entity associated with the human immunodeficiency virus infection. Blood. 1997;89:1413–20.
2. Swerdlow SH, Campo E, Harris NL, Jaffe ES, Pileri SA, Stein H, World Health Organization. WHO classification of tumours of haematopoietic and lymphoid tissues. Lyon: International Agency for Research on Cancer; 2008.
3. Bibas M, Castillo JJ. Current knowledge on HIV-associated plasmablastic lymphoma. Mediterr J Hematol Infect Dis. 2014;6(1):e2014064.
4. Castillo JJ, Bibas M, Miranda RN. The biology and treatment of plasmablastic lymphoma. Blood. 2015;125:2323–30.
5. Carbone A, Gloghini A, Larocca LM, Capello D, Pierconti F, Canzonieri V, Tirelli U, Dalla-Favera R, Gaidano G. Expression profile of MUM1/IRF4, BCL-6, and CD138/syndecan-1 defines novel histogenetic subsets of human immunodeficiency virus-related lymphomas. Blood. 2001;97(3):744–51.
6. Colomo L, Loong F, Rives S, et al. Diffuse large B-cell lymphomas with plasmablastic differentiation represent a heterogeneous group of disease entities. Am J Surg Pathol. 2004;28(6):736–47.
7. Teruya-Feldstein J, Chiao E, Filippa DA, Lin O, Comenzo R, Coleman M, Portlock C, Noy A. CD20-negative large-cell lymphoma with plasmablastic features: a clinically heterogenous spectrum in both HIV-positive and -negative patients. Ann Oncol. 2004;15:1673–9.
8. Castillo J, Pantanowitz L, Dezube BJ. HIV-associated plasmablastic lymphoma: lessons learned from 112 published cases. Am J Hematol. 2008;83:804–9.

9. Shiels MS, Pfeiffer RM, Gail MH, Hall HI, Li J, Chaturvedi AK, et al. Cancer burden in the HIV-infected population in the United States. J Natl Cancer Inst. 2011;103(9):753–62.
10. Shiels MS, Pfeiffer RM, Hall HI, Li J, Goedert JJ, Morton LM, Hartge P, Engels EA. Proportions of Kaposi sarcoma, selected non-Hodgkin lymphomas, and cervical cancer in the United States occurring in persons with AIDS, 1980–2007. JAMA. 2011;305(14): 1450–9.
11. Guech-Ongey M, Simard EP, Anderson WF, Engels EA, Bhatia K, Devesa SS, et al. AIDS-related Burkitt lymphoma in the United States: what do age and CD4 lymphocyte patterns tell us about etiology and/or biology? Blood. 2010;116:5600–4.
12. Magrath I. Epidemiology: clues to the pathogenesis of Burkitt lymphoma. Br J Haematol. 2012;156(6):744.
13. Carbone A, Gloghini A. Plasmablastic lymphoma: one or more entities? Am J Hematol. 2008;83:763–4.
14. Schommers P, Hentrich M, Hoffmann C, Gillor D, Zoufaly A, Jensen B, et al. Survival of AIDS-related diffuse large B-cell lymphoma, Burkitt lymphoma, and plasmablastic lymphoma in the German HIV lymphoma cohort. Br J Haematol. 2014. doi:10.1111/bjh.13221.
15. Gupta S, Jain S, Sandhu S, Sreenivasappa S, Pattali S, Braik T, et al. A retrospective analysis of all hematological malignancies in patients infected with HIV, a subset analysis of the CHAMP study (Cook County Hospital (CCH) AIDS malignancy project). Blood (ASH Annu Meet Abstr). 2011;118:3693.
16. Castillo JJ, Winer ES, Stachurski D, Perez K, Jabbour M, Milani C, Colvin G, Butera JN. Clinical and pathological differences between human immunodeficiency virus-positive and human immunodeficiency virus-negative patients with plasmablastic lymphoma. Leuk Lymphoma. 2010;51:2047–53.
17. Castillo JJ, Furman M, Beltrán BE, Bibas M, Bower M, Chen W, et al. Human immunodeficiency virus-associated plasmablastic lymphoma: poor prognosis in the era of highly active antiretroviral therapy. Cancer. 2012;118(21):5270–7.
18. Chang H, Samiee S, Yi QL. Prognostic relevance of CD56 expression in multiple myeloma: a study including 107 cases treated with high-dose melphalan-based chemotherapy and autologous stem cell transplant. Leuk Lymphoma. 2006;47(1):43–7.
19. Vega F, Chang CC, Medeiros LJ, Udden MM, Cho-Vega JH, Lau CC, Finch CJ. Plasmablastic lymphomas and plasmablastic plasma cell myelomas have nearly identical immunophenotypic profiles. Mod Pathol. 2005;18(6):806–15.
20. Rubinstein PG, Aboulafia DM, Zloza A. Malignancies in HIV/AIDS: from epidemiology to therapeutic challenges. AIDS. 2014;28(4):453–65.
21. Folk GS, Abbondanzo SL, Childers EL, Foss RD. Plasmablastic lymphoma: a clinicopathologic correlation. Ann Diagn Pathol. 2006;10(1):8–12.
22. Bogusz AM, Seegmiller AC, Garcia R, Shang P, Ashfaq R, Chen W. Plasmablastic lymphomas with MYC/IgH rearrangement: report of three cases and review of the literature. Am J Clin Pathol. 2009;132(4):597–605.
23. Taddesse-Heath L, Meloni-Ehrig A, Scheerle J, Kelly JC, Jaffe ES. Plasmablastic lymphoma with MYC translocation: evidence for a common pathway in the generation of plasmablastic features. Mod Pathol. 2010;23(7):991–9.
24. Valera A, Balague O, Colomo L, et al. IG/MYC rearrangements are the main cytogenetic alteration in plasmablastic lymphomas. Am J Surg Pathol. 2010;34(11):1686–94.
25. Ott G, Rosenwald A, Campo E. Understanding MYC-driven aggressive B-cell lymphomas: pathogenesis and classification. Blood. 2013;122(24):3884–91.
26. McLaughlin-Drubin ME, Munger K. Viruses associated with human cancer. Biochim Biophys Acta. 2008;1782:127–50.
27. Ambinder RF. Epstein-Barr virus associated lymphoproliferations in the AIDS setting. Eur J Cancer. 2001;37:1209–16.
28. Carbone A, Tirelli U, Gloghini A, Volpe R, Boiocchi M. Human immunodeficiency virus-associated systemic lymphomas may be subdivided into two main groups according to Epstein-Barr viral latent gene expression. J Clin Oncol. 1993;11:1674–81.

29. Bartel DP. MicroRNAs: target recognition and regulatory functions. Cell. 2009;136:215–33.
30. Qi P, Han JX, Lu YQ, Wang C, Bu FF. Virus-encoded microRNAs: future therapeutic targets? Cell Mol Immunol. 2006;3:411–9.
31. Yeung ML, Bennasser Y, Le SY, Jeang KT. siRNA, miRNA and HIV: promises and challenges. Cell Res. 2005;15:935–46.
32. Lu J, Getz G, Miska EA, Alvarez-Saavedra E, Lamb J, Peck D, et al. MicroRNA expression profiles classify human cancers. Nature. 2005;435:834–8.
33. Pfeffer S, Voinnet O. Viruses, microRNAs and cancer. Oncogene. 2006;25:6211–9.
34. Montes-Moreno S, Gonzalez-Medina AR, Rodriguez-Pinilla SM, et al. Aggressive large B-cell lymphoma with plasma cell differentiation: immunohistochemical characterization of plasmablastic lymphoma and diffuse large B-cell lymphoma with partial plasmablastic phenotype. Haematologica. 2010;95(8):1342–9.
35. Schmelz M, Montes-Moreno S, Piris M, et al. Lack and/or aberrant localization of major histocompatibility class II (MHCII) protein in plasmablastic lymphoma. Haematologica. 2012;97(10):1614–6.
36. Hart LS, Cunningham JT, Datta T, et al. ER stress-mediated autophagy promotes myc-dependent transformation and tumor growth. J Clin Invest. 2012;122(12):4621–34.
37. Avet-Loiseau H, Gerson F, Magrangeas F, et al. Rearrangements of the c-myc oncogene are present in 15% of primary human multiple myeloma tumors. Blood. 2001;98(10):3082–6.
38. Noy A, Cahdburn A, Lensing SY, Moore P. Plasmablastic lymphoma is curable the HAART Era. A 10 year retrospective by the AIDS malignancy consortium (AMC). American Society of Hematology National meeting. Blood. 2013;122:1801.
39. Ibrahim IF, Shapiro GA, Naina HVK. Treatment of HIV-associated plasmablastic lymphoma: a single-center experience with 25 patients. J Clin Oncol. 2014;32:5s. suppl; abstr 8583.
40. Lee LX, Konda B, Assal A, Zell MI, Braunshweig I, Derman O, et al. Plasmablastic lymphoma: a case series of the changing epidemiology of a rare extramedullary plasmacytoid neoplasm, diagnostic challenges, and therapeutic implications. Blood. 2014;124:2995.
41. Schommers P, Wyen C, Hentrich M, Gillor D, Zoufaly A, Jensen B, et al. Poor outcome of HIV-infected patients with plasmablastic lymphoma: results from the German AIDS-related lymphoma cohort study. AIDS. 2013;27(5):842–5.
42. Barta SK, Xue X, Wang D, Tamari R, Lee JY, Mounier N, Kaplan LD, et al. Treatment factors affecting outcomes in HIV-associated non-Hodgkin lymphomas: a pooled analysis of 1546 patients. Blood. 2013;122(19):3251–62.
43. Castillo JJ, Winer ES, Stachurski D, Perez K, Jabbour M, Milani C, et al. Prognostic factors in chemotherapy-treated patients with HIV-associated plasmablastic lymphoma. Oncologist. 2010;15(3):293–9.
44. Reid EG. Bortezomib-induced Epstein-Barr virus and Kaposi sarcoma herpesvirus lytic gene expression: oncolytic strategies. Curr Opin Oncol. 2011;23(5):482–7.
45. Hui KF, Ho DN, Tsang CM, Middeldorp JM, Tsao GS, Chiang AK. Activation of lytic cycle of Epstein-Barr virus by suberoylanilide hydroxamic acid leads to apoptosis and tumor growth suppression of nasopharyngeal carcinoma. Int J Cancer. 2012;131(8):1930–40.
46. Moreau P, Richardson PG, Cavo M, Orlowski RZ, San Miguel JF, Palumbo A, et al. Proteasome inhibitors in multiple myeloma: 10 years later. Blood. 2012;120(5):947–59.
47. Dunleavy K, Pittaluga S, Czuczman MS, Dave SS, Wright G, Grant N, et al. Differential efficacy of bortezomib plus chemotherapy within molecular subtypes of diffuse large B-cell lymphoma. Blood. 2009;113:6069–76.
48. Copeland A, Buglio D, Younes A. Histone deacetylase inhibitors in lymphoma. Curr Opin Oncol. 2010;22(5):431–6.
49. https://clinicaltrials.gov/ct2/show/NCT00598169?term=aids+malignancy+consortium&rank=20.
50. https://clinicaltrials.gov/ct2/show/NCT01193842?term=amc+075&rank=1.
51. Bhatt V1, Alejandro L, Michael A, Ganetsky A. The promising impact of ibrutinib, a Bruton's tyrosine kinase inhibitor, for the management of lymphoid malignancies. Pharmacotherapy. 2014;34:303–14.

# HIV-Associated Primary Effusion Lymphoma

6

Heather A. Leitch and Eric Oksenhendler

## Contents



## 6.1 Introduction

In 1995, Cesarman and colleagues examined the DNA of 193 lymphomas from 42 patients with AIDS to 151 patients who did not have HIV infection. KSHV/HHV-8 DNA sequences were identified in eight lymphomas from HIV-infected patients. All eight, and only these eight, were body-cavity-based lymphomas as characterized by pleural, pericardial, and/or peritoneal lymphomatous effusions, defining an unusual subgroup of AIDS-associated B-cell lymphomas [1]. They also showed that in all

H.A. Leitch, MD, PhD (✉)
Hematology, St. Paul's Hospital and the University of British Columbia,
440-1144 Burrard Street, Vancouver, BC V6Z 2A5, Canada
e-mail: drhleitch@providencehematology.com

E. Oksenhendler, MD
Department of Clinical Immunology, Hôpital Saint-Louis, AP-HP, and EA3963,
University Paris Diderot, Paris, France
e-mail: eric.oksenhendler@sls.aphp.fr



M. Hentrich, S.K. Barta (eds.), *HIV-associated Hematological Malignancies*,
DOI 10.1007/978-3-319-26857-6_6

cases, the neoplastic cells were coinfected with EBV [2] and designated this entity as primary effusion lymphoma (PEL). In 2001, PEL was included as a distinct entity in the World Health Organization (WHO) classification of neoplastic diseases of the hematopoietic and lymphoid tissues [3]. PEL may also present as "extracavitary mass lesions without effusions" [4–6], commonly in the gastrointestinal tract [4, 6]. This is referred to as the solid variant of PEL which shares morphologic, immunophenotypic, and virologic features with classic PEL, allowing the recognition of these entities as part of the spectrum of PEL [7–9]. PEL comprises about 4 % of all HIV-related NHL non-Hodgkin lymphomas [9, 10]. While even less common, it can also occur in HIV-negative patients, usually in elderly or immunosuppressed patients [3]. Patients with HIV-related PEL often have advanced immunosuppression, with a CD4 count less than 150 cells/mL and a history of prior AIDS-defining illnesses [10–14].

## 6.2 Pathology and Diagnosis

PEL usually lacks a tumor mass, and the diagnosis is mainly based on cytology which demonstrates immunoblastic or plasmablastic morphology (see Fig. 6.1a) [3]. Lymphoma cells are often mixed with normal small lymphocytes and macrophages. Analysis of HIV-PEL cell markers by flow cytometry usually reveals expression of CD45 with null cell phenotype, and non-lineage associated antigens, including CD30, may be expressed. Markers of advanced stage of B-cell differentiation ("preplasma" cells) such as CD138/syndecan-1 and MUM1/IRF4 are frequently expressed, as are markers associated with activation such as CD38 and CD71. Expression of the CD20 B-cell antigen and cytoplasmic immunoglobulin is low or absent. The neoplastic cells always derive from a monoclonal B-cell population, even in the presence of aberrant T-cell antigen expression in some cases. Epstein-Barr virus (EBV) is present in PEL cells in about 70 % of cases [2]. However, PEL cells in HIV are uniformly infected with human herpes virus 8 (HHV-8), formerly known as Kaposi sarcoma herpes virus (KSHV). Confirmation of the PEL diagnosis requires cellular expression of HHV-8, which is usually detected by immunostaining for open reading frame (ORF) 73/latency-associated nuclear antigen (LANA) (see Fig. 6.1b ) [2, 3]. Other disorders in HIV involving HHV-8 include multicentric Castleman disease (MCD), HHV8-positive plasmablastic lymphoma (PBL), and Kaposi sarcoma (KS). However, the combined presence of EBV and HHV-8 appears to be unique to PEL [2, 8, 9, 15].

## 6.3 Pathogenesis

HHV-8 infected cells express cellular and viral interleukin-6 (vIL-6) and viral cyclin (v-Cyc), which support cell survival and progression through the cell cycle [16]. Like all herpes viruses, HHV-8 infection has a latent and a lytic phase. In MCD, lytic gene products predominate [17], while in PEL, PBL, and KS, latent infection predominates. About 2 % of PEL cells, however, express lytic gene products at any one time [18].

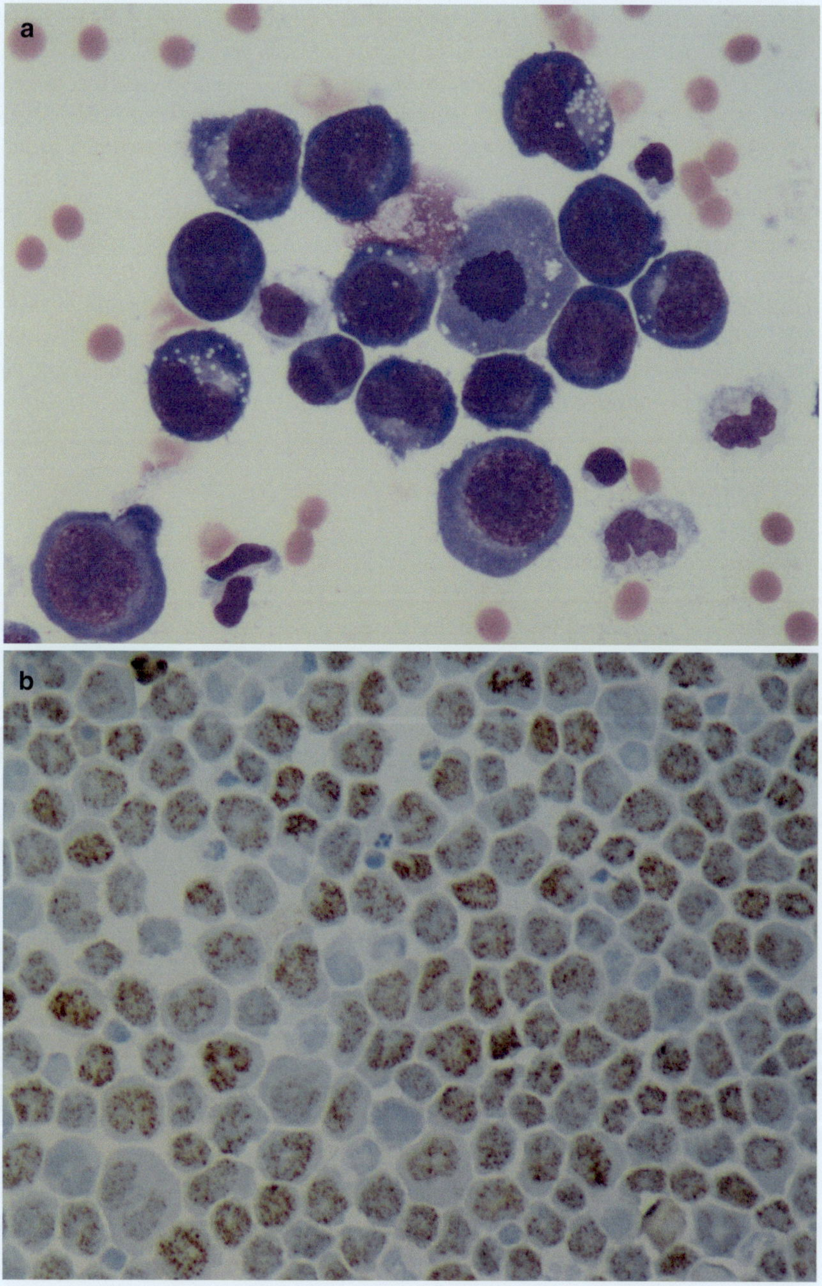


**Fig. 6.1** Cytological features of primary effusion lymphoma (PEL). (**a**) Immunoblastic/plasmablastic morphology of PEL cells. These show features of actively proliferating cells, such as cytoplasmic vacuoles, dispersed chromatin, numerous nucleoli, and frequent mitotic figures. (**b**) Immunohistochemical stain of PEL cells for human herpesvirus-8 (HHV-8) latent nuclear antigen (LANA) (Photomicrographs courtesy of Dr. Deborah Griswold)

Further, only a limited number of latent genes are expressed in PEL cell lines [19]. Among those genes, five are thought to play a possible role in PEL pathogenesis: LANA, v-Cyc, viral Fas-associated death domain-like interleukin-1β-converting enzyme inhibitory protein (v-FLIP), viral interferon regulatory factor (vIRF)-3, and vIL-6. The latter is considered to be a lytic viral protein but is expressed in a variable proportion of PEL cells. The true role of transient expression of lytic genes during neoplastic transformation is unknown [20]. To be effective, antiviral therapies require lytic gene expression, and treatment aimed at abrogating HHV-8 replication has been examined mainly in MCD [21] but also in PEL (see below). In addition, PEL cells produce and release IL-6 and IL-10, and both have been shown to support the growth of PEL cells. Several cell lines also produce high levels of vascular endothelial growth factor (VEGF), and this is consistent with the marked degree of angiogenesis and vascular permeability observed in this neoplasm [22, 23].

## 6.4 Clinical Presentation

In most cases of PEL occurring in HIV-infected patients, severe immunosuppression and low CD4+ T-cell counts are common. PEL can be the first manifestation of KSHV/HHV-8 infection. However, other complications such as Kaposi sarcoma or multicentric Castleman disease may precede or occur concurrently with PEL [11, 24].

Patients often present with constitutional symptoms such as fever, night sweats, or weight loss. Other symptoms are related to effusions involving the pleura, pericardium, and/or peritoneum. As suggested by distinctive imaging features or demonstrated during surgery or at autopsy, PEL presents with multiple small tumor foci and thickening of the serous membranes. These features indicate a primary serous membrane neoplasm that can spread to body cavities, adjacent lymph nodes, and various organs in some cases [2, 6, 11].

In some cases, PEL appears to originate in extranodal, non-serous sites with a clinical presentation closer to that observed in classic aggressive B-cell lymphomas involving the gastrointestinal tract, lung, central nervous system, or skin [5–9]. In such cases, the phenotype and especially virological studies demonstrating the presence of KSHV/HHV-8 with or without EBV in the tumor cells are decisive for the diagnosis [3, 25].

## 6.5 Treatment

The optimal treatment for HIV-PEL is undefined. As PEL is an uncommon NHL, it is difficult to develop treatment approaches with enough patients to evaluate optimal strategies. It is well documented, however, in other NHL that both early and long-term outcomes are superior in patients receiving antiretroviral therapy (ART) [26–33]. Although holding ART short term with some chemotherapy regimens appears to be safe [34], this should probably be done in the context of a clinical trial. Although there are case reports of patients with HIV-PEL responding to

ART alone [12, 14, 35], this treatment approach should only be taken in patients unable to accept or tolerate chemotherapy. Many patients with HIV-PEL receive standard combination chemotherapy regimens such as CHOP. However, while the complete response (CR) rates using this approach arc in the range of 40–50 %, the reported median survival is suboptimal at around 6 months [10, 11, 36]. With improved supportive care, this may be improving; in a series of seven patients treated at the University of British Columbia, five of whom received CHOP, all with ART with or without other prophylaxis, at a median follow-up of 24 (range 1–15) months, five patients were alive, a considerably superior result to that usually reported (see Table 6.1). Although there are as yet no published data in PEL, there is optimism that infusional regimens such as EPOCH or CDE may yield superior outcomes to standard regimens [34, 37, 38]. The use of more intensive chemotherapy in PEL has also been reported, as discussed below.

Although HHV-8 infection is universally present in PEL, it has only recently been considered as a target for PEL therapy, and anti-HHV8 therapy is not currently

**Table 6.1** Baseline characteristics of seven patients with HIV-associated primary effusion lymphoma seen at St. Paul's Hospital in Vancouver, Canada

| Characteristic (units) | *N* or median (range) |
|---|---|
| Age [years; median (range)] | 60 (41–66) |
| Gender (male) | 6 |
| Histology | |
| PEL | 6 |
| Solid variant | 1 |
| ECOG PS | |
| 0–1 | 4 |
| 3–4 | 3 |
| IPI | |
| Low/intermediate-1 | 4 |
| Intermediate-2/high | 3 |
| CD4 count [cells/mL; median (range)] | 250 (50–560) |
| HIV VL (copies/mL) | |
| <40 | 2 |
| On ART at PEL dx ($n=6$) | 4 |
| Prior ON | KS in 3 |
| Coinfections | Hepatitis B in 2 |
| Primary treatment | |
| CHOP | 4 |
| CHOP-R | 1 |
| Declined chemotherapy | 2 |
| Secondary treatment | |
| ART | 7 |
| Valganciclovir | 2 |

*ECOG* Eastern Cooperative Oncology Group, *IPI* International Prognostic Index, *ON* opportunistic neoplasm, *PEL* primary effusion lymphoma, *PS* performance status, *VL* viral load

considered standard treatment. Antiviral medications targeting HHV-8 have been used successfully in the treatment of other HHV-8 associated disorders, including KS [39] and MCD [40], and have been shown to reduce HHV-8 replication [21]. Only a handful of reports have been published on the use of antiviral therapy in PEL specifically, alone or in combination with chemotherapy or other agents, though some long-term remissions have been reported [13, 14, 41, 42]. Three of the above-described seven HIV-PEL patients received valganciclovir in combination with chemotherapy and ART ($n=2$) and with ART alone ($n=1$, declined chemotherapy). Though one of the patients receiving chemotherapy (CHOP) had progressive disease, the second attained long-term remission. The patient who declined chemotherapy also discontinued valganciclovir after 1 month of therapy but remained clinically well without evidence of lymphoma at 9 months on ART alone, which had been instituted at PEL diagnosis. With such small numbers, the benefit of anti-HHV-8 therapy remains unproven, but in our experience appears to be tolerated reasonably well.

There are reports of outcomes using more intensive chemotherapy. Although one patient receiving combination chemotherapy including high-dose methotrexate (HDMTX) remained in complete remission (CR) at 78 months, only three of seven patients receiving this treatment achieved CR [43], and one report of high-dose chemotherapy followed by autologous stem cell transplantation showed no benefit [44]. These limited data likely indicate that intensifying chemotherapy in these patients is of limited benefit. For a summary of chemotherapy-based approaches to HIV-PEL, see Table 6.2.

**Table 6.2** Clinical data on treatment approaches to HIV-associated primary effusion lymphoma

| Treatment | Outcome | Type of report | Comments | References |
|---|---|---|---|---|
| ART alone | CR at 55 months | Case series<br>Case reports | | [12, 14, 35] |
| Cidofovir + interferon | CR at 53 months | Case report<br>Case series | | [13, 74] |
| CHOP | CR 42 %, median OS 6 months | Case series | ART use not specified | [10] |
| Chemotherapy + GCV | CR at 68 months | Case report | Associated HLH<br>ART use not specified | [14, 75] |
| EPOCH | PEL not reported separately | | | [34] |
| CDE | PEL not reported separately | | | [38] |
| Combination chemotherapy including HDMTX | CR in 3 of 7<br>CR at 28 months in one patient | Case series | ART in 6 | [11, 43] |
| ASCT | No benefit in one patient | Case report | | [44] |

*ART* antiretroviral therapy, *ASCT* autologous stem cell transplantation, *CDE* cyclophosphamide, doxorubicin, and etoposide, *CHOP* cyclophosphamide, doxorubicin, vincristine, and prednisone, *CR* complete remission, *EPOCH* etoposide, prednisone, vincristine, cyclophosphamide, and doxorubicin, *GCV* ganciclovir, *HDMTX* high-dose methotrexate, *HLH* hemophagocytic lymphohistiocytosis, *OS* overall survival, *PEL* primary effusion lymphoma

**Table 6.3** Potential treatment approaches to HIV-associated primary effusion lymphoma showing promise in preclinical studies and the molecular mechanism targeted

| Molecular target | Treatment under evaluation in preclinical models | Comment | References |
|---|---|---|---|
| CD30/microtubules | Brentuximab vedotin | ↓ Proliferation<br>↑ G2/M arrest, apoptosis, and OS of PEL-injected mice | [45] |
| NFκB/HIF-1α | Proteasome inhibitors<br>PI + HDAC inhibitors | | [46–52]<br>[53] |
| VEGF | Anti-VEGF antibodies<br>Rapamycin | Involved in angiogenesis and formation of gap junctions with endothelial cells | [16, 54–56] |
| Angiogenin | Neomycin<br>Neamine | | [57] |
| Interleukin-6 | Anti-IL6 antibodies<br>Antisense | v-IL6 is intracellular | [76, 77]<br>[78] |
| miRs[a] | | | [79] |
| v-cyclin D, v-IL6, v-FLIP+ | MAP30 | An anti-HIV agent, inactivates ribosomes | [80] |
| LANA[b] | COX-2 inhibitors<br>Gamma secretase inhibitor | LANA induces chromosomal instability and downregulates TS genes P53 and P73 | [58–69] |
| P53 activation | Nutlin-3a | | [81] |
| Chemotherapy sensitivity | Assay-guided individual therapy | | [82] |
| Tumor growth and angiogenesis | Protease inhibitors | | [70] |
| HHV8 replication | Nelfinavir | | [70] |
| Early lytic genes | Oligomers | | [83] |
| Lytic replication | Valproate + ganciclovir | | [71] |

*AP1* activator protein 1, *c-* cellular, *COX-2* cyclooxygenase-2, *DHMEQ* dehydroxymethylepoxyquinomicin, *EBV* Epstein-Barr virus, *FLIP* FLICE inhibitory protein, *HDAC* histone deacetylase inhibitor, *HIF-1α* hypoxia inducible factor 1 alpha, *HHV8* human herpesvirus 8, *IL-6* interleukin 6, *LANA* latency-associated nuclear antigen, *MAP30* Momordica antiviral protein 30 kDa, *miRs* micro-RNAs, NFκB nuclear factor kappa-B, *OS* overall survival, *P* protein, *PI* proteasome inhibitor, *TS* tumor suppressor, *v-* viral-, *VEGF* vascular endothelial growth factor

[a]Inhibit P21 + inhibits caspases

[b]Maintains the viral episome, induces chromosomal instability, binds tumor suppressor genes P53 and P73, stabilizes c-myc, activates c-JUN, AP1, increases beta-catenin levels, and suppresses EBV

## 6.6 Future Directions

As the molecular mechanisms by which HHV-8 cellular infection results in malignant outgrowth are elucidated, future therapies may become increasingly targeted; potential treatment approaches showing promise in preclinical studies targeting cell surface antigens, cellular and viral proto-oncogenes, tumor suppressor genes, and cytokines are shown in Table 6.3. Cellular or molecular mechanisms with targeting substances that may be particularly amenable to clinical development include the cell surface antigen CD30 (brentuximab vedotin) [45] nuclear transcription factor nuclear factor kappa-B (NFkB; proteasome inhibitors) [46–53]; vascular endothelial growth factor (VEGF)/angiogenin (anti-VEGF antibodies/neomycin) [16, 54–57]; latency-associated nuclear antigen (LANA; cyclooxygenase [COX]-2 inhibitors); tumor growth, angiogenesis, and HHV8 replication (HIV-protease inhibitors, nelfinavir) [58–70]; and lytic HHV8 replication (valproate plus ganciclovir) [71]. In regard to the latter, it is possible to induce lytic replication and apoptosis by cellular stress [72], including with the antiseizure medication valproate [71]. Interestingly, the concentration of valproate used in this experiment was similar to plasma levels that would be present in patients taking this medication for neurologic disorders. In a study by Shaw et al. [73], valproate increased HHV-8 viral load and therefore had potential for activating or exacerbating disease. However, if ganciclovir is concomitantly used with valproate in vitro, HHV-8 replication was blocked without preventing viral entry into the lytic cycle [71]. Administered together, ganciclovir and valproate may potentially prove beneficial, though this has yet to be evaluated in clinical studies. Particularly interesting is a recent report of the in vitro inhibition of proliferation, induction of G2/M arrest and apoptosis, and improvement in overall survival of mice engrafted with PEL cell lines on treatment with brentuximab vedotin [45]. These effects were seen at concentrations that were well tolerated and were similar to those used for treatment of Hodgkin or anaplastic large cell lymphomas.

**Conclusions**

Primary effusion lymphoma comprises a minority of systemic non-Hodgkin lymphoma occurring in HIV infection, making it difficult to accumulate sufficient numbers of patients to delineate its presenting characteristics, optimal treatment approach, and outcomes with certainty. Remissions have been described with the institution of ART, which should however be considered adjunctive therapy until more definitive information is available. Similarly, antiviral approaches to HHV-8 have been employed, which may be adjunctive or possibly useful for secondary prophylaxis. Though standard chemotherapeutic regimens such as CHOP yield short median survivals, some patients do achieve long-term remissions; however, predictive factors for favorable response are not currently delineated. More intensive chemotherapy appears to be less than promising in limited numbers of patients. There is optimism that infusional regimens such as EPOCH or CDE may be effective; however, this remains to be demonstrated in prospective series of patients. Newer approaches targeting cellular pathways disrupted by HHV-8 are under evaluation in preclinical studies; inhibition of NFκB by proteasome inhibition and targeting of lytic HHV-8 infection with valproate in combination with anti-HHV-8 medications may prove to be particularly promising approaches. Anti-CD30 directed treatment with brentuximab vedotin also showed promise in preclinical models.

**Acknowledgments** Dr. Laura Kuyper described the features, treatment, and outcome of five patients with HIV-NHL treated at St. Paul's Hospital in the ART era in 2009.

Dr. Musa Al-Zahrani described the features, treatment, and outcome of 12 patients with HIV/(HHV-8)-related multicentric Castleman disease in 2012 and critically reviewed this manuscript.

## References

1. Cesarman E, Chang Y, Moore PS, et al. Kaposi's sarcoma-associated herpesvirus-like DNA sequences in AIDS-related body-cavity-based lymphomas. N Engl J Med. 1995;332(18): 1186–91.
2. Nador RG, Cesarman E, Chadburn A, et al. Primary effusion lymphoma: a distinct clinicopathologic entity associated with the Kaposi's sarcoma-associated herpes virus. Blood. 1996;88(2):645–56.
3. Said J, Cesarman E. Primary effusion lymphoma. In: Swerdlow SH, Campo E, Harris NL, Jaffe ES, Pileri SA, Stein H, et al., editors. WHO classification of tumours of haematopoietic and lymphoid tissues (4th ed). Lyon: International Agency for Research on Cancer; 2008.
4. Levine AM. Management of AIDS-related lymphoma. Curr Opin Oncol. 2008;20(5):522–8.
5. Carbone A, Gloghini A, Vaccher E, et al. Kaposi's sarcoma-associated herpesvirus/human herpesvirus type 8-positive solid lymphomas: a tissue-based variant of primary effusion lymphoma. J Mol Diagn. 2005;7(1):17–27.
6. Mylona E, Baraboutis IG, Georgiou O, et al. Solid variant of primary effusion lymphoma in successfully treated HIV infection: a case report. Int J STD AIDS. 2008;19(8):570–2.
7. Chadburn A, Hyjek E, Mathew S, et al. KSHV-positive solid lymphomas represent an extracavitary variant of primary effusion lymphoma. Am J Surg Pathol. 2004;28(11):1401–16.
8. Carbone A, Gloghini A. KSHV/HHV8-associated lymphomas. Br J Haematol. 2008; 140(1):13–24.
9. Gloghini A, Dolcetti R, Carbone A. Lymphomas occurring specifically in HIV-infected patients: from pathogenesis to pathology. Semin Cancer Biol. 2013;23(6):457–67.
10. Simonelli C, Spina M, Cinelli R, et al. Clinical features and outcome of primary effusion lymphoma in HIV-infected patients: a single-institution study. J Clin Oncol. 2003;21(21):3948–54.
11. Boulanger E, Gerard L, Gabarre J, et al. Prognostic factors and outcome of human herpesvirus 8-associated primary effusion lymphoma in patients with AIDS. J Clin Oncol. 2005; 23(19):4372–80.
12. Oksenhendler E, Clauvel JP, Jouveshomme S, Davi F, Mansour G. Complete remission of a primary effusion lymphoma with antiretroviral therapy. Am J Hematol. 1998;57(3).
13. Hocqueloux L, Agbalika F, Oksenhendler E, Molina JM. Long-term remission of an AIDS-related primary effusion lymphoma with antiviral therapy. AIDS. 2001;15(2):280–2.
14. Crum-Cianflone NF, Wallace MR, Looney D. Successful secondary prophylaxis for primary effusion lymphoma with human herpesvirus 8 therapy. AIDS. 2006;20(11):1567–9.
15. Carbone A, Cesarman E, Spina M, Gloghini A, Schulz TF. HIV-associated lymphomas and gamma-herpesviruses. Blood. 2009;113(6):1213–24.
16. Gasperini P, Sakakibara S, Tosato G. Contribution of viral and cellular cytokines to Kaposi's sarcoma-associated herpesvirus pathogenesis. J Leukoc Biol. 2008;84(4):994–1000.
17. Sunil M, Reid E, Lechowicz MJ. Update on HHV-8-associated malignancies. Curr Infect Dis Rep. 2010;12(2):147–54.
18. Miller G, Heston L, Grogan E, et al. Selective switch between latency and lytic replication of Kaposi's sarcoma herpesvirus and Epstein-Barr virus in dually infected body cavity lymphoma cells. J Virol. 1997;71(1):314–24.
19. Carbone A. Emerging pathways in the development of AIDS-related lymphomas. Lancet Oncol. 2003;4(1):22–9.
20. Carbone A, Ceserman E, Gloghini A, Drexler H. Understanding pathogenetic aspects and clinical presentation of primary effusion lymphoma through its derived cell lines. AIDS. 2010;24(4):479–90.
21. Casper C, Krantz EM, Corey L, et al. Valganciclovir for suppression of human herpesvirus-8 replication: a randomized, double-blind, placebo-controlled, crossover trial. J Infect Dis. 2008;198(1):23–30.
22. Aoki Y, Tosato G, Nambu Y, Iwamoto A, Yarchoan R. Detection of vascular endothelial growth factor in AIDS-related primary effusion lymphomas. Blood. 2000;95(3):1109–10.
23. Aoki Y, Yarchoan R, Braun J, Iwamoto A, Tosato G. Viral and cellular cytokines in AIDS-related malignant lymphomatous effusions. Blood. 2000;96(4):1599–601.

24. Ammari ZA, Mollberg NM, Abdelhady K, Mansueto MD, Massad MG. Diagnosis and management of primary effusion lymphoma in the immunocompetent and immunocompromised hosts. Thorac Cardiovasc Surg. 2013;61(4):343–9.
25. Simonelli C, Tedeschi R, Gloghini A, et al. Plasma HHV-8 viral load in HHV-8-related lymphoproliferative disorders associated with HIV infection. J Med Virol. 2009;81(5):888–96.
26. Antinori A, Cingolani A, Alba L, et al. Better response to chemotherapy and prolonged survival in AIDS-related lymphomas responding to highly active antiretroviral therapy. AIDS. 2001;15(12):1483–91.
27. Besson C, Goubar A, Gabarre J, et al. Changes in AIDS-related lymphoma since the era of highly active antiretroviral therapy. Blood. 2001;98(8):2339–44.
28. Chow KU, Mitrou PS, Geduldig K, et al. Changing incidence and survival in patients with aids-related non-Hodgkin's lymphomas in the era of highly active antiretroviral therapy (HAART). Leuk Lymphoma. 2001;41(1–2):105–16.
29. Ezzat H, Filipenko D, Vickars L, et al. Improved survival in HIV-associated diffuse large B-cell lymphoma with the addition of rituximab to chemotherapy in patients receiving highly active antiretroviral therapy. HIV Clin Trials. 2007;8(3):132–44.
30. Kirk O, Pedersen C, Cozzi-Lepri A, et al. Non-Hodgkin lymphoma in HIV-infected patients in the era of highly active antiretroviral therapy. Blood. 2001;98(12):3406–12.
31. Matthews GV, Bower M, Mandalia S, et al. Changes in acquired immunodeficiency syndrome-related lymphoma since the introduction of highly active antiretroviral therapy. Blood. 2000; 96(8):2730–4.
32. Navarro JT, Ribera JM, Oriol A, et al. Improved outcome of AIDS-related lymphoma in patients with virologic response to highly active antiretroviral therapy. J Acquir Immune Defic Syndr. 2003;32(3):347–8.
33. Vaccher E, di Gennaro G, Shioppa O, et al. Highly active antiretroviral therapy (HAART) significantly improves disease free survival (DFS) in patients (pts) with HIV-related non-Hodgkin's lymphoma (HIV-NHL) treated with chemotherapy (CT). Proc ASCO. 2001;20(2):294a.
34. Little RF, Pittaluga S, Grant N, et al. Highly effective treatment of acquired immunodeficiency syndrome-related lymphoma with dose-adjusted EPOCH: impact of antiretroviral therapy suspension and tumor biology. Blood. 2003;101(12):4653–9.
35. Ripamonti D, Marini B, Rambaldi A, Suter F. Treatment of primary effusion lymphoma with highly active antiviral therapy in the setting of HIV infection. AIDS. 2008;22(10):1236–7.
36. Chen Y-B, Rahemtullah A, Hochberg E. Primary effusion lymphoma. Oncologist. 2007; 12(5):569–76.
37. Okada S, Goto H, Yotsumoto M. Current status of treatment for primary effusion lymphoma. Intractable Rare Dis Res. 2014;3(3):65–74.
38. Sparano JA, Lee S, Chen MG, et al. Phase II trial of infusional cyclophosphamide, doxorubicin, and etoposide in patients with HIV-associated non-Hodgkin's lymphoma: an Eastern Cooperative Oncology Group Trial (E1494). J Clin Oncol. 2004;22(8):1491–500.
39. Little RF, Merced-Galindez F, Staskus K, et al. A pilot study of cidofovir in patients with kaposi sarcoma. J Infect Dis. 2003;187(1):149–53.
40. Casper C, Nichols WG, Huang ML, Corey L, Wald A. Remission of HHV-8 and HIV-associated multicentric Castleman disease with ganciclovir treatment. Blood. 2004;103(5):1632–4.
41. Halfdanarson TR, Markovic SN, Kalokhe U, Luppi M. A non-chemotherapy treatment of a primary effusion lymphoma: durable remission after intracavitary cidofovir in HIV negative PEL refractory to chemotherapy. Ann Oncol. 2006;17(12):1849–50.
42. Luppi M, Trovato R, Barozzi P, et al. Treatment of herpesvirus associated primary effusion lymphoma with intracavity cidofovir. Leukemia. 2005;19(3):473–6.
43. Boulanger E, Daniel MT, Agbalika F, Oksenhendler E. Combined chemotherapy including high-dose methotrexate in KSHV/HHV8-associated primary effusion lymphoma. Am J Hematol. 2003;73(3):143–8.
44. Waddington TW, Aboulafia DM. Failure to eradicate AIDS-associated primary effusion lymphoma with high-dose chemotherapy and autologous stem cell reinfusion: case report and literature review. AIDS Patient Care STDS. 2004;18(2):67–73.

45. Bhatt S, Ashlock BM, Natkunam Y, et al. CD30 targeting with brentuximab vedotin: a novel therapeutic approach to primary effusion lymphoma. Blood. 2013;122(7):1233–42.
46. Haque M, Kousoulas KG. The Kaposi's sarcoma-associated herpesvirus ORF34 protein binds to HIF-1alpha and causes its degradation via the proteasome pathway. J Virol. 2013;87(4):2164–73.
47. Saji C, Higashi C, Niinaka Y, et al. Proteasome inhibitors induce apoptosis and reduce viral replication in primary effusion lymphoma cells. Biochem Biophys Res Commun. 2011; 415(4):573–8.
48. Abou-Merhi R, Khoriaty R, Arnoult D, et al. PS-341 or a combination of arsenic trioxide and interferon-alpha inhibit growth and induce caspase-dependent apoptosis in KSHV/HHV-8-infected primary effusion lymphoma cells. Leukemia. 2007;21(8):1792–801.
49. Matta H, Chaudhary PM. The proteasome inhibitor bortezomib (PS-341) inhibits growth and induces apoptosis in primary effusion lymphoma cells. Cancer Biol Ther. 2005;4(1):77–82.
50. An J, Sun Y, Fisher M, Rettig MB. Antitumor effects of bortezomib (PS-341) on primary effusion lymphomas. Leukemia. 2004;18(10):1699–704.
51. Wu FY, Wang SE, Tang QQ, et al. Cell cycle arrest by Kaposi's sarcoma-associated herpesvirus replication-associated protein is mediated at both the transcriptional and posttranslational levels by binding to CCAAT/enhancer-binding protein alpha and p21(CIP-1). J Virol. 2003;77(16):8893–914.
52. Dabaghmanesh N, Matsubara A, Miyake A, et al. Transient inhibition of NF-kappaB by DHMEQ induces cell death of primary effusion lymphoma without HHV-8 reactivation. Cancer Sci. 2009;100(4):737–46.
53. Bhatt S, Ashlock BM, Toomey NL, et al. Efficacious proteasome/HDAC inhibitor combination therapy for primary effusion lymphoma. J Clin Invest. 2013;123(6):2616–28.
54. Goto H, Kudo E, Kariya R, et al. Targeting VEGF and interleukin-6 for controlling malignant effusion of primary effusion lymphoma. J Cancer Res Clin Oncol. 2015;141(3):465–74.
55. Haddad L, El Hajj H, Abou-Merhi R, et al. KSHV-transformed primary effusion lymphoma cells induce a VEGF-dependent angiogenesis and establish functional gap junctions with endothelial cells. Leukemia. 2008;22(4):826–34.
56. Aoki Y, Tosato G. Vascular endothelial growth factor/vascular permeability factor in the pathogenesis of primary effusion lymphomas. Leuk Lymphoma. 2001;41(3–4):229–37.
57. Bottero V, Sadagopan S, Johnson KE, et al. Kaposi's sarcoma-associated herpesvirus-positive primary effusion lymphoma tumor formation in NOD/SCID mice is inhibited by neomycin and neamine blocking angiogenin's nuclear translocation. J Virol. 2013;87(21):11806–20.
58. Paul AG, Sharma-Walia N, Chandran B. Targeting KSHV/HHV-8 latency with COX-2 selective inhibitor nimesulide: a potential chemotherapeutic modality for primary effusion lymphoma. PLoS One. 2011;6(9):e24379.
59. Sun Z, Xiao B, Jha HC, et al. Kaposi's sarcoma-associated herpesvirus-encoded LANA can induce chromosomal instability through targeted degradation of the mitotic checkpoint kinase Bub1. J Virol. 2014;88(13):7367–78.
60. Santag S, Jager W, Karsten CB, et al. Recruitment of the tumour suppressor protein p73 by Kaposi's Sarcoma Herpesvirus latent nuclear antigen contributes to the survival of primary effusion lymphoma cells. Oncogene. 2013;32(32):3676–85.
61. Chen W, Hilton IB, Staudt MR, Burd CE, Dittmer DP. Distinct p53, p53:LANA, and LANA complexes in Kaposi's Sarcoma – associated Herpesvirus lymphomas. J Virol. 2010; 84(8):3898–908.
62. Lan K, Murakami M, Bajaj B, et al. Inhibition of KSHV-infected primary effusion lymphomas in NOD/SCID mice by gamma-secretase inhibitor. Cancer Biol Ther. 2009;8(22):2136–43.
63. Liu J, Martin HJ, Liao G, Hayward SD. The Kaposi's sarcoma-associated herpesvirus LANA protein stabilizes and activates c-Myc. J Virol. 2007;81(19):10451–9.
64. Bubman D, Guasparri I, Cesarman E. Deregulation of c-Myc in primary effusion lymphoma by Kaposi's sarcoma herpesvirus latency-associated nuclear antigen. Oncogene. 2007; 26(34):4979–86.
65. An J, Sun Y, Rettig MB. Transcriptional coactivation of c-Jun by the KSHV-encoded LANA. Blood. 2004;103(1):222–8.

66. Fujimuro M, Hayward SD. The latency-associated nuclear antigen of Kaposi's sarcoma-associated herpesvirus manipulates the activity of glycogen synthase kinase-3beta. J Virol. 2003;77(14):8019–30.
67. Katano H, Sato Y, Sata T. Expression of p53 and human herpesvirus-8 (HHV-8)-encoded latency-associated nuclear antigen with inhibition of apoptosis in HHV-8-associated malignancies. Cancer. 2001;92(12):3076–84.
68. Krithivas A, Young DB, Liao G, Greene D, Hayward SD. Human herpesvirus 8 LANA interacts with proteins of the mSin3 corepressor complex and negatively regulates Epstein-Barr virus gene expression in dually infected PEL cells. J Virol. 2000;74(20):9637–45.
69. Ballestas ME, Chatis PA, Kaye KM. Efficient persistence of extrachromosomal KSHV DNA mediated by latency-associated nuclear antigen. Science. 1999;284(5414):641–4.
70. Gantt S, Casper C. Human herpesvirus 8-associated neoplasms: the roles of viral replication and antiviral treatment. Curr Opin Infect Dis. 2011;24(4):295–301.
71. Klass CM, Krug LT, Pozharskaya VP, Offermann MK. The targeting of primary effusion lymphoma cells for apoptosis by inducing lytic replication of human herpesvirus 8 while blocking virus production. Blood. 2005;105(10):4028–34.
72. Yu Y, Black JB, Goldsmith CS, et al. Induction of human herpesvirus-8 DNA replication and transcription by butyrate and TPA in BCBL-1 cells. J Gen Virol. 1999;80(Pt 1):83–90.
73. Shaw RN, Arbiser JL, Offermann MK. Valproic acid induces human herpesvirus 8 lytic gene expression in BCBL-1 cells. AIDS. 2000;14(7):899–902.
74. Boulanger E, Agbalika F, Maarek O, et al. A clinical, molecular and cytogenetic study of 12 cases of human herpesvirus 8 associated primary effusion lymphoma in HIV-infected patients. Hematol J. 2001;2(3):172–9.
75. Pastore RD, Chadburn A, Kripas C, Schattner EJ. Novel association of haemophagocytic syndrome with Kaposi's sarcoma-associated herpesvirus-related primary effusion lymphoma. Br J Haematol. 2000;111(4):1112–5.
76. Drexler HG, Meyer C, Gaidano G, Carbone A. Constitutive cytokine production by primary effusion (body cavity-based) lymphoma-derived cell lines. Leukemia. 1999;13(4):634–40.
77. Asou H, Said JW, Yang R, et al. Mechanisms of growth control of Kaposi's sarcoma-associated herpes virus-associated primary effusion lymphoma cells. Blood. 1998;91(7):2475–81.
78. Zhang YJ, Bonaparte RS, Patel D, Stein DA, Iversen PL. Blockade of viral interleukin-6 expression of Kaposi's sarcoma-associated herpesvirus. Mol Cancer Ther. 2008;7(3):712–20.
79. Thapa DR, Li X, Jamieson BD, Martinez-Maza O. Overexpression of microRNAs from the miR-17-92 paralog clusters in AIDS-related non-Hodgkin's lymphomas. PLoS One. 2011;6(6):e20781.
80. Sun Y, Huang PL, Li JJ, et al. Anti-HIV agent MAP30 modulates the expression profile of viral and cellular genes for proliferation and apoptosis in AIDS-related lymphoma cells infected with Kaposi's sarcoma-associated virus. Biochem Biophys Res Commun. 2001;287(4):983–94.
81. Sarek G, Kurki S, Enback J, et al. Reactivation of the p53 pathway as a treatment modality for KSHV-induced lymphomas. J Clin Invest. 2007;117(4):1019–28.
82. Otvos R, Skribek H, Kis LL, et al. Drug sensitivity patterns of HHV8 carrying body cavity lymphoma cell lines. BMC Cancer. 2011;11:441.
83. Zhang YJ, Patel D, Nan Y, Fan S. Inhibition of primary effusion lymphoma engraftment in SCID mice by morpholino oligomers against early lytic genes of Kaposi's sarcoma-associated herpesvirus. Antivir Ther. 2011;16(5):657–66.

# Primary Central Nervous System Lymphoma

# 7

Panagiotis Papanastasopoulos, Mark Bower, and Thomas S. Uldrick

## Contents



## 7.1 Introduction

Primary central nervous system lymphoma (PCNSL) is an extra-nodal form of non-Hodgkin's lymphoma (NHL) that is confined to the cranio-spinal axis

P. Papanastasopoulos
National Centre for HIV Malignancy, Chelsea and Westminster Hospital, London, UK
e-mail: pan_papas@yahoo.com

M. Bower, PhD, FRCP, FRCPath (✉)
National Centre for HIV Malignancy, Chelsea and Westminster Hospital, London, UK

Department of Oncology, Chelsea and Westminster Hospital,
369 Fulham Road, London SW10 9NH, UK
e-mail: m.bower@imperial.ac.uk

T.S. Uldrick
HIV and AIDS Malignancy Branch, Center for Cancer Research, NCI, Bethesda, MD, USA
e-mail: uldrickts@mail.nih.gov



M. Hentrich, S.K. Barta (eds.), *HIV-associated Hematological Malignancies*,
DOI 10.1007/978-3-319-26857-6_7

without systemic involvement. PCNSL occurs in both immunocompetent and immunodeficient individuals, and the two groups share some features but differ in biology, clinical management and outcomes.

## 7.2 Epidemiology

Early in the HIV pandemic, before the advent of effective antiretroviral therapy, registry linkage studies confirmed a markedly increased relative risk of PCNSL amongst patients with AIDS with an incidence as high as 2–6 % in one early report [1]. This vastly elevated risk of PCNSL was estimated to be over 3,600-fold in people living with HIV (PLWH) [2]. PLWH who developed PCNSL generally had advanced immunosuppression and for the most part a prior AIDS defining illness. Shortly after the introduction of effective combination antiretroviral therapy (cART) in 1996, a substantial decline in the incidence of PCNSL was recognised by many clinicians, and a meta-analysis of cohort studies that compare the pre- and post-cART eras confirmed this significant reduction in incidence (relative risk 0.42; 99 % confidence interval 0.24–0.75) [3]. Indeed this fall is more dramatic than that seen for systemic AIDS-related lymphomas [4–7]. Over the same recent decades that the incidence of PCNSL has declined in PLWH, the incidence of PCNSL in immunocompetent individuals, particularly the elderly, has risen [8].

## 7.3 Histology

PCNSL are B-cell NHL of diffuse large B-cell lymphoma (DLBCL) subtype that express pan-B-cell markers with a post-germinal centre phenotype [9]. The immunophenotype of PCNSL differs between immunocompetent patients and PLWH and between PCNSL and systemic DLBCL [10]. The immunophenotype of PCNSL in PLWH resembles that found in post-transplant lymphoproliferative disorder (PTLD) [11, 12]. Indeed there are a number of similarities between PCNSL in PLWH and PTLD; both are associated with profound immunosuppression, and both are proliferations of B lymphocytes latently infected with Epstein-Barr virus (EBV).

## 7.4 Virology

The gammaherpes virus EBV is almost always detectable in the lymphoma cells in PCNSL in PLWH using immunohistochemical staining for EBV-encoded small RNA (EBER) transcripts [13], although it is rarely present in PCNSL in immunocompetent individuals. PLWH who develop PCNSL usually have profound immunosuppression and CD4 T-cell counts below 50 cells/mm$^3$ and have been found to lack EBV-specific CD4 T-cells [14]. PCNSL in PLWH express a number of EBV proteins including EBV-associated nuclear antigens (EBNA) 1, 2, 3A, 3B and 3C and latent membrane proteins (LMP) 1 and 2. The production of this range of viral proteins is known as latency III and would offer a variety of targets to an intact immune system.

## 7.5 Clinical Presentation

Patients with PCNSL invariably present with neurological symptoms and signs but rarely B symptoms [15]. The clinical presentation of 35 PLWH and PCNSL enrolled in a prospective study included motor deficits (37 %), altered mental status (31 %), headache (29 %), visual disturbance (26 %), cranial nerve deficits (23 %), speech impairment (23 %), cerebellar deficits (20 %), sensory deficits (17 %) and papilledema (4 %) [16]. PLWH and PCNSL are usually profoundly immunosuppressed with CD4 T-cell counts below 50 cells/mm$^3$ [16–18], and the differential diagnosis includes opportunistic infections, especially cerebral toxoplasmosis and less commonly cryptococcal meningoencephalitis and tuberculosis.

## 7.6 Investigation and Diagnosis

The most common causes of cerebral mass lesions in PLWH are toxoplasmosis and primary cerebral lymphoma, and the differential diagnosis often proves difficult [19]. Both diagnoses occur in the context of advanced immunodeficiency and present with headaches and focal neurological deficits. The features that favour PCNSL include a more gradual onset of symptoms over 2–8 weeks and the absence of a fever. CT and MRI scanning usually show solitary or multiple ring-enhancing lesions with prominent mass effect and oedema (Fig. 7.1). Again these findings occur in both diagnoses although PCNSL lesions are frequently periventricular, whilst toxoplasmosis more often affects the basal ganglia [20–23]. Hence, clinical findings and standard radiological investigations, whilst suggestive, cannot provide a definitive diagnosis (see Table 7.1). Moreover, toxoplasma serology (IgG) is falsely negative in 10–15 % of patients with cerebral toxoplasmosis. Over 85 %

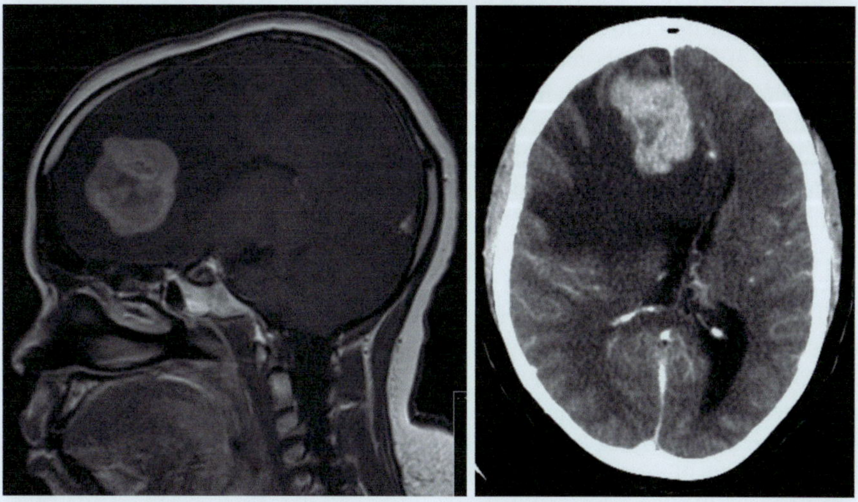

**Fig. 7.1** MRI scan showing frontal PCNSL in a person living with HIV (PLWH)

**Table 7.1** Comparison of clinic-radiological features of cerebral toxoplasmosis and primary CNS lymphoma in people living with HIV

| Feature | Cerebral toxoplasmosis | PCNSL |
|---|---|---|
| CD4 cell count | <100/mm$^3$ | <50/mm$^3$ |
| Onset of symptoms | Days | Weeks |
| Nonfocal symptoms | Fever, headache, reduced cognition | Afebrile, headache, meningism |
| Localising symptoms | Focal deficits 80 %, seizures 30 % | Behavioural changes, diminished mental state, seizures 15 % |
| Location | Basal ganglia, brain stem | Periventricular anywhere |
| Number of lesions | Usually multiple | One or many |
| Contrast enhancement | Prominent, ring enhancing | Prominent, often irregular |
| Mass effect/oedema | Usual | Prominent |
| MRI T1 | Low signal | Low to isodense |
| MRI T2 | High signal | Variable |

patients with cerebral toxoplasmosis will respond clinically and radiologically to 2 weeks of anti-toxoplasma therapy.

In AIDS patients with CNS ring-enhancing lesions, historically it has been common practice to start empirical anti-toxoplasmosis therapy for 2 weeks' duration and resort to a brain biopsy if there is no clinical or radiological improvement. This approach, established in the pre-cART era, excludes routine brain biopsy in a patient population who frequently had a very poor performance status, often due to CNS disease, and without effective HIV medications, and had a very poor prognosis. Whilst starting empiric anti-toxoplasmosis therapy is still reasonable in patients with positive toxoplasmosis serology, the approach of evaluating the effects of therapy after a 2-week course is ineffective in diagnosing PCNSL early and may compromise the long-term outcomes of therapy. Furthermore, there is a disinclination to treat patients with radiotherapy or chemotherapy empirically based exclusively on the failure of anti-toxoplasmosis treatment without a definitive histological diagnosis. Hence, in the cART era, many clinicians adopt a more definitive approach to establishing a diagnosis with early neuroimaging and cerebrospinal fluid (CSF) virology (described below) and brain biopsy. It should be recalled that steroids have a lympholytic effect and often induce a temporary regression of the lymphoma with clinical and radiological improvement. Moreover, they can obscure the histopathologic findings making the diagnosis challenging [24]; hence, their use is strongly discouraged prior to establishing a tissue diagnosis.

The discovery that nearly all HIV-associated PCNSL are associated with EBV infection [13, 25] has led to the development of a polymerase chain reaction (PCR) method that can detect EBV-DNA in CSF. This has become established as a diagnostic test with a high sensitivity (83–100 %) and specificity in the presence of a cerebral space-occupying lesion (93–100 %) [13, 26–28]. In addition, radionuclide imaging by $^{201}$thallium single-photon emission computed tomography ($^{201}$Th-SPECT) [29–36] and $^{18}$F-fluorodeoxyglucose-positron emission tomography (FDG-PET) [37–40] may be able to differentiate between PCNSL and cerebral toxoplasmosis.

PCNSL are thallium avid and demonstrate increased FDG uptake on PET scanning. Although both nuclear imaging techniques have high specificity for differentiating PCNSL from infections in appropriate patient populations [41, 42], neither are highly sensitivity and thus are generally performed in combination with evaluation of CSF for EBV by PCR as a diagnostic alternative to brain biopsy [34]. The application of PCR and $^{201}$Th-SPECT in the diagnosis of contrast-enhancing brain lesions in 27 patients was shown to result in a positive and a negative predictive value of 100 % and 88 %, respectively [43].

Stereotactic brain biopsy has a high diagnostic yield in PLWH who have space-occupying brain lesions, and whilst it has become a safer procedure, biopsies of deep lesions may still be associated with significant morbidity [44–47]. Hence, the combination of low CD4 cell count, detectable EBV in CSF and a consistent $^{201}$Th-SPECT or $^{18}$FDG-PET and lack of systemic lymphoma may be sufficient to establish the diagnosis of PCNSL in PLWH without recourse to brain biopsy.

## 7.7 Clinical Management

The introduction cART has not only led to a decline in the incidence of PCNSL amongst PLWH but also a modest improvement in overall survival [7, 48–52], but outcomes remain dismal with fewer than two in ten patients alive 2 years after diagnosis [53–56]. On the other hand, there are case reports of complete remission of PCNSL in PLWH treated with cART alone [57]. Aside from the value of cART, there is no consensus on the management of PCNSL in PLWH, and there has not been a dramatic improvement in survival that has been achieved through prospective clinical studies in systemic NHL in PLWH. Nonetheless, in addition to cART, administration of some form of lymphoma therapy, either radiation or chemotherapy, has been independently associated with improved survival in database studies [18, 55] and is often warranted.

In immunocompetent patients with PCNSL, upfront induction chemotherapy with high-dose methotrexate and cytarabine followed by consolidation with whole-brain radiotherapy or further chemotherapy with or without autologous haematopoietic stem cell transplantation has become established as the standard of care. In contrast, PLWH who develop PCNSL often present with very poor performance status, severe cognitive and neurological impairment, concurrent opportunistic infections and very low CD4 counts, making the administration of highly toxic treatments impossible in a large proportion of patients [58]. This led to the use of whole-brain radiotherapy as the most commonly used treatment strategy for PCNSL in PLWH in the pre-cART era, but the outcomes were dismal. Whilst the median survival using this approach in immunocompetent patients is 12 months [59], retrospective studies of this approach in PLWH reported median survivals of 2–4.5 m [60, 61]. More encouraging results have been reported recently using the combination of whole-brain radiotherapy and cART. This achieved a 3-year overall survival rate of 64 % (95 % CI, 41.0–80.3 %) in a cohort of 23 PLWH, although a worrying 21 % of those who survived a year developed leucoencephalopathy [62]. The concerns over late neurotoxicity resulted in the increasing use of induction systemic chemotherapy in the management of PCNSL in immunocompetent patients, but the results in PLWH in the cART era are limited. A phase II study in the pre-cART era studied sequential combination chemotherapy followed by whole-brain radiotherapy and enrolled 35 PLWH. The median survival was 2.4 months (95 % confidence interval: 1.1–3.2) and only four (11 %) survived 1 year [16]. Two other small studies have addressed the role of chemotherapy in PCNSL in PLWH. In a small study before the introduction of cART, 15 patients (10 with histological documentation of PCNSL) received high-dose (3 g/m$^2$) methotrexate with leucovorin rescue, and the median survival was 9.6 months (range: 0.3–19) [17]. In the second study, ten patients were treated with high-dose methotrexate-based combination chemotherapy followed by whole-brain radiotherapy. Median survival was 3.5 months and two (20 %) patients survived 1 year [63].

The recognition that Epstein-Barr virus plays a pathogenetic role in PCNSL in PLWH led to studies of targeted antiviral treatments. Two very small studies have used a combination of parenteral zidovudine, ganciclovir and interleukin 2. Significant tumour regression and occasional long-term survival have been reported [64, 65]. Finally, in a small retrospective study, eight patients treated with ganciclovir were found to have significantly lower CSF EBV-DNA levels and somewhat improved survival compared to 17 patients who did not receive ganciclovir (6.0 vs. 2.4 months) [66]. The limited number of small retrospective studies of targeted antiviral treatments does not allow for safe conclusions with regards to their efficacy, and therefore such treatments are not routinely included in the current management guidelines. The US National Cancer Institute is currently prospectively evaluating radiation-sparing immunochemotherapy employing rituximab, high-dose methotrexate with leucovorin and concurrent cART; mature data from this protocol may inform future approaches to management of this disease (Table 7.2).

**Table 7.2** Outcomes of treatment schedules for PCL in PLWH and immunocompetent individuals.

| | No. of patients | Treatment | Outcome |
|---|---|---|---|
| *PLWH* | | | |
| Ambinder et al. [16] | 34 | Cyclophosphamide, doxorubicin, vincristine, IT Ara-C, WBRT | Median OS: 2.4 months, ORR: 12 % |
| Jacometi et al. [17] | 15 | HD MTX, followed by WBRT on progression | Median OS: 9.7 months, ORR: 47 % |
| Forsyth et al. [63] | 10 | HD MTX-based regimens (thiotepa, procarbazine), WBRT | Median OS: 3.5 months, ORR : 86 % |
| *Immunocompetent* | | | |
| De Angelis et al. [67] | 102 | HD MTX, vincristine, procarbazine, IT MTX, followed by WBRT and HD Ara-C | Median OS: 36.9 months, median PFS: 24 months, ORR: 94 % |
| Ferreri et al. [68] | 79 | HD MTX vs. HD MTX and Ara-C (randomised) both followed by WBRT | 3-year OS:32 % vs. 46 % |
| | | | 3-year FFS: 21 % vs. 38 % |
| | | | ORR: 40 % vs. 69 % |

*IT* intrathecal, *WBRT* whole-brain radiotherapy, *OS* overall survival, *ORR* overall response rate, *HD* high dose, *MTX* methotrexate, *PFS* progression-free survival, *FFS* failure-free survival

**Conclusion**

AIDS-related PCNSL remains the most common malignancy of the CNS in PLWH, although cART has substantially reduced the incidence and seems to have modestly improved the survival. An early stereotactic biopsy is recommended in PLWH presenting with ring-enhancing brain lesions not responding to a short course of anti-toxoplasma treatment. The lack of clinical trials in the cART era, which is partly a consequence of the declining incidence, precludes the development of evidence-based algorithms of care. Simply adopting protocols that are employed in immunocompetent individuals may not be appropriate because of the differences in the biology of the tumours in PLWH. Consequently there is an urgent need for multicentred prospective randomised clinical trials to define optimal management in AIDS-related PCNSL.

## References


1. Snider WD, Simpson DM, Nielsen S, Gold JW, Metroka CE, Posner JB. Neurological complications of acquired immune deficiency syndrome: analysis of 50 patients. Ann Neurol. 1983;14(4):403–18.
2. Cote TR, Manns A, Hardy CR, Yellin FJ, Hartge P. Epidemiology of brain lymphoma among people with or without acquired immunodeficiency syndrome. AIDS/Cancer Study Group. J Natl Cancer Inst. 1996;88(10):675–9. Epub 1996/05/15.
3. International Collaboration on HIV and Cancer. Highly active antiretroviral therapy and incidence of cancer in human immunodeficiency virus-infected adults. J Natl Cancer Inst. 2000;92(22):1823–30.
4. Ammassari A, Cingolani A, Pezzotti P, De Luca DA, Murri R, Giancola ML, et al. AIDS-related focal brain lesions in the era of highly active antiretroviral therapy. Neurology. 2000;55(8):1194–200. Epub 2000/11/09.
5. Wolf T, Brodt HR, Fichtlscherer S, Mantzsch K, Hoelzer D, Helm EB, et al. Changing incidence and prognostic factors of survival in AIDS-related non-Hodgkin's lymphoma in the era of highly active antiretroviral therapy (HAART). Leuk Lymphoma. 2005;46(2):207–15.
6. Pipkin S, Scheer S, Okeigwe I, Schwarcz S, Harris DH, Hessol NA. The effect of HAART and calendar period on Kaposi's sarcoma and non-Hodgkin lymphoma: results of a match between an AIDS and cancer registry. AIDS. 2011;25(4):463–71. Epub 2010/12/09.
7. Bower M, Powles T, Nelson M, Mandalia S, Gazzard B, Stebbing J. Highly active antiretroviral therapy and human immunodeficiency virus-associated primary cerebral lymphoma. J Natl Cancer Inst. 2006;98(15):1088–91. Epub 2006/08/03.
8. Olson JE, Janney CA, Rao RD, Cerhan JR, Kurtin PJ, Schiff D, et al. The continuing increase in the incidence of primary central nervous system non-Hodgkin lymphoma: a surveillance, epidemiology, and end results analysis. Cancer. 2002;95(7):1504–10. Epub 2002/09/19.
9. Deckert M, Engert A, Bruck W, Ferreri AJ, Finke J, Illerhaus G, et al. Modern concepts in the biology, diagnosis, differential diagnosis and treatment of primary central nervous system lymphoma. Leukemia. 2011;25(12):1797–807. Epub 2011/08/06.
10. Larocca LM, Capello D, Rinelli A, Nori S, Antinori A, Gloghini A, et al. The molecular and phenotypic profile of primary central nervous system lymphoma identifies distinct categories of the disease and is consistent with histogenetic derivation from germinal center-related B cells. Blood. 1998;92(3):1011–9. Epub 1998/07/29.
11. Carbone A, Gaidano G, Gloghini A, Larocca LM, Capello D, Canzonieri V, et al. Differential expression of BCL-6, CD138/syndecan-1, and Epstein-Barr virus-encoded latent membrane protein-1 identifies distinct histogenetic subsets of acquired immunodeficiency syndrome-related non-Hodgkin's lymphomas. Blood. 1998;91:747–55.

12. Abed N, Casper JT, Camitta BM, Margolis D, Trost B, Orentas R, et al. Evaluation of histogenesis of B-lymphocytes in pediatric EBV-related post-transplant lymphoproliferative disorders. Bone Marrow Transplant. 2004;33(3):321–7. Epub 2003/12/23.
13. MacMahon EM, Glass JD, Hayward SD, Mann RB, Becker PS, Charache P, et al. Epstein-Barr virus in AIDS-related primary central nervous system lymphoma. Lancet. 1991; 338(8773):969–73.
14. Gasser O, Bihl FK, Wolbers M, Loggi E, Steffen I, Hirsch HH, et al. HIV patients developing primary CNS lymphoma lack EBV-specific CD4+ T cell function irrespective of absolute CD4+ T cell counts. PLoS Med. 2007;4(3):e96.
15. Bataille B, Delwail V, Menet E, Vandermarcq P, Ingrand P, Wager M, et al. Primary intracerebral malignant lymphoma: report of 248 cases. J Neurosurg. 2000;92(2):261–6. Epub 2000/02/05.
16. Ambinder RF, Lee S, Curran WJ, Sparano JA, Krigel RL, McArthur JC, et al. Phase II intergroup trial of sequential chemotherapy and radiotherapy for AIDS-related primary central nervous system lymphoma. Cancer Ther. 2003;1:215–21.
17. Jacomet C, Girard P, Lebrette M, Farese V, Monfort L, Rozenbaum W. Intravenous methotrexate for primary central nervous system non-Hodgkin's lymphoma in AIDS. AIDS. 1997;11:1725–30.
18. Bower M, Fife K, Sullivan A, Kirk S, Phillips RH, Nelson M, et al. Treatment outcome in presumed and confirmed AIDS-related primary cerebral lymphoma. Eur J Cancer. 1999; 35(4):601–4.
19. Cheung TW. AIDS-related cancer in the era of highly active antiretroviral therapy (HAART): a model of the interplay of the immune system, virus, and cancer. "On the offensive – the Trojan Horse is being destroyed" – part B: malignant lymphoma. Cancer Invest. 2004; 22(5):787–98.
20. Morgello S, Petito CK, Mouradian JA. Central nervous system lymphoma in the acquired immunodeficiency syndrome. Clin Neuropathol. 1990;9(4):205–15. Epub 1990/07/01.
21. Chang L, Cornford ME, Chiang FL, Ernst TM, Sun NC, Miller BL. Radiologic-pathologic correlation. Cerebral toxoplasmosis and lymphoma in AIDS. AJNR Am J Neuroradiol. 1995;16(8):1653–63. Epub 1995/09/01.
22. Gildenberg PL, Gathe Jr JC, Kim JH. Stereotactic biopsy of cerebral lesions in AIDS. Clin Infect Dis Off Publ Infect Dis Soc Am. 2000;30(3):491–9. Epub 2000/03/18.
23. Bakshi R. Neuroimaging of HIV and AIDS related illnesses: a review. Front Biosci J Virtual libr. 2004;9:632–46. Epub 2004/02/10.
24. Pirotte B, Levivier M, Goldman S, Brucher JM, Brotchi J, Hildebrand J. Glucocorticoid-induced long-term remission in primary cerebral lymphoma: case report and review of the literature. J Neurooncol. 1997;32(1):63–9. Epub 1997/03/01.
25. Bashir R, Luka J, Cheloha K, Chamberlain M, Hochberg F. Expression of Epstein-Barr virus proteins in primary CNS lymphoma in AIDS patients. Neurology. 1993;43(11):2358–62. Epub 1993/11/01.
26. Cinque P, Brytting M, Vago L, Castagna A, Parravicini C, Zanchetta N, et al. Epstein-Barr virus DNA in cerebrospinal fluid from patients with AIDS-related primary lymphoma of the central nervous system. Lancet. 1993;342:398–401.
27. Arribas J, Clifford D, Fichtenbaum C, Roberts R, Powderly W, Storch G. Detection of Epstein-Barr virus DNA in cerebrospinal fluid for diagnosis of AIDS-related central nervous system lymphoma. J Clin Microbiol. 1995;33(6):1580–3.
28. Bossolasco S, Cinque P, Ponzoni M, Vigano MG, Lazzarin A, Linde A, et al. Epstein-Barr virus DNA load in cerebrospinal fluid and plasma of patients with AIDS-related lymphoma. J Neurovirol. 2002;8(5):432–8. Epub 2002/10/29.
29. Ruiz A, Ganz W, Post M, et al. Use of thallium-201 brain SPECT to differentiate cerebral lymphoma from Toxoplasma encephalitis in AIDS patients. AmJ Neuroradiol. 1994;15: 1885–94.
30. Lorberboym M, Estok L, Machac J, Germano I, Sacher M, Feldman R, et al. Rapid differential diagnosis of cerebral toxoplasmosis and primary central nervous system lymphoma by thallium-201 SPECT. J Nucl Med. 1996;37(7):1150–4.

31. D'Amico A, Messa C, Castagna A, Zito F, Galli L, Pepe G, et al. Diagnostic accuracy and predictive value of 201T1 SPET for the differential diagnosis of cerebral lesions in AIDS patients. Nucl Med Commun. 1997;18(8):741–50. Epub 1997/08/01.
32. Miller RF, Hall-Craggs MA, Costa DC, Brink NS, Scaravilli F, Lucas SB, et al. Magnetic resonance imaging, thallium-201 SPET scanning, and laboratory analyses for discrimination of cerebral lymphoma and toxoplasmosis in AIDS. Sex Transm Infect. 1998;74(4):258–64. Epub 1999/01/30.
33. Lorberboym M, Wallach F, Estok L, Mosesson RE, Sacher M, Kim CK, et al. Thallium-201 retention in focal intracranial lesions for differential diagnosis of primary lymphoma and nonmalignant lesions in AIDS patients. J Nucl Med. 1998;39(8):1366–9. Epub 1998/08/26.
34. Antinori A, De Rossi G, Ammassari A, Cingolani A, Murri R, Di Giuda D, et al. Value of combined approach with thallium-201 single-photon emission computed tomography and Epstein-Barr virus DNA polymerase chain reaction in CSF for the diagnosis of AIDS-related primary CNS lymphoma. J Clin Oncol Off J Am Soc Clin Oncol. 1999;17(2):554–60. Epub 1999/03/18.
35. Skiest DJ, Erdman W, Chang WE, Oz OK, Ware A, Fleckenstein J. SPECT thallium-201 combined with Toxoplasma serology for the presumptive diagnosis of focal central nervous system mass lesions in patients with AIDS. J Infect. 2000;40(3):274–81. Epub 2000/07/25.
36. Licho R, Litofsky NS, Senitko M, George M. Inaccuracy of Tl-201 brain SPECT in distinguishing cerebral infections from lymphoma in patients with AIDS. Clin Nucl Med. 2002;27(2):81–6. Epub 2002/01/12.
37. Hoffman J, Waskin H, Schifter T, Hanson M, Gray L, Rosenfeld S, et al. FDG-PET in differentiating lymphoma from nonmalignant central nervous system lesions in patients with AIDS. J Nucl Med. 1993;34(4):567–75.
38. Villringer K, Jager H, Dichgans M, Ziegler S, Poppinger J, Herz M, et al. Differential diagnosis of CNS lesions in AIDS patients by FDG-PET. J Comput Assist Tomogr. 1995; 19(4):532–6.
39. Heald A, Hoffman J, Bartlett J, Waskin H. Differentiation of central nervous system lesions in AIDS patients using positron emission tomography (PET). Int J STD AIDS. 1996; 7(5):337–46.
40. O'Doherty MJ, Barrington SF, Campbell M, Lowe J, Bradbeer CS. PET scanning and the human immunodeficiency virus-positive patient. J Nucl Med. 1997;38(10):1575–83.
41. Kasamon YL, Ambinder RF. AIDS-related primary central nervous system lymphoma. Hematol Oncol Clin North Am. 2005;19(4):665–87. vi–vii. Epub 2005/08/09.
42. Lewitschnig S, Gedela K, Toby M, Kulasegaram R, Nelson M, O'Doherty M, et al. (1)(8) F-FDG PET/CT in HIV-related central nervous system pathology. Eur J Nucl Med Mol Imaging. 2013;40(9):1420–7. Epub 2013/05/21.
43. Castagna A, Cinque P, d'Amico A, Messa C, Fazsio F, Lazzarin A. Evaluation of contrast-enhancing brain lesions in AIDS patients by means of Epstein-Barr virus detection in cerebrospinal fluid and 201thallium single photon emission tomography. AIDS. 1997;11:1522–3.
44. Iacoangeli M, Roselli R, Antinori A, Ammassari A, Murri R, Pompucci A, et al. Experience with brain biopsy in acquired immune deficiency syndrome-related focal lesions of the central nervous system. Br J Surg. 1994;81(10):1508–11. Epub 1994/10/01.
45. Davies MA, Pell MF, Brew BJ. Stereotactic biopsy of cerebral lesions in acquired immunodeficiency syndrome. J Clin Neurosci Off J Neurosurg Soc Australasia. 1995;2(1):40–4. Epub 1995/01/01.
46. Luzzati R, Ferrari S, Nicolato A, Piovan E, Malena M, Merighi M, et al. Stereotactic brain biopsy in human immunodeficiency virus-infected patients. Arch Intern Med. 1996;156(5):565–8. Epub 1996/03/11.
47. Skolasky RL, Dal Pan GJ, Olivi A, Lenz FA, Abrams RA, McArthur JC. HIV-associated primary CNS lymorbidity and utility of brain biopsy. J Neurol Sci. 1999;163(1):32–8. Epub 1999/05/01.
48. Hoffmann C, Tabrizian S, Wolf E, Eggers C, Stoehr A, Plettenberg A, et al. Survival of AIDS patients with primary central nervous system lymphoma is dramatically improved by HAART-induced immune recovery. AIDS. 2001;15(16):2119–27.

49. Skiest DJ, Crosby C. Survival is prolonged by highly active antiretroviral therapy in AIDS patients with primary central nervous system lymphoma. AIDS. 2003;17(12):1787–93.
50. Newell ME, Hoy JF, Cooper SG, DeGraaff B, Grulich AE, Bryant M, et al. Human immunodeficiency virus-related primary central nervous system lymphoma: factors influencing survival in 111 patients. Cancer. 2004;100(12):2627–36.
51. Diamond C, Taylor TH, Im T, Miradi M, Wallace M, Anton-Culver H. Highly active antiretroviral therapy is associated with improved survival among patients with AIDS-related primary central nervous system non-Hodgkin's lymphoma. Curr HIV Res. 2006;4(3):375–8. Epub 2006/07/18.
52. Bayraktar S, Bayraktar UD, Ramos JC, Stefanovic A, Lossos IS. Primary CNS lymphoma in HIV positive and negative patients: comparison of clinical characteristics, outcome and prognostic factors. J Neurooncol. 2011;101(2):257–65. Epub 2010/06/08.
53. Achenbach CJ, Cole SR, Kitahata MM, Casper C, Willig JH, Mugavero MJ, et al. Mortality after cancer diagnosis in HIV-infected individuals treated with antiretroviral therapy. AIDS. 2011;25(5):691–700. Epub 2010/12/17.
54. Norden AD, Drappatz J, Wen PY, Claus EB. Survival among patients with primary central nervous system lymphoma, 1973–2004. J Neurooncol. 2011;101(3):487–93. Epub 2010/06/18.
55. Uldrick TS, Pipkin S, Scheer S, Hessol NA. Factors associated with survival among patients with AIDS-related primary central nervous system lymphoma. AIDS. 2014;28(3):397–405. Epub 2013/10/01.
56. Gopal S, Patel MR, Yanik EL, Cole SR, Achenbach CJ, Napravnik S, et al. Temporal trends in presentation and survival for HIV-associated lymphoma in the antiretroviral therapy era. J Natl Cancer Inst. 2013;105(16):1221–9. Epub 2013/07/31.
57. Aboulafia DM, Puswella AL. Highly active antiretroviral therapy as the sole treatment for AIDS-related primary central nervous system lymphoma: a case report with implications for treatment. AIDS Patient Care STDS. 2007;21(12):900–7. Epub 2007/12/25.
58. Chamberlain MC, Kormanik PA. AIDS-related central nervous system lymphomas. J Neurooncol. 1999;43(3):269–76. Epub 1999/11/24.
59. Nelson DF, Martz KL, Bonner H, Nelson JS, Newall J, Kerman HD, et al. Non-Hodgkin's lymphoma of the brain: can high dose, large volume radiation therapy improve survival? Report on a prospective trial by the Radiation Therapy Oncology Group (RTOG): RTOG 8315. Int J Radiat Oncol Biol Phys. 1992;23(1):9–17. Epub 1992/01/01.
60. Baumgartner JE, Rachlin JR, Beckstead JH, Meeker TC, Levy RM, Wara WM, et al. Primary central nervous system lymphomas: natural history and response to radiation therapy in 55 patients with acquired immunodeficiency syndrome. J Neurosurg. 1990;73(2):206–11. Epub 1990/08/01.
61. Donahue B, Sullivan J, Cooper J. Additional experience with empiric radiotherapy for presumed human immunodeficiency virus-associated primary central nervous system lymphoma. Cancer. 1995;76:328–32.
62. Nagai H, Odawara T, Ajisawa A, Tanuma J, Hagiwara S, Watanabe T, et al. Whole brain radiation alone produces favourable outcomes for AIDS-related primary central nervous system lymphoma in the HAART era. Eur J Haematol. 2010;84(6):499–505. Epub 2010/02/06.
63. Forsyth PA, Yahalom J, DeAngelis LM. Combined-modality therapy in the treatment of primary central nervous system lymphoma in AIDS. Neurology. 1994;44(8):1473–9. Epub 1994/08/01.
64. Raez L, Cabral L, Cai JP, Landy H, Sfakianakis G, Byrne Jr GE, et al. Treatment of AIDS-related primary central nervous system lymphoma with zidovudine, ganciclovir, and interleukin 2. AIDS Res Hum Retroviruses. 1999;15(8):713–9. Epub 1999/06/05.
65. Aboulafia DM, Ratner L, Miles SA, Harrington Jr WJ. Antiviral and immunomodulatory treatment for AIDS-related primary central nervous system lymphoma: AIDS Malignancies Consortium pilot study 019. Clin Lymphoma Myeloma. 2006;6(5):399–402. Epub 2006/04/28.
66. Bossolasco S, Falk KI, Ponzoni M, Ceserani N, Crippa F, Lazzarin A, et al. Ganciclovir is associated with low or undetectable Epstein-Barr virus DNA load in cerebrospinal fluid of patients with HIV-related primary central nervous system lymphoma. Clin Infect Dis Off Publ Infect Dis Soc Am. 2006;42(4):e21–5. Epub 2006/01/20.

67. DeAngelis LM, Seiferheld W, Schold SC, Fisher B, Schultz CJ. Combination chemotherapy and radiotherapy for primary central nervous system lymphoma: Radiation Therapy Oncology Group Study 93-10. J Clin Oncol. 2002;20(24):4643–8. Epub 2002/12/19.
68. Ferreri AJ, Reni M, Foppoli M, Martelli M, Pangalis GA, Frezzato M, et al. High-dose cytarabine plus high-dose methotrexate versus high-dose methotrexate alone in patients with primary CNS lymphoma: a randomised phase 2 trial. Lancet. 2009;374(9700):1512–20. Epub 2009/09/22.

# HIV and Indolent Lymphoma

# 8

Nadia Khan, Dipesh Uprety, Jenny Seo, and Mark Leick

## Contents




N. Khan, MD (✉)
Department of Oncology, Fox Chase Cancer Center, Temple University School of Medicine, Philadelphia, PA, USA
e-mail: Nadia.Khan@fccc.edu

D. Uprety, MD
Department of Internal Medicine, Abington Memorial Hospital, Abington Jefferson Health System, Abington, PA, USA

J. Seo, DO
Department of Internal Medicine, Philadelphia College of Osteopathic Medicine (PCOM), Philadelphia, PA, USA

M. Leick, MD
Department of Internal Medicine, Johns Hopkins Hospital, Johns Hopkins University School of Medicine, Baltimore, MD, USA







M. Hentrich, S.K. Barta (eds.), *HIV-associated Hematological Malignancies*, DOI 10.1007/978-3-319-26857-6_8

The incidence of non-Hodgkin's lymphoma (NHL) is at least 100 times higher in the human immunodeficiency virus (HIV)-infected population as compared with the general population [1, 2]. Approximately 3 % of HIV/AIDS patients develop NHL [3]. Among them, the risk increases with older age, duration of infection, and with a history of AIDS-defining events [4]. Data supporting a decline in NHL in the post-HAART era are inconsistent [5–7]. A prolonged immunocompromised state, with reduced immune surveillance, and chronic antigen stimulation, in the setting of infection with HIV, are contributors to the pathogenesis of NHL. Studies suggest that there are increased p53 gene abnormalities in HIV-1-related NHL [8]. In this chapter, we will focus on the indolent subset of NHL in the HIV-infected population. Of the AIDS-defining illnesses, there are two subtypes of aggressive NHL including Burkitt lymphoma and DLBCL, which are disproportionately more prevalent among HIV lymphoma subtypes. There is a contradistinction in the prevalence of indolent subtypes of NHL in the HIV population, with the incidence rates of these lymphomas being lower as compared with the indolent subtypes in the general population, as described in SEER database analysis of patients from 1992 to 2009, suggesting less of an association with HIV [9]. When looking at incidence of indolent subtypes of NHL in the AIDS subgroup of patients (patients with a prior AIDS-defining illness), the risk of developing an indolent NHL is significantly higher than in the HIV population at large, with a 20-fold increased risk [10]. In patient with advanced AIDS, mortality is impacted by causes other than indolent NHL, in the vast majority of cases [11]. Nevertheless, the presence of a lymphoma in an HIV patient poses distinct challenges for the clinician, because of the need for regimens that are immunosuppressive, in patients with an already suppressed immune systems. Indolent lymphomas are typically considered incurable, with relapses after disease-free intervals following treatment courses and less aggressive clinical behavior as compared to the aggressive subtypes. The indolent subsets represent only 2–7 % of lymphomas occurring in people living with HIV (PLWH) [12–14]. Herein, we review the major indolent NHL subsets and describe the disease features as reported in the HIV population.

## 8.1 CLL/SLL

Chronic lymphocytic leukemia (CLL) and small lymphocytic lymphoma (SLL) are biologically indistinguishable diseases, characterized by the clonal proliferation and expansion of mature CD5+, CD23+ B lymphocytes in the blood, lymph nodes, bone marrow, and spleen. CLL is the most common adult leukemia in the Western world [15].

CLL is most prevalent in the elderly, with a median age of 70 years at diagnosis, and men are twice as likely to develop CLL as women [16]. Most patients present with asymptomatic disease, with the incidental finding of lymphocytosis on routine laboratory assessment. Besides this, patients may present with adenopathy, hepato-/splenomegaly, anemia, and thrombocytopenia. The diagnosis of CLL requires the presence of at least $5 \times 10^9$ B clonal lymphocytes/L in the peripheral blood [17]. The circulating lymphocytes are small with scant cytoplasm and round nuclei. The expression of surface markers and thereby diagnosis are confirmed by flow cytometry. The established treatment of CLL varies according to the mutational profile and concomitant medical comorbidities of the patient, with a number of novel targeted therapies now available for consideration. There is a paucity of literature on the efficacy of novel therapies in the HIV population, as HIV infection is a common exclusion criterion for clinical trial enrollment. Older therapies, such as fludarabine, a highly immunosuppressive chemotherapy should not be foremost in the treatment of an HIV-positive patient with CLL/SLL, and consideration of less immunosuppressive therapies would be appropriate. Therefore, the need for inclusion of HIV patients in clinical trials utilizing novel agents in the treatment of indolent lymphomas is an unmet need, with the caveats of appropriate viral load and CD4 counts for treatment consideration.

There are few case reports of CLL in the HIV population, summarized in Tables 8.1 and 8.2 [18–23]. Cases reported suggest that HIV-infected patients had preserved CD4 counts when diagnosed with CLL; all patients reported had been on combination antiretroviral therapy (CART) and the average CD4 count was greater than 500 cells/mm$^3$. The average life expectancy of a 20-year-old in the USA on CART approaches that of the normal population and yet the median age at CLL diagnosis was 61 years, one decade earlier as compared to the HIV-negative CLL population [24]. Four patients among the cases outlined were treated with chemotherapies, and two of the four had a rituximab-containing regimen. Progressive multifocal leukoencephalopathy (PML) was described in one patient with a CD4 count of 498 cell/mm$^3$ who had been treated with fludarabine, cyclophosphamide, and rituximab (FCR). Bendamustine was used to treat two patients with relapsed/relapsed CLL, while still on CART, with significant cytopenias in one patient and the consideration of transformation to DLBCL as an unproven outcome in another patient [21]. Given the paucity of available literature on HIV patients with CLL, it is not surprising that the data on risk and outcomes of CLL transformation to DLBCL (Richter's syndrome) or transformation to prolymphocytic leukemia, PLL, is also lacking.

There is a well-described risk of secondary malignancies in CLL patients at large, a suspected result of altered immune surveillance in this disease [25, 26]. Given the increased incidence of secondary malignancies in the HIV population, considered attention to malignancy screening in the HIV-infected CLL population is warranted.

## 8.2 Marginal Zone Lymphoma

Marginal zone lymphomas (MZL) include nodal marginal zone lymphoma (NMZL), extranodal MZL of the mucosa-associated lymphoid tissue (MALT), and splenic marginal zone lymphoma (SMZL). Arising from the marginal zone of the lymph node, they are marked by expression for the B cell antigens CD19 and CD20 and are typically negative for CD5, CD10, and CD23. Patients with HIV have an increased incidence of MZL [27]. NOTCH2 mutations are not uncommon and can be identified in almost 20 % of cases [28].

**Table 8.1** Clinical characteristics of CLL patients with HIV infection

| Study | Study type | Age | Sex | CD4+ cell count (cells/mm$^3$) | On ARV therapy | Treatment offered | CLL vs SLL | Complication |
|---|---|---|---|---|---|---|---|---|
| Ravandi et al. [18] | CR | 65 | M | 1100 | Yes | Chlorambucil, F, Alemtuzumab | CLL | CLL-related renal failure |
| Cole et al. [19] | CS | 76 | M | 396 | Yes | None | CLL | None |
| | | 68 | M | 1374 | Yes | BR | CLL | Autoimmune hemolytic anemia |
| | | 55 | M | 487 | Yes | Chlorambucil | CLL | Hypogammaglobulinemia, recurrent pneumonia |
| | | 55 | F | 497 | Yes | F(6), RC(4) | SLL | Progressive multifocal leukoencephalopathy (PML) |
| Sewell et al. [20] | CR | 50 | M | 1100 | No | None | CLL | None |
| Shimada et al. [21][a] | CR | 61 | M | 252 | Yes | F(1), FCR(2),R-CHOP(8), RCOP(6), BR(4) | CLL | Cytopenias |
| Knowles et al. [22] | CS | 31 | M | AIDS by OI criteria | No | None | | |
| | | 34 | M | <200 | No | None | | Death 2/2 PCP pneumonia |
| | | 45 | F | <200 | No | None | | |

*CR* case report, *CS* case series, *M* male, *F* female, *ARV* antiretroviral, *CLL* chronic lymphocytic leukemia, *SLL* small lymphocytic lymphoma, *F* fludarabine, *C* cyclophosphamide, *B* bendamustine, *R* rituximab, *O* vincristine; (#cycles)

[a]High likelihood of transformed disease

**Table 8.2** Clinical course of patient with splenic marginal zone lymphoma patients with HIV infection

| Study | Study type | Age | Sex | On ARV therapy | Cell picture | B-symptoms | LDH | Treatment offered | Disease activity |
|---|---|---|---|---|---|---|---|---|---|
| Cagliuso et al. [39] | CR | 50 | F | Yes | Anemia, pancytopenia | Fever, night sweats | High 317 U/L | Splenectomy | Stable at 2 years |
| Genet et al. [40] | CS | 40 | F | Yes | No anemia, no thrombocytopenia | NA | NA | None | Stable at 2 years |
| | | 28 | M | Yes | NA | NA | NA | None | Stable at 5 years f/u |
| | | 42 | M | Yes | NA | NA | NA | None | Stable, at 2 years f/u |
| Arcaini et al. [41] | CR | 47 | M | Yes | Anemia, thrombocytosis | Hyperthermia, weight loss | High 818 | Splenectomy | Stable at 18 months f/u |

*CR* case report, *CS* case series, *F* female, *M* male, *NA* data not available, *f/u* follow-up

## 8.3 MALT Lymphoma

MALT is the most frequent subtype of MZL, accounting about 5–7 % of all NHL [29]. The stomach is the most common site of involvement. There is a well-known association between *Helicobacter pylori* infection and gastric MALT lymphoma [30, 31]. Other sites commonly involved are the lungs, salivary glands, skin, ocular adnexa, soft tissues, and thyroid gland, with the most common chromosomal translocation identified as t(11; 18) (q21; q21) in this subtype of MZL [32].

The disease typically affects patients in their 60s and with no gender predominance [33]. Clinical presentation is defined by the site of involvement. Patients with gastric MALT lymphomas typically present with peptic ulcer disease symptoms, including epigastric pain or discomfort, dyspepsia, nausea, and vomiting, with B-symptoms (such as fever, drenching night sweats, and weight loss) and raised LDH, being rarely manifested. Treatment of early disease includes eradication of *Helicobacter pylori* with oral antibiotics and endoscopic follow-up and radiation for advanced disease.

Few cases have been described of MALT lymphoma in the HIV population. Wotherspoon et al. described a case of MALT lymphoma in an HIV patient that demonstrated classic morphologic features, with *H. pylori* presence noted and the clinical course resembling that of immunocompetent patients [34]. In a retrospective study of ten cases of indolent NHL coincident with HIV infection, one patient with MALT lymphoma was identified [12]. Although the individual patient description was not given, the patient with indolent lymphoma had a high CD4+ cell count (median 531/mm3), and the clinical course was comparable with the non-HIV population as well.

## 8.4 Splenic Marginal Zone Lymphoma (SMZL)

SMZL is a rare low-grade B-cell NHL that usually involves the spleen. It comprises of less than 1 % of all NHL [35]. The disease typically affects patients with a median age at diagnosis in the seventh decade of life [36]. Kruppel-like factor 2 or KLF2 mutation is the most frequent genetic change in SMZL (42 %) and uncommon in other lymphomas [37]. There is increased association with hepatitis C virus infection, yet the numbers of cases reported in the HIV population are few [38].

Most patients present with splenomegaly (moderate to massive), anemia, and thrombocytopenia, with lymphocytosis present in about one-third of the cases, thus illustrating some potential overlap in the clinical manifestations of advanced HIV/AIDS itself. Leukopenia can also be present, due to splenic sequestration or bone marrow infiltration. Hepatomegaly is described in some cases, with lymphadenopathy presenting rarely. B-symptoms (such as fever, drenching night sweats, and weight loss) and raised LDH are very rare. The identification of a monocolonal paraproteinemia is not unusual in this disease. Examination of the peripheral smear reveals a typical tumor cell, with a round nucleus, condensed chromatin, and basophilic cytoplasm with characteristic villous projections. In advanced disease, intrasinusoidal and/or nodular infiltration of the bone marrow can be seen which is highly characteristic. Splenic pathology will reveal a micronodular pattern formed by small lymphoma cells. The tumor cells express surface immunoglobulins (IgM, IgD); are positive for CD19, CD20, CD22, Pax5, and BCL2; and are characteristically negative for CD3, CD5, CD10, CD23, cyclin D1, and BCL6.

For symptomatic patients, several therapeutic options are available including splenectomy, single-agent rituximab, and chemotherapies combined with rituximab. In those with hepatitis C, treatment of the viral infection is recommended if feasible.

Splenic marginal zone lymphoma is rare in patients with HIV. Several cases have been described in the literature [39–41]. Interestingly, the patients described were relatively young at the time of diagnosis (28–50 years). The lymphoma was stable up to approximately 2 years of follow-up with splenectomy performed in two cases and no case of chemo-immunotherapy administration.

## 8.5 Nodal Marginal Zone Lymphoma (NMZL)

NMZL comprises 2 % of all NHL [42]. Primarily affecting the lymph nodes, involvement of bone marrow or peripheral blood is rare in NMZL. Most patients are asymptomatic and usually present with enlarged lymph nodes. With nodal biopsy, histology resembles with that of other marginal zone lymphomas described. The tumor cells express IgD. There is a paucity of published reports of NMZL in the HIV-positive population. Of the four cases reported in the literature, there was one case of NMZL in a patient with a CD4 count of 261 cells/mm$^3$, not on HAART, who was treated with chemotherapies, including CHOP and then for relapsed disease, fludarabine, cyclophosphamide, and mitoxantrone (FCM) [43]. The patient had no coinfection with HCV. Two additional cases reported did also not demonstrate coinfection with HCV or reported infection with EBV [44, 45].

## 8.6 Follicular Lymphoma

Follicular lymphoma is the most common subtype of indolent NHL and comprises 20 % of NHL cases [46]. The median age at the time of diagnosis is in the seventh decade of life and the t(14;18) translocation is a genetic hallmark of this disease, resulting in the overexpression of the BCL2 oncogene. The most common presenting complaint is painless peripheral lymphadenopathy, yet some patients present with abdominal discomfort due to the development of bulky intra-abdominal nodal disease. The diagnosis is made by excisional lymph node biopsy, and CT imaging or PET/CT is required for staging the disease activity. A strategy of active surveillance is employed for most patients, until symptoms or complications from the disease arise, warranting treatment. The treatment options may differ on the basis of disease stage. Patients with localized disease (stage I or II) may be treated with radiation therapy. Several options are available for patients with advanced disease including R-CHOP (rituximab, cyclophosphamide, doxorubicin, vincristine, and prednisone), R-CVP (rituximab, cyclophosphamide, vincristine, and prednisone), bendamustine with rituximab, and single-agent rituximab.

Follicular lymphoma in HIV patients is comparatively rare. An evaluation of ten large SEER databases comprising patient data from 1992 to 2009 shows that the proportion of follicular lymphoma was 2.4 % among HIV patients with an NHL diagnosis, out of a cohort of 6,784 patients, versus its occurrence in 17.9 % of 108,859 patients without a diagnosis of HIV [9]. Levine et al. reported two cases of follicular lymphoma in a retrospective study of ten cases of indolent NHL in HIV patients [12]. As anticipated, the CD4 count was significantly higher, and the median survival was also longer compared to intermediate- to high-grade lymphomas. However, bone marrow involvement was more common. Ziegler et al. described three cases of small cleaved cell follicular lymphoma among 90 homosexual men [14]. Although the individual patient detail was not mentioned in the study, it is surmised that low histologic grade is predictive of favorable outcome.

## 8.7 Waldenstrom's Macroglobulinemia/ Lymphoplasmacytic Lymphoma (WM/LPL)

WM/LPL is characterized by the finding of LPL in the bone marrow and its secreted IgM paraprotein in the peripheral blood, with 64 years being the median age at diagnosis [47]. Common symptoms include a normocytic anemia and resultant fatigue. WM/LPL is characterized by the presence of a commonly occurring (90 %) MYD88 mutation [48]. An important consideration in this disease is the IgM concentration and hyperviscosity that can occur, due to high blood content of the large protein, leading to sequelae of neurologic and cardiovascular compromise in some cases. Hyperviscosity is managed with plasma exchange, for the emergent filtration of IgM from the blood. Symptomatic or progressive disease may be managed with a variety of chemo-immunotherapies or with the FDA-approved Bruton's tyrosine kinase inhibitor ibrutinib.

An evaluation of patients from the HIV/AIDS Cancer Match (HACM) Study, spanning patient data from 1991 to 2004, and over 200,000 HIV+ patients, discovered an increased risk of WM/LPL in PLWH with a standard incidence ratio of observed cases in the HIV population versus expected cases in the general population of 3.6 [27]. Surprisingly, there was no increased incidence of WM/LPL in the AIDS subpopulation of patients in this study. Another evaluation of US Veterans identified an increased relative risk of 12.05 (CI 2.83–51.46) in patients with HIV, based on evaluation of 361 WM patients, from 1969 to 1996 [49]. The mean exposure time from HIV infection to the development of WM was found to be 1.6 years (1.1–2.7 years). IgM levels and history of antiretroviral therapy (ART) were not provided for analysis within these large cohort studies. Despite reports that the incidence of WM/LPL is increased in PLWH, there are remarkably few case reports in the literature. A single French patient with HIV, diagnosed with LPL in the bone marrow, and found to have a high IgM of 61 g/L, and a synchronously diagnosed

EBV-positive plasmablastic lymphoma, has been described. The patient had a complication from hyperviscosity that led to cardiac-ischemia-related death prior to the initiation of chemotherapy [50]. This patient had coinfection with HCV, a CD4 count of 550, and undetectable HIV and HCV viral loads. Given the higher incidence of this indolent lymphoma reported in the two large patient cohorts referenced above, a potential causal relationship between HIV infection and the appearance of WM/LPL is suggested.

**Conclusions**

In general, HIV patients with indolent lymphoma demonstrate a benign course, similar to that of the HIV-negative population. The mean CD4+ cell counts are relatively higher as compared to those patients who develop intermediate- to high-grade lymphomas, and therefore, their genesis may not be as dependent on immune deregulation, with a notable exception. WM/LPL is reportedly more prevalent in the HIV population as compared with the non-HIV population. Given the increased risk of WM/LPL in PLWH, timely diagnosis and screening may be possible with heightened awareness of this entity.

In the majority of cases identified and outlined herein, mortality was not impacted by the presence of the indolent lymphoma. In cases requiring therapy, special attention to the prevention of opportunistic infection as a compound result of both therapy and the underlying HIV is appropriate, with the use of prophylactic antibiotics. Extremely immunosuppressive agents, such as fludarabine, should be avoided in favor of newer, less immunosuppressive agents given their availability. Since evidence regarding the safety and efficacy of novel therapies in the management of indolent NHL is lacking in the HIV population, inclusion of HIV patients in these ongoing and future studies is highly encouraged, with considered attention to CD4 counts and viral load for inclusion consideration.

## References


1. Patel P, et al. Incidence of types of cancer among HIV-infected persons compared with the general population in the United States, 1992–2003. Ann Intern Med. 2008;148:728–36.
2. Biggar RJ, Curtis RE, Cote TR, Rabkin CS, Melbye M. Risk of other cancers following Kaposi's sarcoma: relation to acquired immunodeficiency syndrome. Am J Epidemiol. 1994;139:362–8.
3. Beral V, Peterman T, Berkelman R, Jaffe H. AIDS-associated non-Hodgkin lymphoma. Lancet (London, England). 1991;337:805–9.
4. Biggar RJ, Rabkin CS. The epidemiology of AIDS – related neoplasms. Hematol Oncol Clin North Am. 1996;10:997–1010.
5. Buchbinder SP, et al. Combination antiretroviral therapy and incidence of AIDS-related malignancies. J Acquir Immune Defic Syndr. 1999;21 Suppl 1:S23–6.
6. Rabkin CS, Testa MA, Huang J, Von Roenn JH. Kaposi's sarcoma and non-Hodgkin's lymphoma incidence trends in AIDS Clinical Trial Group study participants. J Acquir Immune Defic Syndr. 1999;21 Suppl 1:S31–3.
7. Jacobson LP, et al. Impact of potent antiretroviral therapy on the incidence of Kaposi's sarcoma and non-Hodgkin's lymphomas among HIV-1-infected individuals. Multicenter AIDS Cohort Study. J Acquir Immune Defic Syndr. 1999;21 Suppl 1:S34–41.

8. De Re V, et al. p53 protein over-expression and p53 gene abnormalities in HIV-1-related non-Hodgkin's lymphomas. Int J Cancer J Int Cancer. 1994;56:662–7.
9. Shiels MS, et al. The epidemic of non-Hodgkin lymphoma in the United States: disentangling the effect of HIV, 1992–2009. Cancer Epidemiol Biomark Prev: Publ Am Assoc Cancer Res Am Soc Prev Oncol. 2013;22:1069–78.
10. Cote TR, et al. Non-Hodgkin's lymphoma among people with AIDS: incidence, presentation and public health burden. AIDS/Cancer Study Group. Int J Cancer J Int Cancer. 1997;73:645–50.
11. Biggar RJ, Rosenberg PS, Cote T. Kaposi's sarcoma and non-Hodgkin's lymphoma following the diagnosis of AIDS. Multistate AIDS/Cancer Match Study Group. Int J Cancer J Int Cancer. 1996;68:754–8.
12. Levine AM, Sadeghi S, Espina B, Tulpule A, Nathwani B. Characteristics of indolent non-Hodgkin lymphoma in patients with type 1 human immunodeficiency virus infection. Cancer. 2002;94:1500–6.
13. Lowenthal DA, et al. AIDS-related lymphoid neoplasia. The Memorial Hospital experience. Cancer. 1988;61:2325–37.
14. Ziegler JL, et al. Non-Hodgkin's lymphoma in 90 homosexual men. Relation to generalized lymphadenopathy and the acquired immunodeficiency syndrome. N Engl J Med. 1984;311:565–70.
15. Maurer C, Hallek M. Chronic lymphocytic leukemia. Dtsch Med Wochenschr (1946). 2013;138:2153–66.
16. Ghia P, Caligaris-Cappio F. The origin of B-cell chronic lymphocytic leukemia. Semin Oncol. 2006;33:150–6.
17. Hallek M, et al. Guidelines for the diagnosis and treatment of chronic lymphocytic leukemia: a report from the International Workshop on Chronic Lymphocytic Leukemia updating the National Cancer Institute-Working Group 1996 guidelines. Blood. 2008;111:5446–56.
18. Ravandi F, Verma A, Ridgeway J, Pursell K. Chronic lymphocytic leukemia (B-CLL) occurring with human immunodeficiency virus (HIV) infection: implications. Leuk Res. 2003;27:853–7.
19. Cole J, Pantanowitz L, Aboulafia D. Human immunodeficiency virus and chronic lymphocytic leukemia. Leuk Lymphoma. 2009;50:1885–8.
20. Sewell HF, Walker F, Bennett B, Dawson AA. Chronic lymphocytic leukaemia contemporaneous with HIV infection. Br Med J (Clin Res Ed). 1987;294:938–9.
21. Shimada N, et al. Treatment of chronic lymphocytic leukemia with bendamustine in an HIV-infected patient on antiretroviral therapy: a case report and review of the literature. Clin Case Rep. 2015;3:453–60.
22. Knowles DM, et al. Lymphoid neoplasia associated with the acquired immunodeficiency syndrome (AIDS). The New York University Medical Center experience with 105 patients (1981–1986). Ann Intern Med. 1988;108:744–53.
23. Kaplan MH, et al. Neoplastic complications of HTLV-III infection. Lymphomas and solid tumors. Am J Med. 1987;82:389–96.
24. Samji H, et al. Closing the gap: increases in life expectancy among treated HIV-positive individuals in the United States and Canada. PLoS One. 2013;8:e81355.
25. Callea V, et al. Incidence of second neoplasia in patients with B-cell chronic lymphocytic leukemia treated with chlorambucil maintenance chemotherapy. Leuk Lymphoma. 2006;47:2314–20.
26. Tsimberidou AM, Wen S, McLauaghlin P, et al. Other malignancies in chronic lymphocytic-leukemia/small lymphocytic lymphoma. J Clin Oncol. 2008;27:1–9.
27. Gibson TM, Morton LM, Shiels MS, Clarke CA, Engels EA. Risk of non-Hodgkin lymphoma subtypes in HIV-infected people during the HAART era: a population-based study. AIDS (London, England). 2014;28:2313–8.
28. Rossi D, et al. The coding genome of splenic marginal zone lymphoma: activation of NOTCH2 and other pathways regulating marginal zone development. J Exp Med. 2012;209:1537–51.

29. Armitage JO, Weisenburger DD. New approach to classifying non-Hodgkin's lymphomas: clinical features of the major histologic subtypes. Non-Hodgkin's Lymphoma Classification Project. J Clin Oncol: Off J Am Soc Clin Oncol. 1998;16:2780–95.
30. Radaszkiewicz T, Dragosics B, Bauer P. Gastrointestinal malignant lymphomas of the mucosa-associated lymphoid tissue: factors relevant to prognosis. Gastroenterology. 1992;102:1628–38.
31. Parsonnet J, et al. Helicobacter pylori infection and gastric lymphoma. N Engl J Med. 1994;330:1267–71.
32. Auer IA, et al. t(11;18)(q21;q21) is the most common translocation in MALT lymphomas. Ann Oncol: Off J Eur Soc Med Oncol ESMO. 1997;8:979–85.
33. Zucca E, Bertoni F, Roggero E, Cavalli F. The gastric marginal zone B-cell lymphoma of MALT type. Blood. 2000;96:410–9.
34. Wotherspoon AC, et al. Low grade gastric B-cell lymphoma of mucosa associated lymphoid tissue in immunocompromised patients. Histopathology. 1996;28:129–34.
35. Liu L, et al. Splenic marginal zone lymphoma: a population-based study on the 2001–2008 incidence and survival in the United States. Leuk Lymphoma. 2013;54:1380–6.
36. Berger F, et al. Non-MALT marginal zone B-cell lymphomas: a description of clinical presentation and outcome in 124 patients. Blood. 2000;95:1950–6.
37. Clipson A, et al. KLF2 mutation is the most frequent somatic change in splenic marginal zone lymphoma and identifies a subset with distinct genotype. Leukemia. 2015;29:1177–85.
38. Zuckerman E, et al. Hepatitis C virus infection in patients with B-cell non-Hodgkin lymphoma. Ann Intern Med. 1997;127:423–8.
39. Cagliuso M, et al. Splenic marginal zone lymphoma in a HIV-1 infected patient: evidence favouring a pathogenetic role of HIV-1 itself in the lymphomagenesis. Infection. 2013;41:255–8.
40. Genet P, et al. Splenic marginal zone lymphoma with villous lymphocytes in patients with human immunodeficiency virus. Leuk Lymphoma. 2013;54:181–3.
41. Arcaini L, et al. Splenic marginal zone B-cell lymphoma in a HIV-positive patient: a case report. Ann Hematol. 2009;88:379–81.
42. Conconi A, et al. Nodal marginal zone B-cell lymphomas may arise from different subsets of marginal zone B lymphocytes. Blood. 2001;98:781–6.
43. Abella E, et al. Nodal marginal zone lymphoma in AIDS patients: a casual association? AIDS (London, England). 2002;16:2232–4.
44. Charton-Bain MC, Le Tourneau A, Weiss L, Bruneval P, Diebold J. Rare non-Hodgkin's lymphoma in the course of infection with human immunodeficiency virus. Two cases with bone marrow invasion. Ann Pathol. 1997;17:38–40.
45. Sheibani K, et al. Monocytoid B-cell lymphoma in a patient with human immunodeficiency virus infection. Demonstration of human immunodeficiency virus sequences in paraffin-embedded lymph node sections by polymerase chain reaction amplification. Arch Pathol Lab Med. 1990;114:1264–7.
46. A clinical evaluation of the International Lymphoma Study Group classification of non-Hodgkin's lymphoma. The Non-Hodgkin's Lymphoma Classification Project. Blood. 1997;89:3909–18.
47. Gertz MA, Fonseca R, Rajkumar SV. Waldenstrom's macroglobulinemia. Oncologist. 2000;5:63–7.
48. Treon SP, et al. MYD88 L265P somatic mutation in Waldenström's macroglobulinemia. N Eng J Med. 2012;367:826–33.
49. Koshiol J, Gridley G, Engels EA, McMaster ML, Landgren O. Chronic immune stimulation and subsequent Waldenstrom macroglobulinemia. Arch Intern Med. 2008;168:1903–9.
50. Terrier B, et al. Characteristics of B-cell lymphomas in HIV/HCV-coinfected patients during the combined antiretroviral therapy era: an ANRS CO16 LYMPHOVIR cohort study. J Acquir Immune Defic Syndr (1999). 2013;63:249–53.

# HIV-Associated Hodgkin Lymphoma

# 9

Marcus Hentrich, Michele Spina, and Silvia Montoto

## Contents




M. Hentrich, MD (✉)
Department of Hematology and Oncology, Red Cross Hospital, University of Munich, Munich, Germany
e-mail: marcus.hentrich@swmbrk.de

M. Spina
Division of Medical Oncology A, National Cancer Institute, Aviano, Italy
e-mail: mspina@cro.it

S. Montoto, MD
Centre for Haemato-Oncology, St Bartholomew's Hospital, Barts Cancer Institute, Queen Mary University of London, London, UK
e-mail: s.montoto@qmul.ac.uk







M. Hentrich, S.K. Barta (eds.), *HIV-associated Hematological Malignancies*,
DOI 10.1007/978-3-319-26857-6_9

## 9.1 Introduction

Hodgkin lymphoma (HL) is one of the most common non-AIDS-defining malignancies in patients infected with HIV. Unfavorable features such as higher frequency of advanced-stage disease and extranodal involvement are frequently encountered. Prior to the advent of combined antiretroviral therapy (cART), the prognosis of patients with HIV-HL was poor. However, with standard curative-intent therapy and modern cART, the outcome is similar to that reported in the general population.

## 9.2 Epidemiology

Compared with the general population, the incidence of HIV-HL is increased by approximately 10–15-fold with about 45–55 new cases per 100,00 person-years among HIV-infected persons [1–10]. Notably, the incidence has remained stable or may have even further increased in the cART era. An overview of recent studies providing data on standardized incidence ratios is given in Table 9.1.

With a median age of 40–45 years, patients are about 10 years older than their HIV-negative counterparts. In high-prevalence areas such as South Africa, 61 % of HL cases were reported to be attributed to HIV between 2007 and 2009 [11], while incidence rates in the USA are highest among African Americans. A recent study on the prevalence of HIV infection among US Hodgkin lymphoma cases showed that between 2000 and 2010, 17 % of HL cases among African Americans were HIV related [12].

**Table 9.1** Studies providing standardized incidence ratios (SIR) for HL in persons with HIV/AIDS

| Country | Period | *N* | SIR | Reference |
|---|---|---|---|---|
| Switzerland | 1985–2003 | 7304 | 17.3 | Clifford [1] |
| | | | 36.2 (prior cART) | |
| USA | 1996–2002 | 317,428 (AIDS only) | 9.4 | Biggar [2] |
| | | | 13.2 (1996–2002) | |
| France/Italy | 1985–2005 | 8074 | 10.8 | Serraino [3] |
| USA | 1991–2002 | 57,350 | 5.6 | Engels [4] |
| USA | 1992–2003 | 54,730 | 14.7 | Patel [5] |
| | | | 17.9 (2000–2003) | |
| UK | 1983–2007 | 11,112 | 13.9 | Powles [6] |
| | | | 32.4 (2002–2007) | |
| USA | 1984–2007 | 6949 | 7.3 | Seaberg [7] |
| Switzerland | 1985–2006 | 9429 | 9.2 (1985–1996) | Franceschi [8] |
| | | | 21 (1997–2001) | |
| | | | 28.1 (2002–2006) | |
| USA | 1996–2008 | 20,775 | 18.7 | Silverberg [9] |
| Italy | 1999–2009 | 5090 | 12.3 | Calabresi [10] |

### 9.2.1 CD4 T-Cell Counts and Risk of HIV-HL

Median CD4 cell counts at HL diagnosis are roughly between 150 and 260 cells/μl [2, 13–18]. However, data on the relationship of CD4 cell counts and the risk of HIV-HL are somewhat inconsistent. Although the risk of HIV-HL is generally increased at CD4+ T-cell counts below 500 cells/μl, it was shown to be highest in CD4 counts between 50 and 100 cells/μl [19–21]. By contrast, the US HIV/AIDS Cancer Match Study found that the incidence of HL decreased in persons with AIDS and falling CD4 cell counts [2]. This finding is in line with data from the German HIV lymphoma cohort study showing HL to be as common as non-Hodgkin lymphoma in patients with sustained viral suppression and limited immune deficiency defined as HIV RNA <50 copies/ml for more than 12 months and CD4 cell counts of >200/μl [22]. However, in an analysis of 16 European cohorts, the risk of HL declined as the most recent (time updated) CD4 count increased with an adjusted hazard ratio of 0.27 for patients with more than 350 compared to less than 50 cells/μl [20].

The first 6 months after initiating cART are the period with the highest risk of HIV-HL diagnosis [17, 21, 23], but there is also some evidence of a higher risk within 12 months after cART initiation [24]. The increased risk within 6 months after initiating cART may, at least in part, be explained by the occurrence of an immune reconstitution inflammatory syndrome (IRIS) [24]. Unmasking lymphoma IRIS, defined as lymphoma within 6 months after ART accompanied by a $\geq 0.5\ \log_{10}$ copies/ml HIV RNA reduction, was recently observed in 15 % of HL cases documented in the Centers for AIDS Research Network of Integrated Clinical Systems (CNICS) cohort from 1996 until 2011 [25]. Data from the US Veterans Affairs cohort also suggests HIV-HL incidence may be highest in the first year of cART exposure with a steady decline over 10 years of cART use [26]. Notably, HIV-1 viral replication is not associated with the risk of HL [20].

Case control studies of HIV patients showed a marked decline of CD4 cells by approximately 100 cells/μl over 12 months prior to HL diagnosis [17, 20, 27]. However, as a major decline in CD4+ T-cell count is not unique to HL, the predictive value of declining CD4+ T cells as a marker for an impending HL neither appears sensitive nor specific enough to be suitable as a diagnostic marker for HL [27, 28].

## 9.3 Pathology

There are some remarkable differences in the pathology between HIV-HL and HL in the general population. First, the mixed cellularity subtype is most commonly observed in HIV-HL [2, 29–31], a finding which is in contrast to HL in HIV-negative patients where the nodular sclerosis subtype predominates (Figs. 9.1 and 9.2). Although a higher proportion of classical HL not otherwise specified (NOS) may have been diagnosed in recent years [12, 17], the MC predominance has not changed over the last decades [2, 14, 15].

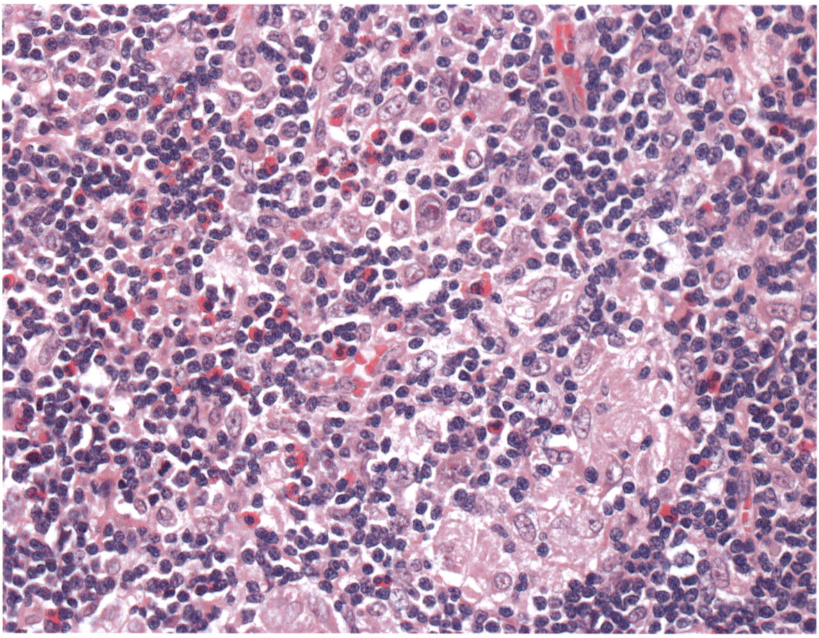

**Fig. 9.1** This photomicrograph shows a case of HIV-related Hodgkin lymphoma. In between a mixed "reactive" cell infiltrate, Hodgkin and Reed-Sternberg (H/RS) cells are shown with prominent central nucleoli. Hematoxylin and eosin stain. Original magnification, ×400

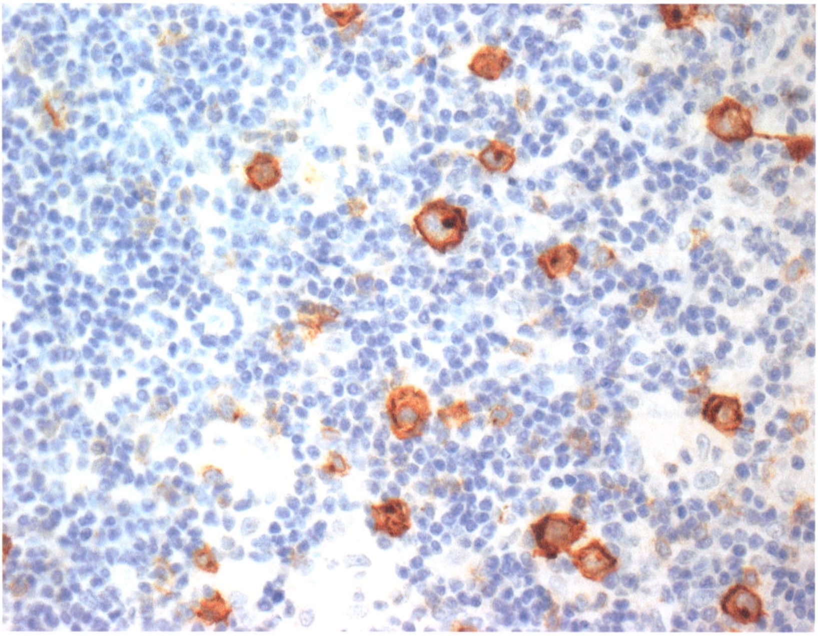

**Fig. 9.2** Immunohistochemical staining of CD30 in H/RS cells of HIV-HL. Note the membranous and Golgi staining. Original magnification, ×400

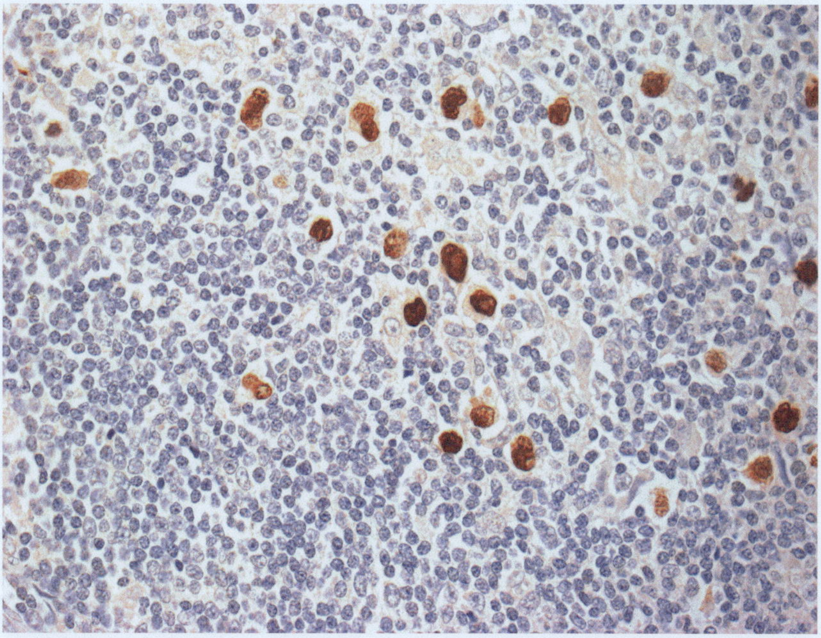

**Fig. 9.3** In situ hybridization for EBV-encoded RNA (EBER) in H/RS cells of HIV-HL. The EBER signal is located to the nucleus. Original magnification, ×400 (Images kindly provided by Marcus Kremer, Institute of Pathology, Staedtisches Klinikum Muenchen, Germany)

Second, HIV-HL has been shown to be associated with EBV in 80–100 % of cases (Fig. 9.3). This contrasts to HIV-negative HL in which EBV genome is observed in 20–50 % only according to histological subtype and age at diagnosis [32, 33]. EBV-infected Hodgkin Reed-Sternberg cells (HRS) mainly express EBV-encoded genes such as Epstein-Barr nuclear antigen (EBNA1) and latent membrane proteins (LMP1, LMP2A, LMP2B). LMP1 and LMP2 are important for NF-KB and B-cell receptor signaling as well as for B-cell proliferation [34]. Further, EBV infection induces an increase in T-regulatory cells and associated immunosuppressive cytokines (IL10) that may inhibit an immune response against EBV+ cells [35].

Third, decreased nodal CD4+ T cells and lack of CD4+ rosetting around HRS have been described in HIV-HL as compared to HL in the HIV-negative setting [36, 37]. While CD8+ T cells appear to be preserved, cytotoxic granzyme B expression is decreased, suggesting a defective antitumoral response in HIV-HL [38].

## 9.4 Management

### 9.4.1 Clinical Presentation and Diagnosis

Approximately 65–80 % of patients present with advanced stages or with B symptoms [14, 15, 30]. Compared to HL in the general population, the bone marrow is far more frequently involved and may be the only site of disease.

There is only limited evidence on the role of PET scans in the diagnosis of HIV lymphoma. Findings should be interpreted with caution as baseline $^{18}$FDG-PET can be false positive in particular in ART-naïve viremic patients or those with low CD4 counts [39–43]. Notably, false-negative results were also reported [44].

Apart from obtaining an HIV-related history, CD4 T-cell counts and HIV RNA should be evaluated at HL diagnosis as should be hepatitis B and hepatitis C virus serology.

### 9.4.2 Prognostic Factors

Before the advent of cART results of chemotherapy and long-term outcomes of patients with HIV-HL were poor [45–47]. This was mainly due to a poor tolerance of standard chemotherapy with high rates of opportunistic infections and toxic deaths. However, a number of cohort studies have shown that complete remission (CR) and overall survival rates were significantly higher in patients on cART as compared to those treated in the pre-cART era [48–52]. Of note, response to cART [50, 51], low CD4 counts [51, 52], and CR [50–52] were independently associated with overall survival (OS).

Data on the predictive power of the International Prognostic Score (IPS) in HIV-HL are inconsistent [13, 14, 18, 53], and treatment decisions should not be based on the IPS outside clinical trials. Nevertheless, a large retrospective analysis of 596 HIV-HL patients from 6 European countries that included patients treated in the pre- and post-cART era found 2 parameters independently associated with OS: CD4 counts <200 cells/μl [HR 1.63] and IPS >2 [HR 2.33]. Based on these factors, a new European score was developed that may be considered for future prospective studies [54].

While in the German study, a CD4 cell count <200/μl did not predict the outcome [14], a multi-institutional retrospective study of 229 advanced HIV-HL patients who had received ABVD plus cART showed CD4 cell counts <200/μl to be an independent adverse prognostic factor for PFS and OS [18]. The larger sample size of the latter study may have allowed a more meaningful analysis of CD4 counts as prognostic factor.

### 9.4.3 Primary Chemotherapy

In a retrospective study on patients with stage III/IV HIV-HL, 6–8 cycles of AVBD along with concurrent cART resulted in a CR rate of 87 % and a 5-year OS rate of 76 % [31]. Another large retrospective study from the UK compared the outcome of 93 HIV-positive and 131 HIV-negative HL patients treated with 6 cycles of ABVD [15]. Importantly, HIV status did not adversely affect the outcome with no significant differences in the 5-year event-free survival (66 % versus 59 %) and OS (81 % versus 88 %) between HIV-positive and HIV-negative patients (Fig. 9.4). Data on ABVD in HIV-HL are summarized in Table 9.2.

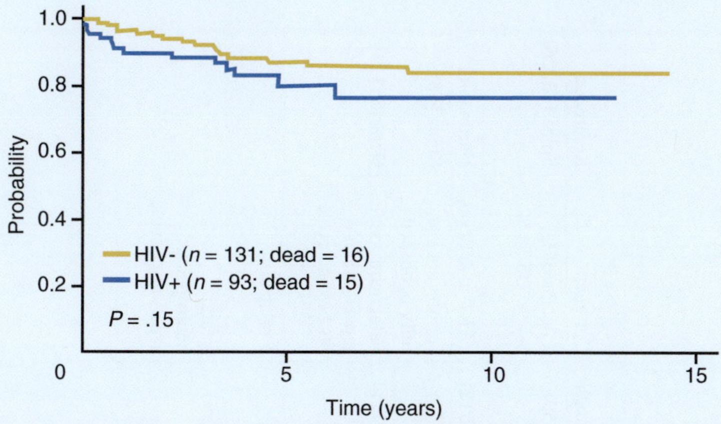


**Fig. 9.4** Overall survival of HIV-HL patients treated with ABVD according to HIV status (Adapted from Montoto et al. [15]. Reprint permission obtained from American Society of Clinical Oncology)

**Table 9.2** Results from retrospective studies on ABVD in HIV-HL in the cART era

| *N* | Recruitment period | Stage III/IV | No cycles | CR rate | OS | Toxic deaths | Comment | Reference |
|---|---|---|---|---|---|---|---|---|
| 62 | 1996–2005 | 100 % | 6: 68 %<br>8: 15 %<br><6: 17 % | 87 % | 76 % (5-years) | 5 % (3/62) | All pts with concurrent cART; median CD4 counts 129/μl | Xicoy [31] |
| 93 | 1997–2010 | 80 % | 6 | 74 % | 81 % (5-years) | 1 % (1/93) | Concurrent cART in 92/93 pts; median CD4 counts 185/μl; no impact of HIV status on OS | Montoto [15] |

*CR* complete remission, *OS* overall survival

While the use of the Stanford V regimen and concomitant cART resulted in a 3-year OS rate of 51 % [13], high cure rates have recently been reported in a large prospective study on a stage-adapted treatment of HIV-HL [14]. Patients with early favorable HL received 2–4 cycles of ABVD followed by involved-field radiation; patients with early unfavorable disease were treated with 4 cycles of BEACOPP baseline or 4 cycles of ABVD; and patients with advanced HIV-HL received 6–8 cycles of BEACOPP baseline. In patients with advanced HIV infection, BEACOPP was replaced by ABVD. Ninety-four percent received concurrent cART while on protocol therapy. The CR rate for patients with early favorable, early unfavorable, and advanced-stage HL was 96 %, 100 %, and 86 %, respectively (Table 9.3). The

**Table 9.3** Results from prospective studies on HIV-HL in the cART era

| Regimen | *N* | Recruitment period | Stage III/IV | No cycles (median) | CR rate | OS | Toxic deaths | Comment | Reference |
|---|---|---|---|---|---|---|---|---|---|
| Stanford V | 59 | 1997–2001 | 71 % | Planned treatment in 69 %[a] | 81 % | 51 % (3 years) | 2 % (1/59) | 2 deaths of OI 5-year OS 54 % | Spina [13, 56] |
| BEACOPP | 12 | 1993–2002 | 92 % | 6 | 100 % | 75 % (3 years) | 17 % (2/12) | cART in 4/12 pts | Hartmann [57] |
| VEBEP | 73 | 2001–2008 | 70 % | NR | 67 % | 66 % (3 years) | 6 % (4/73) | Results not yet fully published | Spina [58] |
| BEACOPP or ABVD | 71 | 2004–2010 | 100 % | 2 | 86 % | 87 % (2 years) | 6 % (4/71) | Fatal neutropenic sepsis in 3 of 4 pts beyond cycle 7 | Hentrich [14] |
| ABVD or BEACOPP | 14 | 2004–2010 | Early unfavorable | 4 | 100 % | 100 % (2 years) | 0 | 1 relapse | |
| ABVD | 23 | 2004–2010 | Early favorable | 2 | 96 % | 96 % (2 years) | 4 % (1/23) | 1 fatal neutropenic sepsis after cycle 1 | |

*VEBEP* vinblastine, epirubicin, bleomycin, etoposide, prednisone, *NR* not reported
[a]12-week chemotherapy without dose reduction or delay in administration

2-year OS of the entire study population was 90.7 % with no significant difference between early favorable (95.7 %), early unfavorable (100 %), and advanced HL (86.8 %) (Fig. 9.5). Treatment-related mortality in patients with advanced disease was 7 %. However, as three of four toxic deaths occurred after the seventh cycle of BEACOPP, chemotherapy should be limited to 6 cycles as has recently been demonstrated in HIV-negative HL patients receiving the more intensified BEACOPP-escalated regimen [55]. An overview of prospective clinical studies in HIV-HL in the cART era is given in Table 9.3.

Taken together, a stage adapted treatment approach is feasible and effective. Two cycles of ABVD followed by involved-field (IF) radiation therapy (RT) can be regarded as standard treatment for early favorable HL. As the use of 20-Gy and 30-Gy doses of RT proved equally effective in HIV-negative early-stage HL, the lower dose of 20-Gy RT may also be given in early-stage HIV-HL [59]. While the use of 4 cycles of ABVD followed by 30 Gy IF-RT may be considered standard of care for patients with early-stage unfavorable HL, 6 cycles of ABVD or BEACOPP baseline may be applied to patients with advanced-stage HIV-HL [14, 15, 60]. Nevertheless, ABVD is most commonly used and regarded as the standard of care for advanced HIV-HL in many parts of the world [61–63].

There is some evidence suggesting that increased viremia during the 6 months after lymphoma diagnosis is associated with an increased risk of death between 6 months and 5 years after diagnosis [64]. As chemotherapy and concurrent cART have been shown to be feasible and effective during chemotherapy for HIV-HL, cART should either be continued or initiated according to current guidelines for the use of ART [14–16, 65]. However, the potential of interactions between cytotoxics and antiretrovirals must be considered. When possible, strong enzyme inhibitors such as ritonavir-boosted protease inhibitors should be avoided because of the reported increased risk of myelotoxicity [66]. More detailed information on interactions between cytotoxics and antiretrovirals is presented in Chap. 17.

### 9.4.4 Relapsed and Resistant Disease

Patients with relapsed or refractory HIV-HL should be considered early for high-dose chemotherapy (HDCT) and autologous stem cell transplantation (ASCT). Peripheral blood stem cells can be effectively mobilized, and autologous stem cell transplantation (ASCT) has been shown to be a useful treatment in HIV-infected lymphoma patients with chemosensitive relapse [67–70]. Further information on HDCT and ASCT in HIV lymphoma is given in Chap. 12.

### 9.4.5 Future Directions

In HIV-negative HL response-adapted therapy based on early interim, $^{18}$FDG-PET is currently being investigated in many prospective trials. Cycle 1 or 2 negative PET scans may be useful in identifying those for whom more limited therapy can be

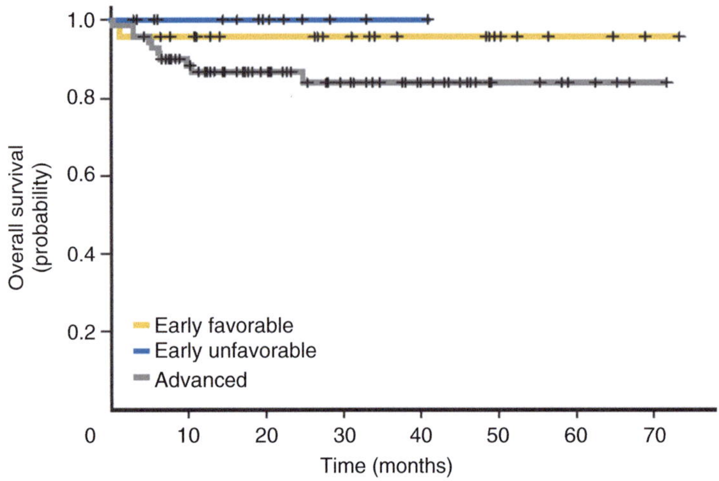


**Fig. 9.5** Overall survival of HIV-HL patients according to Hodgkin stage (Adapted from Hentrich et al. [14]. Reprint permission obtained from American Society of Clinical Oncology)

applied [71, 72]. There is only limited data on interim PET scans in HIV-HL. The predictive value of positive interim scans may be hampered by false-positive results in patients with HIV. However, recent data from a retrospective cohort study indicate a high negative predictive value of a PET scan performed after 2–3 cycles of ABVD (PET-2 or PET-3) [73]. The role of interim PET in HIV-HL should be further investigated in well-designed clinical studies.

Novel agents may change the landscape of treatment of non-HIV-HL in the future. Brentuximab vedotin, a CD30-directed immunoconjugate of the antimitotic agent monomethyl auristatin E, has been shown to be effective in relapsed and resistant HL and is now being incorporated into upfront treatment [74, 75]. Recent case studies indicate that brentuximab vedotin may also be useful in HIV-positive patients with relapsed HL [76]. A combination of brentuximab vedotin, doxorubicin, vinblastine, and dacarbazine is currently being investigated in a study by the AIDS Malignancy Consortium (NCT 01771107). Finally, immunomodulatory approaches such as checkpoint inhibition with anti-programmed death 1 (PD1) agents are currently studied in non-HIV-HL and may also be investigated in HIV-HL in future studies.

## References

1. Clifford GM, Polesel J, Rickenbach M, et al. Cancer risk in the Swiss HIV cohort study: associations with immunodeficiency, smoking, and highly active antiretroviral therapy. J Natl Cancer Inst. 2005;97:425–32.
2. Biggar RJ, Jaffe ES, Goedert JJ, et al. Hodgkin lymphoma and immunodeficiency in persons with HIV/AIDS. Blood. 2006;108:3786–91.
3. Serraino D, Piselli P, Busnach G, et al. Risk of cancer following immunosuppression in organ transplant recipients and in HIV-positive individuals in southern Europe. Eur J Cancer. 2007;43:2117–23.

4. Engels EA, Biggar RJ, Hall HI, et al. Cancer risk in people infected with human immunodeficiency virus in the United States. Int J Cancer. 2008;123:187–94.
5. Patel P, Hanson DL, Sullivan PS, et al. Incidence of types of cancer among HIV-infected persons compared with the general population in the United States, 1992–2003. Ann Intern Med. 2008;148:728–36.
6. Powles T, Robinson D, Stebbing J, et al. Highly active antiretroviral therapy and the incidence of non-AIDS-defining cancers in people with HIV infection. J Clin Oncol. 2009;27(6):884–90.
7. Seaberg EC, Wiley D, Martínez-Maza O, et al. Cancer incidence in the Multicenter AIDS Cohort Study before and during the HAART era: 1984–2007. Cancer. 2010;116:5507–16.
8. Franceschi S, Lise M, Clifford GM, et al. Changing patterns of cancer incidence in the early- and late-HAART periods: the Swiss HIV Cohort Study. Br J Cancer. 2010;103:416–22.
9. Silverberg MJ, Chao C, Leyden WA, et al. HIV infection, immunodeficiency, viral replication, and the risk of cancer. Cancer Epidemiol Biomarkers Prev. 2011;20:2551–9.
10. Calabresi A, Ferraresi A, Festa A, et al. Incidence of AIDS-defining cancers and virus-related and non-virus-related non-AIDS-defining cancers among HIV-infected patients compared with the general population in a large health district of northern Italy, 1999–2009. HIV Med. 2013;14:481–90.
11. Wiggill TM, Mantina H, Willem P, et al. Changing pattern of lymphoma subgroups at a tertiary academic complex in a high-prevalence HIV setting: a South African perspective. J Acquir Immune Defic Syndr. 2011;56:460–6.
12. Shiels MS, Koritzinsky EH, Clarke CA, et al. Prevalence of HIV infection among U.S. Hodgkin lymphoma cases. Cancer Epidemiol Biomarkers Prev. 2014;23:274–81.
13. Spina M, Gabarre J, Rossi G, et al. Stanford V regimen and concomitant HAART in 59 patients with Hodgkin disease and HIV infection. Blood. 2002;100:1984–8.
14. Hentrich M, Berger M, Wyen C, et al. Stage-adapted treatment of HIV-associated Hodgkin lymphoma: results of a prospective multicenter study. J Clin Oncol. 2012;30(33):4117–23.
15. Montoto S, Shaw K, Okosun J, et al. HIV status does not influence outcome in patients with classical Hodgkin lymphoma treated with chemotherapy using doxorubicin, bleomycin, vinblastine, and dacarbazine in the highly active antiretroviral therapy era. J Clin Oncol. 2012;30:4111–6.
16. Gopal S, Patel MR, Yanik EL, et al. Temporal trends in presentation and survival for HIV-associated lymphoma in the antiretroviral therapy era. J Natl Cancer Inst. 2013;105 (16):1221–9.
17. Gotti D, Danesi M, Calabresi A, et al. Clinical characteristics, incidence, and risk factors of HIV-related Hodgkin lymphoma in the era of combination antiretroviral therapy. AIDS Patient Care STDS. 2013;27(5):259–65.
18. Castillo JJ, Bower M, Brühlmann J, et al. Prognostic factors for advanced-stage Human Immunodeficiency Virus-associated classical Hodgkin Lymphoma treated with doxorubicin, bleomycin, vinblastine, and dacarbazine plus combined antiretroviral therapy. Cancer. 2015;121:423–31.
19. Guiguet M, Boue F, Cadranel J, et al. Effect of immunodeficiency, HIV viral load, and antiretroviral therapy on the risk of individual malignancies (FHDH-ANRS CO4): a prospective cohort study. Lancet Oncol. 2009;10(12):1152–9.
20. Bohlius J, Schmidlin K, Boué F, et al. Therapy: incidence and evolution of CD4 + T-cell lymphocytes HIV-1-related Hodgkin lymphoma in the era of combination antiretroviral. Blood. 2011;117(23):6100–8.
21. Lanoy E, Rosenberg PS, Fily F, et al. HIV-associated Hodgkin lymphoma during the first months on combination antiretroviral therapy. Blood. 2011;118:44–9.
22. Hoffmann C, Hentrich M, Gillor D, et al. Hodgkin lymphoma is as common as non-Hodgkin lymphoma in HIV-positive patients with sustained viral suppression and limited immune deficiency: a prospective cohort study. HIV Med. 2015;16:261–4.
23. Yanik EL, Napravnik S, Cole SR, et al. Incidence and timing of cancer in HIV-infected individuals following initiation of combination antiretroviral therapy. Clin Infect Dis. 2013;57(5):756–64.

24. Kowalkowski MA, Mims MP, Amiran ES, et al. Effect of immune reconstitution on the incidence of HIV-related Hodgkin lymphoma. PLoS One. 2013;8(10):e77409.
25. Gopal S, Patel MR, Achenbach CJ, et al. Lymphoma immune reconstitution inflammatory syndrome in the center for AIDS research network of integrated clinical systems cohort. Clin Infect Dis. 2014;59(2):279–86.
26. Kowalkowski MA, Mims MA, Day RS, et al. Longer duration of combination antiretroviral therapy reduces the risk of Hodgkin lymphoma: a cohort study of HIV-infected male veterans. Cancer Epidemiol. 2014;38(4):386–92.
27. Gupta RK, Marks M, Edwards SG, et al. A declining CD4 count and diagnosis of HIV-associated Hodgkin lymphoma: do prior clinical symptoms and laboratory abnormalities aid diagnosis? PLoS One. 2014;9(2):e87442.
28. Helleberg M, Kronborg G, Larsen CS, et al. CD4 Decline is associated with increased risk of cardiovascular disease, cancer, and death in virally suppressed patients with HIV. Clin Inf Dis. 2013;57:314–21.
29. Herndier BG, Sanchez HC, Chang KL, et al. High prevalence of Epstein-Barr virus in the Reed-Sternberg cells of HIV associated Hodgkin's disease. Am J Pathol. 1993;142(4):1073–9.
30. Tirelli U, Errante D, Dolcetti R, et al. Hodgkin's disease and human immunodeficiency virus infection: clinicopathologic and virologic features of 114 patients from the Italian Cooperative Group on AIDS and Tumors. J Clin Oncol. 1995;13(7):1758–67.
31. Xicoy B, Ribera J-M, Miralles P, et al. Results of treatment with doxorubicin, bleomycin, vinblastine and dacarbazine and highly active antiretroviral therapy in advanced stage, human immunodeficiency virus-related Hodgkin's lymphoma. Haematologica. 2007;92:191–8.
32. Carbone A, Gloghini A, Larocca LM, et al. Human immunodeficiency virus associated Hodgkin's disease derives from post-germinal center B cells. Blood. 1999;93:2319–26.
33. Dolcetti R, Boiocchi M, Gloghini A, Carbone A. Pathogenetic and histogenetic features of HIV-associated Hodgkin's disease. Eur J Cancer. 2001;37(10):1276–87.
34. Carbone A, Gloghini A, Dotti G. EBV-associated lymphoproliferative disorders: classification and treatment. Oncologist. 2008;13:577–85.
35. Morales O, Mrizak D, Francois V, et al. Epstein-Barr virus infection induces an increase of T regulatory type 1 cells in Hodgkin lymphoma patients. Br J Haematol. 2014;166(6):875–90.
36. Hartmann S, Jakobus C, Rengstl B, et al. Spindle-shaped CD163+ rosetting macrophages replace CD4+ T-cells in HIV-related classical Hodgkin lymphoma. Mod Pathol. 2013;26(5):648–57.
37. Koulis A, Trivedi P, Ibrahim H, et al. The role of the microenvironment in human immunodeficiency virus-associated classical Hodgkin Lymphoma. Histopathology. 2014;65(6):749–56.
38. Bosch Princep R, Lejeune M, Salvado Usach MT, et al. Decreased number of granzyme B+ activated CD8+ cytotoxic T lymphocytes in the inflammatory background of HIV-associated Hodgkin's lymphoma. Ann Hematol. 2005;84(10):661–6.
39. Goshen E, Davidson T, Avigdor A, et al. PET/CT in the evaluation of lymphoma in patients with HIV-1 with suppressed viral loads. Clin Nucl Med. 2008;33:610–4.
40. Lucignani G, Orunesu E, Cesari M, et al. FDG-PET imaging in HIV-infected subjects: relation with therapy and immunovirological variables. Eur J Nucl Med Mol Imaging. 2009;36(4):640–7.
41. Valour F, Sénéchal A, Chidiac C, Ferry T. Chronic HIV-1 infection mimicking splenic malignant lymphoma on F-18 FDG-PET/CT. BMJ Case Rep. 2012. doi:10.1136/bcr.11.2011.5195.
42. Mhlanga JC, Durand D, Tsai HL, et al. Differentiation of HIV-associated lymphoma from HIV-associated reactive adenopathy using quantitative FDG PET and symmetry. Eur J Nucl Med Mol Imaging. 2014;41(4):596–604.
43. Sathekge M. Differentiation of HIV-associated lymphoma from HIV-reactive adenopathy using quantitative FDG-PET and symmetry. Eur J Nucl Med Mol Imaging. 2014;41(4):593–5.
44. Liu L. Concurrent FDG, avid nasopharyngeal lesion and generalized lymphadenopathy on PET-CT imaging is indicative of lymphoma in patients with HIV infection. AIDS Res Treat. 2012;2012:764291. Epub 2012 Sep 6.

45. Errante D, Tirelli U, Gastaldi R, et al. Combined antineoplastic and antiretroviral therapy for patients with Hodgkin's disease and human immunodeficiency virus infection. A prospective study of 17 patients. The Italian Cooperative Group on AIDS and Tumors (GICAT). Cancer. 1994;73(2):437–44.
46. Errante D, Gabarre J, Ridolfo AL, et al. Hodgkin's disease in 35 patients with HIV infection: an experience with epirubicin, bleomycin, vinblastine and prednisone chemotherapy in combination with antiretroviral therapy and primary use of G-CSF. Ann Oncol. 1999;10(2):189–95.
47. Levine AM, Li P, Cheung T, et al. Chemotherapy consisting of doxorubicin, bleomycin, vinblastine, and dacarbazine with granulocyte colony-stimulating factor in HIV-infected patients with newly diagnosed Hodgkin's disease: a prospective, multi-institutional AIDS clinical trials group study (ACTG 149). J Acquir Immune Defic Syndr. 2000;24(5):444–50.
48. Ribera J-M, Navarro J-T, Oriol A, et al. Prognostic impact of highly active antiretroviral therapy in HIV-related Hodgkin's disease. AIDS. 2002;16:1973–6.
49. Gérard L, Galicier L, Boulanger E, Quint L, Lebrette MG, et al. Improved survival in HIV-related Hodgkin's lymphoma since the introduction of highly active antiretroviral therapy. AIDS. 2003;17:81–7.
50. Hoffmann C, Chow KU, Wolf E, Faetkenheuer G, Stellbrink HJ, et al. Strong impact of highly active antiretroviral therapy on survival in patients with human immunodeficiency virus-associated Hodgkin's disease. Br J Haematol. 2004;124:455–62.
51. Hentrich M, Maretta L, Chow KU, Bogner JR, Schürmann D, et al. Highly active antiretroviral therapy (HAART) improves survival in HIV-associated Hodgkin's disease: results of a multicenter study. Ann Oncol. 2006;17:914–9.
52. Berenguer J, Miralles P, Ribera JM, et al. Characteristics and outcome of AIDS related Hodgkin Lymphoma before and after the introduction of highly active antiretroviral therapy. J Acquir Immune Defic Syndr. 2008;47:422–8.
53. Xicoy B, Ribera J-M, Miralles P, et al. Limited prognostic value of the International Prognostic Score in advanced stage human immunodeficiency virus infection-related Hodgkin lymphoma treated with the doxorubicin, bleomycin, vinblastine, and dacarbazine regimen. Leuk Lymph. 2009;50:1718–20.
54. Spina M, Ribera J-M, Gabarre J, et al. Hodgkin's disease and HIV infection (HD-HIV): prognostic factors in 596 patients (pts) within the European Group for the Study of HIV and Tumours (GECAT). Blood. 2010;116:3883. abstr.
55. Engert A, Haverkamp H, Kobe C, et al. Reduced-intensity chemotherapy and PET-guided radiotherapy in patients with advanced stage Hodgkin's lymphoma (HD15 trial): a randomised, open-label, phase 3 non-inferiority trial. Lancet. 2012;379:1791–9.
56. Spina M, Gabarre J, Mancuso S, et al. Long term results of Stanford V regimen and highly active antiretroviral therapy (HAART) in 59 patients (pts) with HD and HIV-infection (HD-HIV). Haematologica. 2011;96(s2):322. abstr. 0773.
57. Hartmann P, Rehwald U, Salzberger B, et al. BEACOPP therapeutic regimen for patients with Hodgkin's disease and HIV infection. Ann Oncol. 2003;14(10):1562–9.
58. Spina M, Antinori A, Bibas M, et al. VEBEP regimen in patients (pts) with HD and HIV infection (HIV-HD): final results of a phase II study of the italian cooperative group on AIDS and Tumors (GICAT). Haematologica. 2011;96(s2):320. abstr. 0768.
59. Engert A, Plütschow A, Eich HT, et al. Reduced treatment intensity in patients with early-stage Hodgkin's lymphoma. N Engl J Med. 2010;363(7):640–52.
60. Hentrich M, Hoffmann C, Mosthaf F, et al. Therapy of HIV-associated lymphoma -recommendations of the oncology working group of the German Study Group of Physicians in Private Practice Treating HIV-Infected Patients (DAGNÄ), in cooperation with the German AIDS Society (DAIG). Ann Hematol. 2014;93(6):913–21.
61. Bower M, Palfreeman A, Alfa-Wali M, et al. British HIV association guidelines for HIV-associated malignancies 2014. HIV Med. 2014;15 Suppl 2:1–92.
62. Kaplan LD. Management of HIV-associated Hodgkin lymphoma: how far we have come. J Clin Oncol. 2012;30(33):4056–8.
63. Uldrick TS, Little RF. How I treat classical Hodgkin lymphoma in patients infected with human immunodeficiency virus. Blood. 2015;125:1226–35.

64. Gopal S, Patel MR, Yanik EL, et al. Association of early HIV viremia with mortality after HIV-associated lymphoma. AIDS. 2013;27(15):2365–73.
65. European AIDS Clinical Society guidelines Version 7.1 Nov 2014. Part II: ART in HIV-positive persons. http://www.eacsociety.org.
66. Cingolani A, Torti L, Pinnetti C, et al. Detrimental clinical interaction between ritonavir-boosted protease inhibitors and vinblastine in HIV-infected patients with Hodgkin's lymphoma. AIDS. 2010;24:2408–12.
67. Balsalobre P, Diez-Martin JL, Re A, et al. Autologous stem cell transplantation in patients with HIV-related lymphoma. J Clin Oncol. 2009;27:2192–8.
68. Diez-Martin JL, Balsalobre P, Re A, et al. Comparable survival between HIV+ and HIV- non-Hodgkin and Hodgkin lymphoma patients undergoing autologous peripheral blood stem cell transplantation. European Group for Blood and Marrow Transplantation Lymphoma Working Party. Blood. 2009;113:6011–4.
69. Krishnan A, Palmer JM, Zaia JA, et al. HIV status does not affect the outcome of autologous stem cell transplantation (ASCT) for non-Hodgkin lymphoma (NHL). Biol Blood Marrow Transplant. 2010;16:1302–8.
70. Re A, Cattaneo C, Skert C, et al. Stem cell mobilization in HIV seropositive patients with lymphoma. Haematologica. 2013;98:1762–8.
71. Gallamini A, Barrington SF, Biggi A, et al. The predictive role of interim positron emission tomography for Hodgkin lymphoma treatment outcome is confirmed using the interpretation criteria of the Deauville five-point scale. Haematologica. 2014;99(6):1107–13.
72. Hutchings M, Kostakoglu L, Zaucha JM, et al. In vivo treatment sensitivity testing with positron emission tomography/computed tomography after one cycle of chemotherapy for Hodgkin lymphoma. J Clin Oncol. 2014;32(25):2705–11.
73. Okosun J, Warbey V, Shaw K, et al. Interim fluoro-2-deoxy-D-glucose-PET predicts response and progression-free survival in patients with Hodgkin lymphoma and HIV infection. AIDS. 2012;26:861–5.
74. Younes A, Gopal AK, Smith SE, et al. Results of a pivotal phase II study of brentuximab vedotin for patients with relapsed or refractory Hodgkin's lymphoma. J Clin Oncol. 2012;30(18):2183–9.
75. Younes A, Connors JM, Park SI, et al. Brentuximab vedotin combined with ABVD or AVD for patients with newly diagnosed Hodgkin's lymphoma: a phase 1, open-label, dose-escalation study. Lancet Oncol. 2013;14(13):1348–56.
76. Ghandi M, Petrich A. Brentuximab vedotin in patients with relapsed HIV-related lymphoma. J Natl Compr Canc Netw. 2014;12:16–9.

# HIV Infection and Myelodysplastic Syndrome/Acute Myeloid Leukemia 10

Ryan C. Fang and David M. Aboulafia

## Contents



## 10.1 Introduction

Highly active antiretroviral therapy (HAART) is defined as antiviral regimens which combine three or more different drugs such as two nucleoside reverse transcriptase inhibitors (NRTIs) and a protease inhibitor boosted with ritonavir (PI), two NRTIs and a non-nucleoside reverse transcriptase inhibitor (NNRTI), or other such combinations including an integrase inhibitor and an HIV cell surface entry inhibitor (Table 10.1) [1]. Prior to the widespread use of HAART, high-dose combination chemotherapy regimens for the treatment of intermediate- and high-grade B cell lymphoma and acute myeloid leukemia (AML) were perceived as too toxic to administer to patients with the acquired immune deficiency syndrome (AIDS) [2, 3]. However, with the advent of HAART and better supportive care for patients receiving aggressive

R.C. Fang
Section of Hematology and Oncology, Virginia Mason Medical Center, Seattle, WA, USA
e-mail: ryancfang@gmail.com

D.M. Aboulafia, MD (✉)
Division of Hematology, Virginia Mason Medical Center, University of Washington, Seattle, WA, USA
e-mail: hemdma@virginiamason.org



M. Hentrich, S.K. Barta (eds.), *HIV-associated Hematological Malignancies*, DOI 10.1007/978-3-319-26857-6_10

chemotherapy regimens, the prospect of treating these patients with conventional AML induction and consolidation chemotherapy became a reality.

A number of case reports and case series, often derived from the limited experiences of single-center institutions, suggest improved outcomes for patients with both HIV and AML who are treated with standard induction and consolidation regimens, particularly those patients with CD4+ counts >200 cells/mm$^3$ and with well-controlled HIV viremia [4, 5]. As people living with HIV/AIDS (PLWHA) age, it is expected that the incidence of AML will likely rise incrementally in this group as long-term survivors live into their sixth, seventh, and eight decades [6–8]. In this chapter, we briefly review the available literature on frequency, etiology, and treatment of AML and myelodysplastic syndrome (MDS) in the setting of HIV infection.

**Table 10.1** FDA-approved HIV medications

| Nucleoside reverse transcriptase inhibitors (NRTIs) | Non-nucleoside reverse transcriptase inhibitors (NNRTIs) |
|---|---|
| Abacavir sulfate (Ziagen®) | Delavirdine (Rescriptor®) |
| Didanosine (Videx®) | Efavirenz (Sustiva®) |
| Emtricitabine (Emtriva®) | Etravirine (Intelence®) |
| Lamivudine (Epivir®) | Nevirapine (Viramune®) |
| Stavudine (Zerit®) | Rilpivirine (Edurant®) |
| Tenofovir (Viread®) | |
| Zidovudine (Retrovir®) | |
| Protease inhibitors (PIs) | Integrase inhibitors |
| Atazanavir (Reyataz®) | Dolutegravir (Tivicay®) |
| Darunavir (Prezista®) | Elvitegravir (Vitekta®) |
| Fosamprenavir (Lexiva®) | Raltegravir (Isentress®) |
| Indinavir (Crixivan®) | |
| Nelfinavir (Viracept®) | Pharmacokinetic enhancers |
| Ritonavir (Norvir®) | Cobicistat (Tybost®) |
| Saquinavir (Invirase®) | |
| Tipranavir (Aptivus®) | |
| Fusion inhibitors | Entry inhibitors |
| Enfuvirtide (Fuzeon®) | Maraviroc (Selzentry®) |
| Combination HIV medicines | |
| Abacavir and lamivudine (Epzicom®) | |
| Abacavir, dolutegravir, and lamivudine (Triumeq®) | |
| Abacavir, lamivudine, and zidovudine (Trizivir®) | |
| Efavirenz, emtricitabine, and tenofovir (Atripla®) | |
| Elvitegravir, cobicistat, emtricitabine, and tenofovir (Stribild®) | |
| Emtricitabine, rilpivirine, and tenofovir (Complera®) | |
| Emtricitabine and tenofovir (Truvada®) | |
| Lamivudine and zidovudine (Combivir®) | |
| Lopinavir and ritonavir (Kaletra®) | |

Adapted from http://aidsinfo.nih.gov/education-materials/

## 10.2 Frequency

In the United States, 18,000 people are diagnosed with acute leukemia annually, of which over 12,000 are defined as myeloid, and 5000 more without specification on the type of leukemia. More than 10,000 die from the disease, which constitutes approximately 2 % of deaths due to cancer. Leukemia (all forms) is expected to strike 1 % of females and 1.5 % of males during their lifetime and is the leading cause of cancer death in males younger than 40 years and in females younger than 20 years [9]. AML is generally a disease of older people and is uncommon before the age of 45 years. The average age of a patient with AML is 67 years.

With the introduction of HAART, the incidence of AIDS-defining cancers has declined, but non-AIDS-defining hematological malignancies (NADHMs) have emerged including AML [10]. This gradual but significant increase in the incidence of certain NADHMs is expected to continue as PLWHA age. In a recent retrospective review of ten pre-HAART era and nine HAART era HIV-infected patients, the median time from diagnosis of HIV infection to development of hematological malignancy decreased from 9 to 3 years after HAART [11].

The French-American-British (FAB) classification system divides AML into eight subtypes, M0 through to M7, based on the type of cell from which the leukemia developed and its degree of maturity (Table 10.2). This is done by examining the appearance of the malignant cells with light microscopy and/or by using cytogenetics to characterize any underlying chromosomal abnormalities (see Fig. 10.1a–d).

**Table 10.2** French-American-British classification schema

| Type | Name | Cytogenetics | Percentage of adult AML patients |
|---|---|---|---|
| M0 | Acute myeloblastic leukemia, minimally differentiated | | 5 % |
| M1 | Acute myeloblastic leukemia, without maturation | | 15 % |
| M2 | Acute myeloblastic leukemia, with granulocytic maturation | t(8;21)(q22;q22), t(6;9) | 25 % |
| M3 | Promyelocytic, or acute promyelocytic leukemia (APL) | t(15;17) | 10 % |
| M4 | Acute myelomonocytic leukemia | inv(16)(p13q22), del(16q) | 20 % |
| M4eo | Myelomonocytic together with bone marrow eosinophilia | inv(16), t(16;16) | 5 % |
| M5 | Acute monoblastic leukemia (M5a) or acute monocytic leukemia (M5b) | del (11q), t(9;11), t(11;19) | 10 % |
| M6 | Acute erythroid leukemias, including erythroleukemia (M6a) and very rare pure erythroid leukemia (M6b) | | 5 % |
| M7 | Acute megakaryoblastic leukemia | t(1;22) | 5 % |

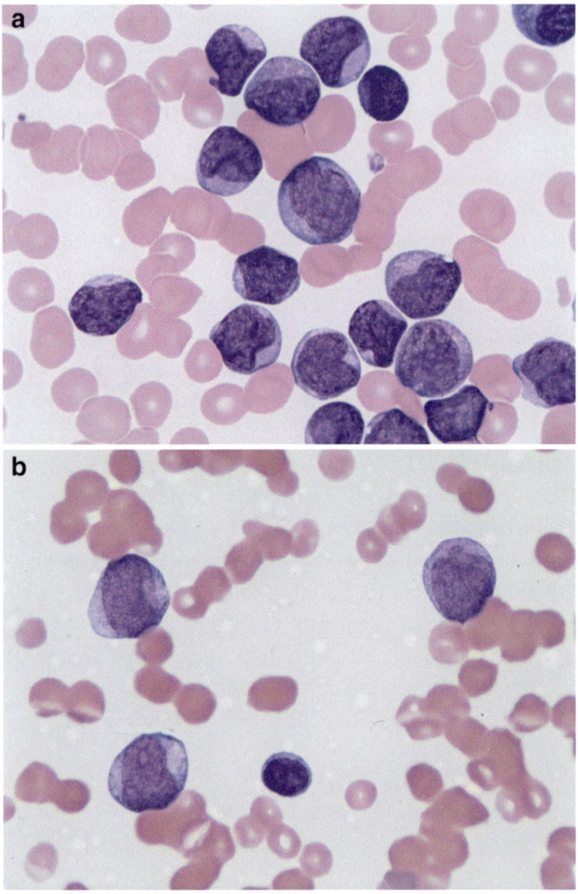


**Fig. 10.1** (**a**) Myeloblasts in a peripheral blood smear from a patient with acute myeloid leukemia without maturation (AML-M1) showing variation in size, amount of cytoplasm, and azurophilic granules. (**b**) Blood smear from a patient with acute myeloid leukemia with maturation (AML-M2) showing occasional Auer rods. (**c**) Blood smear from a patient with acute myelomonocytic leukemia (AML-M4) showing a myeloid blasts with Auer rods and azurophilic granules and promonocytes with delicately convoluted nuclei. (**d**) Blood smear from a patient with acute myeloid leukemia with myelodysplasia-related changes. A myeloid blast is seen together with a dysplastic hypolobated neutrophil (Images and descriptions courtesy of Dr. Dick Hwang, Virginia Mason Medical Center)

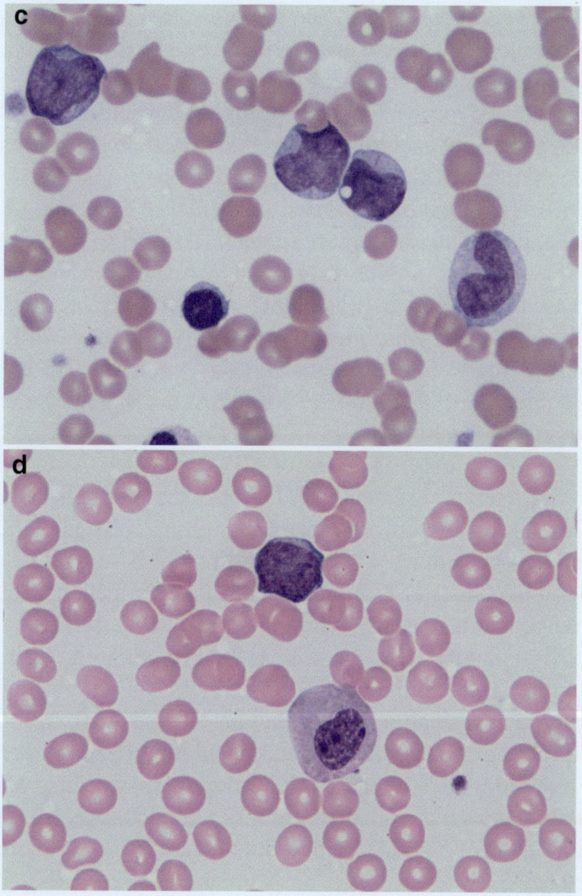


**Fig. 10.1** (continued)

The subtypes have varying prognoses and responses to therapy. Although the WHO classification may be more useful in providing prognostic information, the FAB system is still most widely used. Eight FAB subtypes were proposed in 1976 [12].

The precise frequency at which AML occurs in the setting of HIV infection is uncertain, although several analyses suggest that it may be greater than that seen in the general population [5, 13]. Furthermore, a 2007 meta-analysis of the incidence of cancer in PLWHA found an increased incidence of leukemia in patients with HIV, but identification of an association between HIV and specific classes of leukemia was not evaluated [14]. Similarly, in a nationwide epidemiological study from Japan encompassing the years between 1991 and 2010, the incidence and clinical outcomes of 47 NADHMs were identified, 13 of which had AML. The median patient age was 42 years, and the median CD4+ count was 255 cells/mm$^3$. Most notably, when comparing 1991–2000 to 2001–2009, the estimated incidence of total NADHMs increased 4.5-fold [15].

From 1986 to 2011, only 68 cases of HIV-associated AML were identified through a PubMed literature search [16]. In 2009, the first case of pediatric AML was reported in a 7-year-old boy with parotid swelling, a bleeding diathesis, and a CD4+ count of 900 cells/mm$^3$ [17]. The child received supportive care and succumbed from complications of bleeding and presumed infection 4 weeks later.

In that same year, five cases of therapy-related AML following treatment of HIV-associated lymphoma were reported [18]. Furthermore, of the 13 patients with AML identified through the Japanese National Data set, nine had recurrent or complex karyotype abnormalities [15]. Therapy-related AML accounts for about 10–20 % of all cases of AML in the general population [19]. In fact, patients with Hodgkin's or non-Hodgkin's lymphomas develop therapy-related MDS/AML at a 10-year cumulative incidence rate of 1–10 % [20–22]. This too could have significant implications as PLWHA survive their initial cancer treatment only to develop therapy-related MDS.

## 10.3 Etiology

HIV-related bone marrow changes are common and often include myelodysplastic features (MDF). Their pathogenesis may differ from primary MDS and is associated with various factors including the virus itself and marrow morphologic changes that are induced by particular antiretroviral agents.

The link between HIV infection, antiretroviral medications, and morphologic changes in bone marrow architecture that mimic MDS but do not have the same clinical implications was studied in 158 HIV-infected hemophiliacs, and the results were compared with those of 61 non-HIV-infected patients with primary MDS (31 with refractory anemia, 10 with refractory anemia with ringed sideroblasts, 11 with refractory anemia with excessive blasts [RAEB], 3 with RAEB transformation, and 6 with chronic myelomonocytic leukemia) [23]. The peripheral blood and bone marrow examination revealed MDF in 44 HIV-infected hemophilic patients (28 %). The median time from seroconversion was 12.5 years, and the mean time under therapy with the NRTI zidovudine was 44.1 months. Nineteen of these patients (43 %) had hemoglobin levels <10 g/dL, while neutropenia and thrombocytopenia were observed in 30 % and 25 %, respectively. There were statistically significant morphological alterations between HIV-related MDF and MDS. Hypocellularity, plasmatocytosis, and eosinophilia were more pronounced among HIV-infected hemophiliacs with MDF, while dysplasia of erythroblasts, megakaryocytes, and granulocytes was more frequent in MDS patients. None of the hemophiliacs with MDF had more than 5 % blasts in the bone marrow, nor did any develop RAEB or AML. The cytogenetic analysis was normal in HIV-infected patients with hemophilia, whereas 43 % of the non-HIV-infected patients with MDS had an abnormal karyotype. These data suggest that bone marrow changes in long-term PLWHA have different characteristics and clinical implications than those HIV-seronegative individuals with primary MDS.

The importance of HIV in contributing to the risk of MDS and AML in PLWHA, nonetheless, remains unsettled. HIV infection may play a major role in the transformation of MDS to AML. In a retrospective analysis that compared eight patients with HIV-associated MDS with a historical cohort of HIV-uninfected MDS patients, the HIV-MDS patients had more complex cytogenetic abnormalities, more 7q deletions, and monosomy 7 anomalies and were younger. Additionally, HIV-associated MDS patients may be predisposed to a greater risk of conversion to AML since in that small cohort, 63 % eventually developed AML as opposed to 22 % in the HIV-uninfected MDS population [24].

Several additional mechanisms have been offered to explain why PLWHA may have unique predisposition to develop AML. The first of these mechanisms involves acute infection of CD4+ T lymphocytes. During this process, the HIV-1 *trans*-activator protein *Tat* is released extracellularly. *Tat* plays a major role in angiogenesis, which in turn plays a vital role in the pathogenesis of acute leukemia. Second, the basic domain of *Tat* has the ability to displace preformed basic fibroblast growth factor (bFGF), which has been demonstrated to augment myelopoiesis directly via FGF receptors on myeloid progenitors. Third, by infecting monocytes and macrophages, HIV may alter the bone marrow microenvironment by activating the genes of cytokines involved in leukemogenesis, making it more prone to the growth of leukemic cells [25].

In addition to unique ways that HIV infection may increase a patient's risk of developing AML, receiving treatment for hematologic malignancies such as lymphomas, multiple myeloma, polycythemia vera, essential thrombocythemia, and acute lymphoblastic leukemia might lead to therapy-related AML. Therapy-related AML accounts for 10–20 % of all cases of AML in the general population and is classically recognized to be induced by alkylating agents and topoisomerase II inhibitors. MDS and AML induced by alkylating agents are typically associated with deletions or loss of chromosome arm 5q or 7q or the loss of the entire chromosome. In topoisomerase II inhibitor-induced AML, karyotypic abnormalities include balanced aberrations involving transcription factor genes such as MLL at 11q23, AML1 at 21q22, RARA at 17q21, CBFB at 16q22, and NUP98 at 11p15. These abnormalities lead to chimeric rearrangements between genes encoding hematopoietic transcription factors and their partner genes, which in turn cause loss of function and augment expression of oncogenes [18].

Patients that receive chemotherapy for other hematologic malignancies, which then facilitate the development of therapy-related AML, have unusually poor prognoses. Among five such patients, the median age at the time of AML diagnosis was 39 years, and the median time between chemotherapy treatments of lymphoma to AML was 18 months [18]. Two patients had non-detectable HIV viral loads and CD4+ counts >200 cells/mm$^3$; the other three patients' conditions were not reported [18, 26, 27]. Cytogenetic analysis revealed that these patients exhibited deletions on chromosome 7 and 11q21 and translocations 3:22, 9:11, and 10:11. Four died from progressive leukemia or infection within weeks to 2 months of initiation of induction treatment. The remaining patient achieved a complete remission after receiving standard induction chemotherapy but died 4 weeks after a second cycle of chemotherapy.

## 10.4 Treatment

Before the widespread use of HAART, hematologic malignancies accounted for approximately 10 % of all deaths among HIV-infected patients [28]. Due to their underlying immunodeficiency, those with AML could not tolerate intensive chemotherapy, and they often succumbed from opportunistic infections and other complications induced by protracted cytopenias. In addition, efforts to treat these patients with high-dose chemotherapy and autologous stem cell transplantation (auto-SCT) in the pre-HAART era remained problematic. Infection would continue to be a significant cause of morbidity and mortality until better strategies around supportive care and HAART became available to this group [3].

With better strategies to prevent bacterial, fungal, and opportunistic infections, HIV-infected patients could more safely face the rigors of AML induction chemotherapy. With the widespread use of HAART beginning in 1996, better strategies were employed for patients with AML to prevent opportunistic infections through the use of prophylactic antifungals and antibacterial agents. By using HAART that did not include zidovudine, marrow sparing options could more safely be integrated into HIV-infected patient's regimens, and soon thereafter, it became more feasible to offer PLWHA and AML standard induction and consolidation chemotherapy (Table 10.2). In a report summarizing cases treated within their own group, along with cases found from MEDLINE, CancerLit, and AIDSLINE, Aboulafia and colleagues identified 47 HIV-infected patients with AML, 29 of whom received standard AML induction chemotherapy [25]. The median survival rates of the chemotherapy-treated patients and patients who did not receive chemotherapy were 7.5 months and 1 month, respectively (Table 10.3).

Karyotype and CD4+ count have been proposed as strong predictors of survival for HIV-infected patients with AML. In a retrospective study of 31 HIV-infected patients with AML, the distribution of karyotypes from favorable, intermediate, to unfavorable was similar to that of an HIV-negative AML control group [4]. For those with HIV and AML, the median CD4+ counts at diagnosis were 355 cells/mm$^3$, 196 cells/mm$^3$, and

**Table 10.3** Overview of common induction therapy regimens for acute myeloid leukemia in younger adults

| Drugs | Dosing | Comments |
|---|---|---|
| Cytarabine + daunorubicin | *Cytarabine*: 100–200 mg/m$^2$ daily as a CI × 7 days; *daunorubicin*: 60–90 mg/m$^2$ IVP days 1–3 | "Standard 7 + 3" induction regimen resulting in approximately 60–80 % remission rate and acceptable toxicity in patients <60 years old |
| Cytarabine (HDAC) + daunorubicin | *Cytarabine*: 1–3 g/m$^2$ 2× daily for a total of 12 doses; *daunorubicin*: 45 mg/m$^2$ IVP × 3 days following cytarabine | Yields a 90 % remission rate; however, substantial toxicity precludes post-remission therapy in a high proportion of patients |
| Cytarabine + idarubicin | *Cytarabine*: 100–200 mg/m$^2$ daily as a CI × 7 days; *idarubicin*: 12–13 mg/m$^2$ IVP on days 1–3 | Has produced a greater remission rate (88 versus 70 %) than cytarabine/daunorubicin in younger patients; appears superior to daunorubicin in patients with hyperleukocytosis; overall survival not clearly superior to "standard" regimen |

Adapted from UpToDate, Wolters Kluwer Editors, Induction therapy for AML. Richard Larson accessed April 19, 2015

*CI* continuous infusion, *IVP* intravenous push, *HDAC* high-dose cytarabine

60 cells/mm$^3$ for patients in the favorable, intermediate, and unfavorable karyotype groups, respectively. Median survival for intensively treated favorable and intermediate-risk karyotype patients with CD4+ counts <200 cells/mm$^3$ was 8.5 months compared to 48 months for those with >200 cells/m$^3$. Although the connection between favorable karyotype and higher CD4+ cell count has not been established, this study suggests that favorable karyotype and CD4+ counts >200 cells/mm$^3$ predict better survival compared to unfavorable karyotype and <200 CD4+ cells/mm$^3$.

Because patients with AML and HIV infection are relatively uncommon, there are no clinical trial results to form best practice recommendations, and optimal therapy has not been established. However, a retrospective evaluation of 13 HIV-infected patients with AML, acute lymphoblastic leukemia (ALL), or high-risk MDS suggests that standard chemotherapy followed by auto-SCT or allogeneic (allo)-SCT is feasible in select instances [29]. The median CD4+ count in this patient group was 336 cells/mm$^3$. Three patients received palliative care and died after a median of 51 days, while the remaining ten patients received HAART prior to and during chemotherapy. Eight of these ten were treated with standard induction chemotherapy, one underwent allo-SCT, and 1 received azacytidine but died 4 months later. Eight entered complete remission, two of whom were treated with auto-SCT and another two received allo-SCT. Neutrophil engraftment was established after a median of 10 days and 19 days after auto- and allo-SCT, respectively. The median overall survival of those that received chemotherapy followed by auto- or allo-SCT was 9 months, and 20 % have survived for at least 3 years. In Japan, it has been reported that two HIV-infected patients with AML underwent high-dose chemotherapy and then allo-SCT, and both survived for more than 4 years [15, 30, 31].

The seminal 2009 report that the so-called Berlin patient had been cured of both AML and HIV infection following allo-SCT has sparked enormous interest in both the HIV and transplantation research communities [32]. This individual received myeloablative therapy and allo-SCT from a donor whose cells were resistant to HIV infection due to being homozygous for CCR5-D32, a nonfunctional allele of the CCR5 co-receptor used by HIV to infect human cells. Remarkably, he remains without AML and without detectable HIV despite now greater than 7 years without HAART [33].

**Conclusion**

Over the past two decades, HAART has produced dramatic survival gains among HIV-infected patients. It is currently estimated that newly infected PLWHAs have a life expectancy rivaling that of age-matched HIV-negative individuals. With the widespread use of HAART, the incidence of NADHMs such as AML appears to be increasing. AML will likely be an increasingly important cause of morbidity and mortality as this population ages and approaches the median age of non-HIV-infected AML patients.

HIV infection may play an important role in the transformation of MDS to AML. Possible mechanisms to explain why PLWHA may have unique predisposition to develop AML include acute infection of CD4+ T lymphocytes, HIV-1 *trans*-activator protein *Tat*'s ability to displace preformed bFGF, and the infection of monocytes and macrophages. In addition to these mechanisms, therapies for other hematological malignancies such as topoisomerase II inhibitors and alkylating agents are widely recognized for inducing AML. There are a handful of cases of survivors of hematologic malignancies developing therapy-related MDS and AML. As more patients in the HAART era receive chemotherapy for malignancies and achieve long-term disease-free status, this may become increasingly relevant in the coming years.

Treating HIV-infected patients with AML in the pre-HAART era with induction chemotherapy was thought to be too toxic for those patients with compromised immune systems. Within the HAART era, survival of HIV-infected patients with AML who did and did not receive induction chemotherapy was 7.5 months and 1 month, respectively. Additionally, patients with CD4+ cell counts of >200 cells/mm$^3$ and favorable karyotypes are associated with better survival. Auto- and allo-SCT are currently offered as potential cure options for AML in HIV-infected patients, and a handful of cases demonstrate improved treatment outcomes. In fact, one patient, the "Berlin patient," continues to live free of AML and with undetectable HIV without HAART 7 years after allo-SCT.

## References

1. Panel on Antiretroviral Guidelines for Adults and Adolescents. Guidelines for the use of antiretroviral agents in HIV-1-infected adults and adolescents. Department of Health and Human Services. Availablle at www.aidsinfo.nih.gov/ContentFiles/AdultandAdolescentGL.pdf. Accessed 11-29-2015.
2. Kaplan LD, et al. Low-dose compared with standard-dose m-BACOD chemotherapy for non-Hodgkin's lymphoma associated with human immunodeficiency virus infection. National

Institute of Allergy and Infectious Diseases AIDS Clinical Trials Group. N Engl J Med. 1997;336(23):1641–8.

3. Krishnan A. Stem cell transplantation in HIV-infected patients. Curr Opin HIV AIDS. 2009;4(1):11–5.
4. Evans MW, et al. Risk assessment in human immunodeficiency virus-associated acute myeloid leukemia. Leuk Lymphoma. 2012;53(4):660–4.
5. Sutton L, et al. Acute myeloid leukaemia in human immunodeficiency virus-infected adults: epidemiology, treatment feasibility and outcome. Br J Haematol. 2001;112(4):900–8.
6. Samji H, et al. Closing the gap: increases in life expectancy among treated HIV-positive individuals in the United States and Canada. PLoS One. 2013;8(12):e81355.
7. Wada N, et al. Cause-specific mortality among HIV-infected individuals, by CD4(+) cell count at HAART initiation, compared with HIV-uninfected individuals. AIDS. 2014;28(2):257–65.
8. Miller V, Hodder S. Beneficial impact of antiretroviral therapy on non-AIDS mortality. AIDS. 2014;28(2):273–4.
9. Juliusson G, et al. Acute myeloid leukemia in the real world: why population-based registries are needed. Blood. 2012;119(17):3890–9.
10. Robbins HA, et al. Excess cancers among HIV-infected people in the United States. J Natl Cancer Inst. 2015;107(4):1–8.
11. Ibarrondo P, et al. HIV-related hematologic malignancies pre-HAART (highly active antiretroviral therapy) era and HAART era: experience in one centre. Haematologica. 2013; 98(1):649–50.
12. Bennett JM, et al. Proposals for the classification of the acute leukaemias. French-American-British (FAB) co-operative group. Br J Haematol. 1976;33(4):451–8.
13. Frisch M, et al. Association of cancer with AIDS-related immunosuppression in adults. JAMA. 2001;285(13):1736–45.
14. Grulich AE, et al. Incidence of cancers in people with HIV/AIDS compared with immunosuppressed transplant recipients: a meta-analysis. Lancet. 2007;370(9581):59–67.
15. Hagiwara S, et al. Non-AIDS-defining hematological malignancies in HIV-infected patients: an epidemiological study in Japan. AIDS. 2013;27(2):279–83.
16. Dy IA, et al. Treatment outcome of acute myeloid leukemia (AML) in HIV plus patients. J Clin Oncol. 2012;30(15):1884–91.
17. Tullu MS, et al. Acute myelogenous leukemia in a child with HIV infection. Eur J Pediatr. 2010;169(5):629–31.
18. Mani D, Dorer RK, Aboulafia DM. Therapy-related acute myeloid leukemia following HIV-associated lymphoma. Clin Lymphoma Myeloma. 2009;9(4):316–9.
19. Park DJ, Koeffler HP. Therapy-related myelodysplastic syndromes. Semin Hematol. 1996; 33(3):256–73.
20. Brusamolino E, et al. The risk of acute leukemia in patients treated for Hodgkin's disease is significantly higher aft [see bined modality programs than after chemotherapy alone and is correlated with the extent of radiotherapy and type and duration of chemotherapy: a case-control study. Haematologica. 1998;83(9):812–23.
21. Josting A, et al. Secondary myeloid leukemia and myelodysplastic syndromes in patients treated for Hodgkin's disease: a report from the German Hodgkin's Lymphoma Study Group. J Clin Oncol. 2003;21(18):3440–6.
22. Armitage JO, et al. Treatment-related myelodysplasia and acute leukemia in non-Hodgkin's lymphoma patients. J Clin Oncol. 2003;21(5):897–906.
23. Katsarou O, et al. Myelodysplastic features in patients with long-term HIV infection and haemophilia. Haemophilia. 2001;7(1):47–52.
24. Takahashi K, et al. Clinical and cytogenetic characteristics of myelodysplastic syndrome in patients with HIV infection. Leuk Res. 2012;36(11):1376–9.
25. Aboulafia DM, et al. Acute myeloid leukemia in patients infected with HIV-1. AIDS. 2002;16(6):865–76.
26. Nabil S, et al. Topoisomerase II inhibitor induced leukemia in a patient with AIDS. AIDS. 2001;15(3):421–3.

27. Olalla J, et al. Acute myelocytic leukemia and human immunodeficiency virus infection. Am J Med. 2001;111(1):79.
28. Kravcik S, et al. Causes of death of HIV-infected persons in Ottawa, Ontario, 1984–1995. Arch Intern Med. 1997;157(18):2069–73.
29. Pagani C, et al. Acute leukemia and high-risk myelodysplastic syndromes in HIV-positive patients: a clinical study of the Rete Ematologica Lombarda. Haematologica. 2013;98(3):141.
30. Oka Y, et al. Successful unrelated bone marrow transplantation for a human immunodeficiency virus type-1-seropositive acute myelogenous leukemia patient following HAART. Int J Hematol. 2010;91(1):140–5.
31. Sora F, et al. Highly active antiretroviral therapy and allogeneic CD34(+) peripheral blood progenitor cells transplantation in an HIV/HCV coinfected patient with acute myeloid leukemia. Exp Hematol. 2002;30(3):279–84.
32. Hutter G, et al. Long-term control of HIV by CCR5 Delta32/Delta32 stem-cell transplantation. N Engl J Med. 2009;360(7):692–8.
33. Smiley ST, et al. Progress toward curing HIV infections with hematopoietic stem cell transplantation. Clin Infect Dis. 2015;60(2):292–7.

# Acute Lymphoblastic Leukemia 11

Josep-Maria Ribera

## Contents



## 11.1 Epidemiology

The term "non-AIDS-defining cancers" (NADCs) refers to neoplasms other than AIDS-defining malignancies that occur in individuals with HIV infection. The spectrum and incidence of various neoplasms reported among persons infected with human immunodeficiency virus (HIV) has increased [1–3], and this emerging problem has contributed to the mortality of HIV-infected persons in the current era of potent antiretroviral therapy (ART) [4]. Large, population-based studies involving registry match data have reported a wide range of cancers in association with HIV infection. Incidence of cancer among HIV-infected persons was compared with that of the general population from 1992 to 2003 in a prospective observational study conducted in the United States. Investigators reported that the incidence of leukemia was only slightly higher in HIV-infected people (standardized incidence ratio, SIR: 2.5; 95 % CI: 1.6–3.8) [5] (Table 11.1). Acute lymphoblastic leukemia (ALL) constituted 15 % of NADC in Japan [6], with an estimated incidence of 5.6 cases/100,000 HIV-infected persons and year. An observational cohort study using data from Centers for AIDS Research Network of Integrated Clinical Systems found that rates of other NADCs increased


J.-M. Ribera, MD, PhD
Clinical Hematology Department, ICO-Hospital Germans Trias i Pujol, Jose Carreras Research Institute, Universitat Autònoma de Barcelona, Badalona, Spain
e-mail: jribera@iconcologia.net





M. Hentrich, S.K. Barta (eds.), *HIV-associated Hematological Malignancies*,
DOI 10.1007/978-3-319-26857-6_11

**Table 11.1** Maximum standardized incidence ratios (SIR) for AIDS-defining and non-AIDS-defining cancers in HIV-infected individuals

| SIR | >1.5 | <1.5 |
|---|---|---|
| AIDS-defining cancers | Kaposi's sarcoma (3640) | None |
| | Cervical cancer (22) | |
| | Non-Hodgkin's lymphoma (354) | |
| Non-AIDS-defining cancers | Anal (50) | Breast (1) |
| | Liver (22) | Prostate (1) |
| | Skin (20) | Colorectal (1) |
| | Hodgkin's lymphoma (18) | Melanoma (1) |
| | Penile (8) | |
| | Vulvar/vaginal (7) | |
| | Leukemia (5) | |
| | Myeloma (5) | |
| | Lung (5) | |
| | Brain (4) | |
| | Ovarian (4) | |
| | Bladder cancer (4) | |
| | Small bowel (4) | |
| | Lip (3) | |
| | Thyroid (3) | |
| | Stomach (3) | |
| | Oropharyngeal (3) | |
| | Pancreas (3) | |
| | Larynx (3) | |
| | Uterine (2) | |
| | Esophageal (2) | |
| | Renal (2) | |
| | Eye (2) | |
| | Testicular (2) | |

Modified from Patel et al. [5]

slowly with time on ART [7]. From these epidemiological data, we can conclude that the incidence of leukemias in general, and ALL in particular, in HIV-infected patients is only slightly higher than that observed in the general population. For that reason, the clinical reports of ALL in HIV-infected patients are almost exclusively based on isolated case reports, without major case series being found in the literature.

## 11.2 Acute Lymphoblastic Leukemia in HIV-Infected Patients

In the general population, ALL comprises approximately 25 % of acute leukemia cases and is the most frequent neoplastic disease in children (four to five new cases/100,000 persons and year), with a peak incidence at the age of 5–9 years. This incidence decreases in adolescence, being a rare disease in adults (one to two new cases/100,000 persons and year) [8]. B-cell precursor ALL represents 80 % of ALL cases, being CD10-positive (common) ALL the most frequent subtype. Mature B-(Burkitt-like) ALL only represents 2–3 % of ALL in children and 5–6 % of ALL in adults. In contrast, mature B-ALL is by far the most frequent ALL subtype reported in HIV-infected patients, representing more than 50 % of ALL cases. Given that mature B-ALL constitutes the leukemic form of Burkitt's lymphoma, we refer the reader to the chapter of burkitt's lymphoma, and the present chapter will focus on the remaining subtypes of ALL.

The first case reports of ALL in HIV-infected patients were published in the 1980s [9–13]. At that time ALL was considered among the unusual types of cancer in HIV-infected individuals, representing 5 out of 49 NADC cases in adults in an Italian registry [14], 4 out of 33 cases in a study conducted in the United States by the Pediatric Oncology Group [15], and 5 out of 64 cases in a survey conducted by the Children's Cancer Group and the National Cancer Institute (NCI) [16]. In general, ALL represents 10 % of NADC in both children and adults. ALL cases have been reported at any age (including one case of ALL in an infant exposed to zidovudine in utero and early infancy) [17] and in all risk groups for HIV infection. In most cases ALL was diagnosed in patients with known HIV infection. In almost all patients, the leukemia was of B-cell origin, with the only T-ALL published cases corresponding to T-lymphoblastic lymphomas with bone marrow involvement [18]. Except for the higher frequency of mature B-ALL, no significant clinical and biologic differences were observed in ALL arising in HIV-infected individuals as compared to non-immunosuppressed patients.

## 11.3 Diagnostic and Therapeutic Approach

It is extremely difficult to make recommendations on the therapy of ALL arising in HIV-infected patients based on case reports, most of which were published prior to the potent ART era [19–28]. The most realistic approach in the current era of potent ART would be to try to apply the same diagnostic and therapeutic strategy to that employed in non-immunosuppressed patients. The basic diagnostic workup (Table 11.2) should include morphologic, immunophenotypic, cytogenetic, and molecular studies. This is not only important for an accurate ALL diagnosis but also for adequate stratification of patients into risk groups. Analysis of breakpoint fusion genes or clone-specific Ig and/or T-cell receptor (TCR) gene rearrangements by RT-PCR and RQ-PCR is essential if follow-up of the minimal residual disease (MRD) is to be performed by these methods. Screening for CNS involvement (morphologic study of CSF after cytocentrifugation, ideally complemented with immunophenotypic study) is mandatory. Other studies should include the search for infections by hepatotropic viruses (hepatitis B and C), opportunistic infections, as well as the study of the main basic parameters of HIV infection: HIV viral load and CD4+ lymphocyte count.

The main adverse risk factors of ALL at baseline are advanced age (especially over 50 years), high WBC count, pro-B or early pre-T or mature T phenotype, *MLL*

**Table 11.2** Approach to the HIV-infected patient with acute lymphoblastic leukemia

| | |
|---|---|
| Medical history | Including search for risk factors for HIV infection, prior opportunistic infections, or other cancers |
| Physical examination | |
| General laboratory tests | Full blood count |
| | Coagulation analysis |
| | Liver and kidney function |
| | LDH |
| | Serology for hepatitis B and C |
| | HIV viral load |
| | CD4 lymphocyte count |
| | Other analyses based on the status of the patient |
| Instrumental procedures | Bone marrow aspirate |
| | Lumbar puncture |
| | Chest X-ray |
| | ECG |
| | Assessment of left ventricular function (echocardiography, MUGA scan) in older patients or patients with antecedent heart disease |
| Specific procedures for ALL diagnosis | Morphology: blast percentage in bone marrow |
| | Immunophenotyping |
| | First step: CyMPO, CD117, TdT, cyCD3, CD7, cyCD79a, CD19, CD13, CD33, CD34, HLA-DR |
| | Second step: |
| | B-ALL: CD10, CD22, cyIgM, sIg |
| | T-ALL: CD1a, CD2, CD3, CD5, CD4, CD8 |
| | Cytogenetics (standard, FISH) |
| | Molecular genetics |
| | First step: detection of *BCR-ABL* or *MLL* rearrangements |
| | Second step: |
| | Detection of other fusion genes as required for risk stratification |
| | Detection of Ig/TCR rearrangements |
| | Gene expression profiling (for research/diagnostic purposes) |
| | Storage of cells, DNA, RNA, and serum (for research purposes) |
| HLA typing of patients and close relatives as soon as possible | |

*ECG* electrocardiogram, *MUGA* multigated acquisition, *CyMPO* cytoplasmic myeloperoxidase, *FISH* fluorescent in situ hybridization, *Ig* immunoglobulin, *TCR* T-cell receptor

or *BCR-ABL* rearrangements, and slow response to initial therapy. However, the most powerful prognostic factor is the pattern of MRD clearance assessed either by clone-specific Ig/TCR rearrangements or by detection of aberrant phenotypes by multiparametric flow cytometry.

The general strategy of ALL treatment includes induction chemotherapy, consolidation treatment, CNS prophylaxis, and postconsolidation therapy, the latter including maintenance chemotherapy or allogeneic hematopoietic stem cell transplantation (alloHSCT). In the modern protocols, the level of MRD after induction and consolidation is used for selection of the patients who will receive alloHSCT or chemotherapy (patients with poor MRD clearance are submitted to alloHSCT and those with molecular remission receive maintenance chemotherapy). Several reports have shown that HSCT appears to be a feasible treatment for selected HIV-infected patients with ALL [29], and thus HSCT as part of standard care should be incorporated into therapeutic planning for HIV-infected individuals with ALL. Patients with mature B-ALL should be treated with the same schedules used for the treatment of Burkitt's lymphoma. Recent data have shown the same promising results as those observed in non-immunosuppressed patients [30, 31], but the toxicity was remarkable in HIV-infected patients. Other effective and less toxic regimens could be useful in these patients [32]. Patients with *BCR-ABL*-positive ALL should be treated with tyrosine kinase inhibitors (TKI) together with chemotherapy, although the experience with the combination of TKI, chemotherapy, and potent ART is extremely scarce. Referral to investigational studies for this purpose should be prioritized.

Since the duration of ALL treatment is long, HIV-infected patients must concomitantly receive potent ART and chemotherapy. Clinicians need to be mindful of the fact that combining cytotoxic chemotherapy with antiretrovirals may result in additive cytotoxicity or other drug-drug interactions that may further enhance immunosuppression [33]. Several antiretrovirals induce and inhibit enzymes involved in drug metabolism. For example, protease inhibitors (PI) inhibit CYP3A4, an enzyme that mediates the metabolism of many drugs that undergo hepatic metabolism, including chemotherapy agents. Vinca alkaloids, essential drugs in ALL treatment, may increase the risk of hematologic and neurologic toxicity when coadministered with boosted PI [34, 35]. The concomitant administration of the novel targeted therapies such as TKI with potent ART may impede the efficacy or increase the toxicity of ART. Antiretroviral agents that are likely to interact with the newer targeted anticancer drugs are PI and non-nucleoside reverse transcriptase inhibitors [35]. Thus, adequate selection of ART and chemotherapy is essential and requires close collaboration between hematologists and physicians who treat the HIV infection. In addition, special attention should be given to the prophylaxis and treatment of opportunistic infections and infections during the periods of neutropenia [36, 37]. Supportive therapy with G-CSF can be useful for shortening the duration of neutropenia.

Taking into account the previous considerations, it seems probable that in the potent ART era the prognosis of ALL arising in HIV-infected patients will be similar to that of non-immunosuppressed patients, as currently occurs with other AIDS-related cancers or NADC. However, since HIV-infected patients are not included in the current investigational trials in ALL, the development and implementation of specific global multicenter clinical trials for HIV-infected patients with ALL should be prioritized, as occurs in other AIDS-related lymphoid cancers such as lymphomas.

**Funding** Supported in part by grants from the Red Temática de Investigación Cooperativa en Cáncer (RTICC, FEDER) (RD12/0036/0029); 2014 SGR225 (GRE) Generalitat de Catalunya; PI14/01971 from Fondo de Investigaciones Sanitarias, Instituto de Salud Carlos III; and Fundació Internacional Josep Carreras i Obra Social "la Caixa," Spain.

## References

1. Pantanowitz L, Dezube BJ. Evolving spectrum and incidence of non-AIDS-defining malignancies. Curr Opin HIV AIDS. 2009;4:27–34.
2. Grulich AE, van Leeuwen MT, Falster MO, Vajdic CM. Incidence of cancers in people with HIV/AIDS compared with immunosuppressed transplant recipients: a meta-analysis. Lancet. 2007;370:59–67.
3. Stebbing J, Duru O, Bower M. Non-AIDS-defining cancers. Curr Opin Infect Dis. 2009;22: 7–10.
4. Ingle SM, May MT, Gill MJ, Mugavero MJ, Lewden C, Abgrall S, et al. Impact of risk factors for specific causes of death in the first and subsequent years of antiretroviral therapy among HIV-infected patients. Clin Infect Dis. 2014;59:287–97.
5. Patel P, Hanson DL, Sullivan PS, Novak RM, Moorman AC, Tong TC, et al. Incidence of types of cancer among HIV-infected persons compared with the general population in the United States, 1992–2003. Ann Intern Med. 2008;148:728–36.
6. Hagiwara S, Yotsumoto M, Odawara T, Ajisawa A, Uehira T, Nagai H, et al. Non-AIDS-defining hematological malignancies in HIV-infected patients: an epidemiological study in Japan. AIDS. 2013;27:279–83.
7. Yanik EL, Napravnik S, Cole SR, Achenbach CJ, Gopal S, Olshan A, et al. Incidence and timing of cancer in HIV-infected individuals following initiation of combination antiretroviral therapy. Clin Infect Dis. 2013;57:756–64.
8. Cancer Statistics US Working Group. United States Cancer Statistics: 1999–2010 incidence and mortality web-based report. Atlanta: Department of Health and Human Services. Centers for Disease Control and Prevention, and National Cancer Institute; 2013. Available at: http://www.cdc.gov/uscs. [Last accessed 29 December 2014].
9. Rossi G, Gorla R, Cadeo GP, Stellini R, Marinone G. Acute lymphoblastic leukaemia of B cell origin in an anti-HIV positive intravenous drug abuser. Br J Haematol. 1988;68:140–1.
10. Garavelli PL. Acute lymphoblastic leukemia, L3 type, in a HIV positive patient. Haematologica. 1988;73:89.
11. Brunet S, Rabella N, Aventín A, Soler J. Acute lymphoblastic leukemia of the Burkitt's type in a patient seropositive for the human immunodeficiency virus. Med Clin (Barc). 1987;89:527.
12. Biggar RJ, Horm J, Goedert JJ, Melbye M. Cancer in a group at risk of acquired immunodeficiency syndrome (AIDS) through 1984. Am J Epidemiol. 1987;126:578–86.
13. Berman M, Minowada J, Loew JM, Ramsey MM, Ebie N, Knospe WH. Burkitt cell acute lymphoblastic leukemia with partial expression of T-cell markers and subclonal chromosome abnormalities in a man with acquired immunodeficiency syndrome. Cancer Genet Cytogenet. 1985;16:341–7.
14. Monfardini S, Vaccher E, Pizzocaro G, Stellini R, Sinicco A, Sabbatani S, et al. Unusual malignant tumours in 49 patients with HIV infection. AIDS. 1989;3:449–52.
15. Pollock BH, Jenson HB, Leach CT, McClain KL, Hutchison RE, Garzarella L, et al. Risk factors for pediatric human immunodeficiency virus-related malignancy. JAMA. 2003;289:2393–9.
16. Granovsky MO, Mueller BU, Nicholson HS, Rosenberg PS, Rabkin CS. Cancer in human immunodeficiency virus-infected children: a case series from the Children's Cancer Group and the National Cancer Institute. J Clin Oncol. 1998;16:1729–35.
17. Moschovi M, Theodoridou M, Papaevangelou V, Tzortzatou-Stathopoulou F. Acute lymphoblastic leukaemia in an infant exposed to zidovudine in utero and early infancy. AIDS. 2000;14:2410–1.

18. Lorenzon D, Perin T, Bulian P, De Re V, Caggiari L, Michieli M, et al. Human immunodeficiency virus-associated precursor T-lymphoblastic leukemia/lymphoblastic lymphoma: report of a case and review of the literature. Hum Pathol. 2009;40:1045–9.
19. Bacci MR, Santos JA, Zing NC, Barros DM. Acute lymphocytic leukaemia and AIDS. BMJ Case Rep. 2013. doi:10.1136/bcr-2013-010036.
20. Stefan DC, Dippenaar A, De Bruin G, Uys R, van Toorn R. Challenges to treatment of leukemia in HIV-positive children. J Trop Pediatr. 2012;58:521–2.
21. Ghosh M, Banerjee M, Chakraborty S, Bhattacharyya S. Successful outcome in a HIV infected child presenting with Pre-B Acute Lymphoblastic Leukemia. Indian J Pediatr. 2012;79: 267–9.
22. Tomonari A, Takahashi S, Shimohakamada Y, Ooi J, Takasugi K, Ohno N, et al. Unrelated cord blood transplantation for a human immunodeficiency virus-1-seropositive patient with acute lymphoblastic leukemia. Bone Marrow Transplant. 2005;36:261–2.
23. Girmenia C, Gastaldi R, Martino P. Catheter-related cutaneous aspergillosis complicated by fungemia and fatal pulmonary infection in an HIV-positive patient with acute lymphocytic leukemia. Eur J Clin Microbiol Infect Dis. 1995;14:524–6.
24. Gérinière L, Bastion Y, Dumontet C, Salles G, Espinouse D, Coiffier B. Heterogeneity of acute lymphoblastic leukemia in HIV-seropositive patients. Ann Oncol. 1994;5:437–40.
25. Turner ML, Watson HG, Russell L, Langlands K, Ludlam CA, Parker AC. An HIV positive haemophiliac with acute lymphoblastic leukaemia successfully treated with intensive chemotherapy and syngeneic bone marrow transplantation. Bone Marrow Transplant. 1992;9: 387–9.
26. Batlle M, Ribera JM, Font A, Millà F. Burkitt-type acute lymphoblastic leukemia in a patient with human immunodeficiency virus infection. Sangre (Barc). 1991;36:249–50.
27. Pogliani EM, Rossini F, Pioltelli P, Lanzi E, Casaroli I, Bolis S, et al. A case of acute lymphoblastic leukemia in an anti-HIV positive patient. Allergol Immunopathol (Madr). 1991;19:103.
28. Mansberg R, Rowlings PA, Yip MY, Rozenberg MC. First and second complete remissions in a HIV positive patient following remission induction therapy for acute non-lymphoblastic leukaemia. Aust NZ J Med. 1991;21:55–7.
29. Polizzotto MN, Skinner M, Cole-Sinclair MF, Opat SS, Spencer A, Avery S. Allo-SCT for hematological malignancies in the setting of HIV. Bone Marrow Transplant. 2010;45:584–6.
30. Xicoy B, Ribera JM, Müller M, García O, Hoffmann C, Oriol A, et al. PETHEMA Group and German HIV Lymphoma Cohort. Dose-intensive chemotherapy including rituximab is highly effective but toxic in human immunodeficiency virus-infected patients with Burkitt lymphoma/leukemia: parallel study of 81 patients. Leuk Lymphoma. 2014;55:2341–8.
31. Ribera JM, García O, Grande C, Esteve J, Oriol A, Bergua J, et al. Dose-intensive chemotherapy including rituximab in Burkitt's leukemia or lymphoma regardless of human immunodeficiency virus infection status: final results of a phase 2 study (Burkimab). Cancer. 2013;119:1660–8.
32. Dunleavy K, Pittaluga S, Shovlin M, Steinberg SM, Cole D, Grant C, et al. Low-intensity therapy in adults with Burkitt's lymphoma. N Engl J Med. 2013;369:1915–25.
33. Rudek MA, Flexner C, Ambinder RF. Use of antineoplastic agents in patients with cancer who have HIV/AIDS. Lancet Oncol. 2011;12:905–12.
34. Corona G, Vaccher E, Spina M, Toffoli G. Potential hazard drug-drug interaction between boosted protease inhibitors and vinblastine in HIV patients with Hodgkin's lymphoma. AIDS. 2013;27:1033–5.
35. Deeken JF, Pantanowitz L, Dezube BJ. Targeted therapies to treat non-AIDS-defining cancers in patients with HIV on HAART therapy: treatment considerations and research outlook. Curr Opin Oncol. 2009;21:445–54.
36. Stefan DC. Effect of HIV infection on the outcome of cancer therapy in children. Lancet Oncol. 2014;15:e562–7.
37. Little RF, Dunleavy K. Update on the treatment of HIV-associated hematologic malignancies. Hematol Am Soc Educ Prog. 2013;2013:382–8.

# Autologous Stem Cell Transplantation 12

Alessandro Re, Amrita Krishnan, and Marcus Hentrich

## Contents



## 12.1 Introduction

Autologous stem cell transplantation (ASCT) is a treatment strategy that allows for the administration of higher than usual doses of myelotoxic chemotherapy and/or radiation therapy to treat several hematologic and nonhematologic malignancies. High-dose chemotherapy (HDT) with ASCT is widely performed in HIV-negative patients with Hodgkin (HL) and non-Hodgkin lymphoma (NHL) and is standard therapy for refractory and relapsed patients, based on results of phase III trials [1, 2]. It is also used as part of initial therapy for aggressive NHL, particularly in patients with

A. Re, MD (✉)
Department of Hematology, Spedali Civili, Brescia, Italy
e-mail: sandrore@aruba.it

A. Krishnan
Department of Hematology and Hematopoietic Cell Transplantation, City of Hope Medical Center, Duarte, CA, USA
e-mail: AKrishnan@coh.org

M. Hentrich
Department of Hematology and Oncology, Red Cross Hospital, University of Munich, Munich, Germany
e-mail: marcus.hentrich@swmbrk.de



M. Hentrich, S.K. Barta (eds.), *HIV-associated Hematological Malignancies*,
DOI 10.1007/978-3-319-26857-6_12

poor prognostic factors at diagnosis [3]. In earlier eras, this treatment approach has been considered prohibitive in HIV-positive patients, because of the potential toxicity and risk of worsening immune function, thereby accelerating the course of HIV infection. The introduction of combination antiretroviral therapy (cART) in the mid-1990s has led to improvement of immune function and reduced morbidity of HIV-infected patients, thus allowing more aggressive treatment strategies including HDT and ASCT in cART-treated patients [4, 5]. Moreover, the use of peripheral blood stem cells instead of bone marrow significantly shortens the time to engraftment after HDT and has helped to further reduce transplant-related morbidity and mortality [6].

## 12.2 Feasibility of HDT and ASCT in HIV-Associated Lymphomas

The high incidence of hematopoietic dysfunction in HIV-infected subjects has raised concern about the feasibility of procuring adequate numbers of hematopoietic stem cells for autologous transplantation in these patients [7]. However, antiretroviral therapy has favorable effects on hematologic reserves, and therefore, with the advent of cART, stem cell mobilization and collection in HIV-infected patients are possible [8]. A recent European retrospective study on 155 HIV-positive patients with lymphoma demonstrated that the majority of patients (73 %) were able to mobilize stem cells and that adequate CD34+ cells were collected at the first mobilization attempt to proceed to transplant. Moreover, engraftment kinetics in patients who received ASCT was comparable with the HIV-negative ASCT population [9].

The use of HDT with ASCT has been demonstrated to be feasible in several series of HIV-positive patients with NHL and HL, who had mainly refractory or relapsed disease [4, 5, 10, 11]. These series have shown a good tolerance to myeloablative chemotherapy, with regimen-related and infectious complications during the period of aplasia, similar to those seen in patients without HIV infection. The use of G-CSF as well as anti-infective prophylaxis is strongly recommended after transplant with antibacterial, antifungal, and antiviral prophylaxis with quinolones, fluconazole, and acyclovir being advisable. Trimethoprim-sulfamethoxazole is used to prevent pneumocystis jiroveci pneumonia but has to be withheld from day of stem cell infusion until engraftment due to its known hematologic toxicity. Antiretroviral therapy is usually given throughout the ASCT program, avoiding the use of zidovudine because of its potential myelosuppressive effects. However, in a minority of patients, cART has been reported to be transitorily discontinued because of gastrointestinal toxicity [12], with HIV-viral load becoming at least temporarily detectable in several patients. In these cases, cART should be reassumed as soon as possible to avoid resistance. The CD4+ cell count decreases after HDT with the nadir at approximately 3–6 months after transplantation and subsequently recovers to pretransplant levels within the first year [10, 13]. The thymus-dependent pathway of T-cell reconstitution after ASCT has been demonstrated to be as efficient as in HIV-uninfected individuals [14, 15]. Thus, the underlying HIV infection does not worsen after the transplantation procedure, at least in patients who are compliant with cART.

## 12.3 Clinical Results

Many trials have analyzed the clinical efficacy of ASCT in HIV-associated lymphoma patients not responding to or relapsing after first-line chemotherapy, for whom responses and survival are poor, complete remission rate from 10 to 26 %, and median overall survival of few months with standard-dose salvage chemotherapy [16–19].

Different preparative regimens have been used as salvage/debulking treatment before HDT (mainly platinum-containing regimens) and as conditioning preparation to ASCT (mainly BEAM: BCNU, etoposide, cytarabine, melphalan). No superiority has been demonstrated of one regimen over another even in the HIV-negative population. The results of the main series reported in literature are shown in Table 12.1 [12, 13, 20–24]. These studies showed that transplant-related mortality rates were low and that durable remissions could be obtained. After variable follow-up periods, progression-free survival (PFS) varied from 29 to 85 % and overall survival (OS) from 36 to 87 %, with excellent results in those studies that included patients in first complete remission (variously defined at "high risk"), in partial remission, and in first relapse [13, 24], while the outcome was less satisfactory in series that included patients with primary refractory and salvage-resistant disease [20]. Hence, the efficacy of ASCT in HIV-related lymphoma depends on the status of disease at the time of transplantation, as is the case in HIV-negative patients. The best results are achieved in patients who have minimal disease before the transplant, as reported in a multicenter trial from 20 centers in Europe. In this study, that enrolled 68 patients, a subgroup analysis found that patients not in complete remission or with refractory disease at the time of transplant had a poorer progression-free survival [12]. However, the reported studies on ASCT in HIV-positive patients were mainly retrospective [12, 20] or recruited patients at the time of stem cell collection [11, 13, 22, 24], thus rendering it difficult to understand the real impact of the procedure on the whole population of relapsing/refractory patients who need salvage. Instead, in the Italian study [21], patients were recruited at the time of treatment failure or relapse; 54 % of the entire series of 50 patients were able to proceed to ASCT, a percentage comparable to the HIV-negative population, with satisfactory results in patients receiving transplantation (overall survival 74.6 %) as well as in the entire series, with 49.8 % of patients alive after a median follow-up of 45 months (9–86 months) (Fig. 12.1).

> Response to cART and absence of active opportunistic infections remain essential for the success of ASCT and patient selection is necessary. Moreover, in the Italian study low CD4+ cell count was an adverse prognostic factor regarding the ability of patients to receive a transplant, mainly due to early disease progression and poor stem cell mobilization. [21]

Another potential bias of the studies in this setting is that the reported series include patients with varied histologies, the majority had diffuse large B-cell lymphoma, but also included were Burkitt, plasmablastic, and anaplastic lymphoma and even HL. Indeed, HL in the HIV setting can have aggressive features that are similar to HIV-associated NHL [25], and ASCT remains the standard treatment for relapse/refractory HIV-negative patients with HL. The preliminary experiences of

**Table 12.1** Transplant experience in HIV-positive patients with lymphoma

| Reference | N total ASCT (NHL/HL) | Age (range) | Disease status before salvage therapy (n pts) | Disease status at transplant (n pts) | Conditioning regimen (n pts) | PFS | OS | Follow-up |
|---|---|---|---|---|---|---|---|---|
| Gabarre et al. [20] | 14 (8/6) | 37 years (27–53) | Rel 1 (9)<br>Rel >1 (3)<br>Ref (2) | CR (8)<br>PR (3)<br>Ref (3) | BEAM (5)<br>Bu/Ara-C/Mel (1)<br>TBI-based (8) | 29 % | 36 % | 32 ms (14–49) |
| Krishnan et al. [13] | 20 (18/2) | 44 years (11–68) | Rel 1 (7)<br>Rel >1 (2)<br>PR (5)<br>CR >1 (2)<br>hrCR 1 (4) | CS (16)<br>hrCR 1[a] (4) | CBV (28)<br>TBI/Cy/Eto (4) | 85 % | 85 % | 32 ms (6–70) |
| Re et al. [21] | 27 (19/8) | 39 years (31–59) | Rel 1 (12)<br>Rel >1 (3)<br>Ref (11)<br>PR (1) | CS (26)]<br>PR (1) | BEAM | 76 % | 75 % | 44 ms (4–70) |
| Serrano et al. [24] | 33 (23/10) | 39 years (31–61) | hrCR 1, Rel, Ref | hrCR 1[a] (14)<br>CR >1 (10)<br>PR (9) | BEAM (27)<br>BEAC (3)<br>TBI-based (3) | 53 % | 61 % | 61 ms |
| Balsalobre et al. [12] | 68 (50/18) | 41 years (29–62) | NR | CR 1 (16)<br>CS (44)<br>Ref (8) | BEAM and variants (65)<br>TBI-based (3) | 56 % | 61 % | 32 ms (2–81) |
| Spitzer et al. [22] | 20 (15/5) | 42 years (33–60) | Rel, Ref | CR (6)<br>PR (2)<br>CS (12) | Dose reduced BU/Cy | 49 % | 74 % | 6 ms (1–30) |
| Alvarnas J et al. [23] | 40 (25/15) | 47 years (22–62) | Rel, Ref | CR (30)<br>PR (8)<br>Rel/Progr (2) | BEAM | 82 % at 1 year | 87 % at 1 year | 24 ms |

*NR* not reported, *Rel* relapse, *Ref* refractory disease, *CR* complete remission, *hrCR* high-risk CR, *PR* partial remission, *CS* chemosensitive disease, *TBI* total body irradiation, *Cy* cyclophosphamide, *Mel* melphalan, *Bu* busulfan, *Ara-C* cytarabine, *BEAM/C* (BNCU, etoposide, cytarabine, melphalan/cyclophosphamide), *CBV* (cyclophosphamide, BNCU, etoposide)

[a]These patients received transplant as frontline consolidation for CR defined at high risk (high IPI, 2 treatment lines to achieve CR, undertreated Burkitt lymphoma)

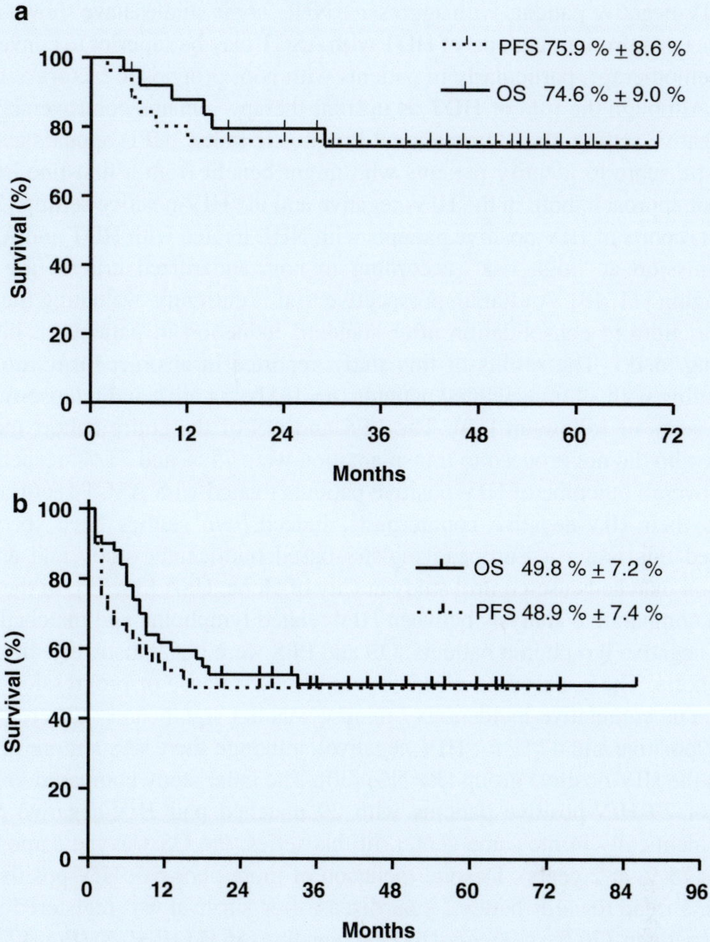


**Fig. 12.1** (**a**) Overall survival and progression-free survival of 27 patients with HIV-related lymphoma after ASCT (Ref. [21]). (**b**) Overall survival and progression-free survival of the entire series of 50 patients with HIV-related lymphoma eligible for the study (Ref. [21])

ASCT in plasmablastic lymphoma in the HIV-positive setting appear promising [26] in both upfront treatment and for relapsed patients. However, NHL histologies other than diffuse large B-cell lymphoma proved to be an adverse prognostic factor on multivariate analysis in a European multicenter series [12]. Furthermore, Burkitt lymphoma is currently treated with specific intensive treatment programs without ASCT, both in the HIV-positive and in the HIV-negative population, and the role of ASCT remains unclear. Future studies evaluating ASCT should be designed for specific histologic entities. Larger studies would also provide more insight into various parameters that may play an important role in influencing outcome, such as type of cART, CD4 cell count, HIV-viral load before ASCT, EBV status, and tumor histogenesis.

In HIV-negative patients with aggressive NHL, some studies have shown that the early use (as upfront treatment) of HDT with ASCT may be superior to conventional dose chemotherapy, particularly in patients with poor prognostic factors at diagnosis [3]. Although the role of HDT as upfront therapy remains controversial in the HIV-negative setting, the "International Prognostic Index" (IPI) appears a suitable prognostic score to identify patients who might benefit from a first-line intensive treatment approach, both in the HIV-negative and the HIV-positive setting [27, 28]. The first reports of HIV-positive patients with NHL treated with HDT and ASCT in first remission at "high risk" according to nonstandardized criteria are highly encouraging [11, 13]. An Italian prospective trial is currently evaluating the role of ASCT as upfront consolidation after standard induction in patients at high risk according to IPI. The results of this study, reported in abstract form, are highly encouraging with all transplanted patients ($n = 14$) being alive and relapse-free after several years of follow-up [29]. The PFS and OS of the entire cohort including patients who did not proceed to transplantation were 75 % and 71 %, respectively.

The overall outcome of HIV-positive patients treated with ASCT seems comparable to their HIV-negative counterparts. Indeed, two studies have specifically addressed this issue, a European registry-based multicenter study and a single-institution matched case-control study at City of Hope, USA [30, 31]. In the former study, a comparative analysis between HIV-related lymphoma and matched cohort of HIV-negative lymphoma patients, OS and PFS were not statistically different in both cohorts. The main cause of death was disease relapse or progression in both groups. The cumulative incidence of relapse was not significantly different (29 % for HIV positive and 42 % for HIV negative), although there was a more favorable trend in the HIV-positive group ($P = \text{NS}$) [30]. The latter study compared long-term results of 29 HIV-positive patients with 29 matched pair HIV-negative patients treated identically in the same center. In this series, the OS was the same in both cohorts (75 % at 2 years). Despite inclusion of more poor-risk HIV-positive NHL patients, a trend towards better 2-year disease-free survival was registered in HIV-positive patients (76 %) compared to HIV negative (56 %) ($P = 0.3$) (Fig. 12.2). The only factor predictive of outcome was disease status at transplant [31].

## 12.4 Toxicity and Antiretroviral Therapy

Several studies on ASCT in patients with relapsed malignant lymphoma have shown that HIV-infected patients experience more infectious complications than patients without HIV. However, this did not translate into a significant difference in non-relapse mortality (NRM) and survival. In the EBMT study [30], the overall cumulative incidence of NRM was reported to be 8 % in HIV-positive lymphoma patients, mainly because of bacterial infections, and 2 % in HIV-negative controls ($P = 0.2$). Age more than 50 years at ASCT was the only independent adverse prognostic factor for NRM found in the multivariate analysis (relative risk 4.5, $P = 0.04$) [30]. Likewise, in the matched control study from City of Hope, NRM was not statistically different between HIV-infected NHL patients (11 %) and HIV-negative NHL

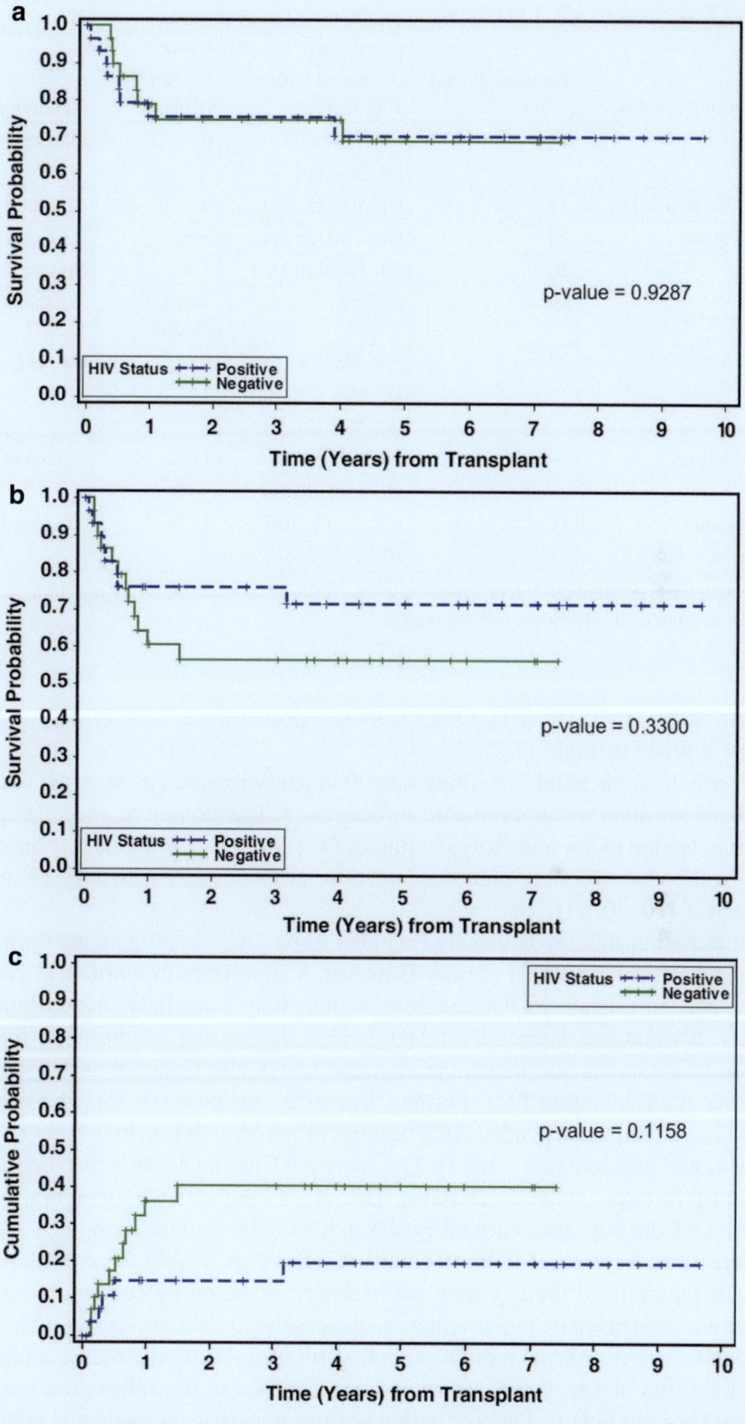


**Fig. 12.2** (**a**) Probability of overall survival by HIV status (Adapted from Ref. [31]). (**b**) Probability of disease-free survival by HIV status. (**c**) Cumulative probability of relapse/progression (**a**–**c**, Adapted from Krishnan et al. [31]. Reprint permission obtained from Elsevier)

**Table 12.2** Toxicity of ASCT in HIV-positive patients with lymphoma

| Study group/country | Pts transplanted (*N*) | Grade 3/4 infections within 100 days | NRM (95 % CI) (n pts) | Reference |
|---|---|---|---|---|
| France | 14 | FN: 1/14 (7 %) | 0 | Gabarre [20] |
| | | OI: 2/14 (14 %) | | |
| GELTAMO/GESIDA | 11 | DI: 8/14 (57 %) | 0 | Serrano [11] |
| City of Hope | 20 | OI: 7/20 (35 %) | 5 % | Krishnan [13] |
| AMC | 20 | DI: 12/20 (60 %) | 5 % | Spitzer [22] |
| EBMT | 69 | NR | 7.6 % (3–20) | Balsalobre [12] |
| Italy | 27 | FN: 9/27 (33 %) | 0 | Re [21] |
| | | DI: 6/27 (22 %) | | |
| | | OI: 3/27 (11 %) | | |
| City of Hope | 29 | 16/29 (55 %) | 11 % (1–20) | Krishnan [31] |
| | | OI: 5/29 (17 %) | | |
| Weill Cornell New York | 12 | FN: 12/12 (100 %) BI: 3/12 (25 %) | 33 % | Morawa [37] |

*NRM* non-relapse mortality, *FN* febrile neutropenia, *BI* bacterial infections, *OI* opportunistic infections, *DI* documented infections, *NR* not reported

controls (4 %) ($P=0.18$) [31]. Other studies reported lower or even higher NRM rates as outlined in Table 12.2.

Nevertheless, bacterial infections were frequently reported as were HIV-related complications such as opportunistic infections or, less common, encephalopathy. This may be due to the transitory decline of the post-ASCT immune response with CD4+ cell counts reaching pretransplantation levels not earlier than 6–12 months after ASCT [10, 20, 21].

Antiretroviral therapy is usually intended to be given to all patients during the pre- and posttransplantation period. However, a significant proportion of patients are not able to tolerate it. For example, in the study from Italy that included 50 patients, two patients suspended cART before starting the conditioning regimen because of cytopenia and hepatotoxicity, and cART was restarted at day +20 and +75 after transplantation [21]. Further, five of 27 patients (19 %) who received BEAM conditioning suspended ART because of intolerance resulting from mucositis ($n=4$) and hepatotoxicity ($n=1$). The same ART regimens were restarted after a median of 16 days (range, 5–28 days). Of note, all patients who temporarily suspended ART did not experience an excess in infectious complication [21].

Interactions between cytotoxics and antiretrovirals should be considered, as chemotherapy-related toxicity may be markedly increased by concomitant use of antiretrovirals. This may, in particular, be the case with antiretroviral combinations that include strong enzyme inhibitors such as ritonavir-boosted protease inhibitors.

Reactivation of hepatitis C virus as a consequence of transplantation has been reported very rarely [13]. Patients with a positive anti-HBc antibody test who were positive for HBV-DNA received appropriate prophylaxis, such as lamivudine or tenofovir, as part of their cART in order to effectively prevent HBV reactivation.

The risk of hepatic veno-occlusive disease (VOD) does not seem to be increased in HIV-positive patients undergoing ASCT with only one case of fatal VOD being reported in the available literature so far [22].

## 12.5 Genetic Manipulation of Stem Cells as Attempt to Eliminate the HIV Reservoir

Many trials have explored the role of autologous hematopoietic stem cell transplantation for HIV-associated lymphoma. Beyond this, the cure of HIV infection remains the ultimate goal of hematopoietic stem cell therapy. This has been achieved with the use of allogeneic stem cell transplantation from a donor genetically resistant to HIV-1 into an AIDS patient with acute myelogenous leukemia. The unrelated donor was homozygous for a 32-base-pair deletion in the chemokine receptor 5 gene (CCR5Δ32/Δ32). Individuals who are homozygous at this locus do not express CCR5 on their cell surface and therefore cannot be infected with CCR5 (R5) tropic HIV-1 [32]. The donor cells were infused after fully ablative conditioning, and the recipient attained complete donor chimerism. Antiretrovirals were suspended early after transplant, and the patient remains with undetectable HIV-1 RNA in blood and undetectable HIV-1 DNA in tissues using single-copy-sensitive PCR methods for more than 7 years after treatment [33]. The rarity of this gene mutation as well as the inherent higher risk of allogeneic stem cell transplantation compared with autologous transplantation limits the widespread applicability of this approach.

Genetic modification of autologous hematopoietic cells circumvents both these issues. A pilot trial at City of Hope treated four relapsed HIV-1 positive NHL patients with stem cells transduced with a lentivirus encoding three anti-HIV-1 RNAs, namely, TAR, siRNA to tat/rev, and a ribozyme targeting CCR5 [34]. Low levels of gene marking were seen (0.35 %), but importantly durability of engraftment was also demonstrated. The low level marking may be in part due to competition with the unmodified stem cells that were concomitantly infused as well as to the total cell dose infused. Likely future success is contingent upon high levels of only genetically modified stem cells being infused or selection of the protected cells after engraftment.

Several new trials are following this approach by infusing only transduced cells and suspending antiretroviral therapy as a method of positive pressure selection. In addition, new conditioning regimens are being utilized. Initial trials used fully ablative conditioning as a treatment for lymphoma. New trials are selecting patients with lymphoma in remission who do not need myeloablative doses of chemotherapy. Genetically modified cells will be infused after completion of frontline lymphoma therapy such as EPOCH or after low-dose busulfan to facilitate engraftment. Clinical trials in human genetic diseases, especially in the pediatric populations using solely gene-modified stem cells, have provided guidance on the use of busulfan-based regimens. Candotti et al. correlated busulfan dosing with area under the curve [AUC] measurements demonstrating doses ranging from 65 to 90 mg/m$^2$ [equivalent to ~4 mg/kg] achieved an AUC in the range of 4000–4800 mU*min which was associated with engraftment [35].

New methods of genetic modification are also under study. Of particular interest is the use of zinc finger nucleases (ZFN) for CCR5 knockout. The zinc finger nuclease construct has already been successfully tested with autologous T lymphocytes [36]. T lymphocytes are attractive targets for gene therapy in that they are easily obtained from the donor's peripheral blood, and they can be expanded to large numbers in vitro. Targeting mature T lymphocytes has the added advantage that the effect of the therapeutic gene can be rapidly monitored for effects on cell survival and HIV-viral loads. The first T-cell trial with zinc fingers included 12 patients who had chronic aviremic HIV-1 infection. No conditioning was used prior to infusion of the CCR5-negative ZFN-edited T-cell product. Patients in cohort 1 ($n=6$) underwent a 12-week analytic treatment interruption (ATI) of antiretrovirals beginning 4 weeks after the T-cell infusion. HIV-1 viral load was undetectable at the start of ATI and became detectable in four of the six patients at 2–4 weeks after cessation of cART. There was a decline of CD4 counts during ATI, but this decline in CCR5-modified cells (1.81 cells/day) was significantly less than unmodified cells (7.25 cells/day) suggestive of a selective advantage to the modified cells. This set the platform to the use of ZFN editing for hematopoietic cell therapy. Future trials will apply this to CD34+ selected hematopoietic cells in conjunction with busulfan-based conditioning to facilitate engraftment.

**Conclusions**

In conclusion, given the beneficial effects of cART, HIV infection should not preclude lymphoma patients from undergoing ASCT. The same eligibility criteria as established for HIV-negative lymphoma patients should be adopted for patients with HIV. However, special attention should be paid to infection prophylaxis and to the immune recovery surveillance during and after ASCT, respectively. Beyond this, manipulation of autologous stem cells by genetic modification may provide a platform towards the goal of ultimately eliminating the HIV reservoir in the future.

## References

1. Philip T, Giglielmi C, Hagenbeek A, et al. Autologous bone marrow transplantation as compared with salvage chemotherapy in relapses of chemotherapy-sensitive non-Hodgkin's lymphoma. N Engl J Med. 1995;333:1540–5.
2. Linch DC, Winfield D, Goldstone AH, et al. Dose intensification with autologous bone marrow transplantation in relapsed and resistant Hodgkin's disease. Lancet. 1993;341:1051–4.
3. Milpied N, Deconinck E, Gaillard F, et al. Initial treatment of aggressive lymphoma with high-dose chemotherapy and autologous stem-cell support. N Engl J Med. 2004;350:1287–95.
4. Gabarre J, Azar N, Autran B, et al. High-dose therapy and autologous haematopoietic stem-cell transplantation for HIV-1-associated lymphoma. Lancet. 2000;355:1071–2.
5. Krishnan A, Molina A, Zaia J, et al. Autologous stem cell transplantation for HIV associated lymphoma. Blood. 2001;98:3857–9.

6. Schmitz N, Linch DC, Dreger P, et al. Randomised trial of filgrastim-mobilised peripheral blood progenitor cell transplantation versus autologous bone-marrow transplantation in lymphoma patients. Lancet. 1996;347:353–7.
7. Moses A, Nelson J, Bagby GC. The influence of human immunodeficiency virus-1 on hematopoiesis. Blood. 1998;91:1479–95.
8. Huang SS, Barobour JD, Deeks SG, et al. Reversal of human immunodeficiency virus type 1 associated hematosuppression by effective antiretroviral therapy. Clin Infect Dis. 2000;30:504–10.
9. Re A, Cattaneo C, Skert C, et al. Stem cell mobilization in HIV seropositive patients with lymphoma. Haematologica. 2013;98:1762–8.
10. Re A, Cattaneo C, Michieli M, et al. High-dose therapy and autologous peripheral-blood stem-cell transplantation as salvage treatment for HIV-associated lymphoma in patients receiving highly active antiretroviral therapy. J Clin Oncol. 2003;21:4423–7.
11. Serrano D, Carrion R, Balsalobre P, et al. HIV-associated lymphoma successfully treated with peripheral blood stem cell transplantation. Exp Hematol. 2005;3:487–94.
12. Balsalobre P, Diez-Martin JL, Re A, et al. Autologous stem-cell transplantation in patients with HIV-related lymphoma. J Clin Oncol. 2009;27:2192–8.
13. Krishnan A, Molina A, Zaia J, et al. Durable remissions with autologous stem cell transplantation for high risk HIV-associated lymphomas. Blood. 2005;105:874–8.
14. Resino S, Perez A, Seoane E, et al. Short communication: immune reconstitution after autologous peripheral blood stem cell transplantation in HIV-infected patients: might be better than expected? AIDS Res Hum Retroviruses. 2007;23:543–8.
15. Simonelli C, Zanussi S, Pratesi C, et al. Immune recovery after autologous stem cell transplantation is not different for HIV-infected versus HIV-uninfected patients with relapsed or refractory lymphoma. Clin Infect Dis. 2010;50:1672–9.
16. Tirelli U, Errante D, Spina M, et al. Second-line chemotherapy in human immunodeficiency virus-related non-Hodgkin's lymphoma. Evidence of activity of a combination of etoposide, mitoxantrone, and prednimustine in relapsed patients. Cancer. 1996;77:2127–31.
17. Levine AM, Tulpule A, Tessman D, et al. Mitoguazone therapy in patients with refractory or relapsed AIDS-related lymphoma: results from a multicenter phase II trial. J Clin Oncol. 1997;15:1094–103.
18. Spina M, Vaccher E, Juzbasic S, et al. Human immunodeficiency virus-related non-Hodgkin lymphoma. Activity of infusional cyclophosphamide, doxorubicin, and etoposide as second-line chemotherapy in 40 patients. Cancer. 2001;92:200–6.
19. Bi J, Espina BM, Tulpule A, et al. High-dose cytosine-arabinoside and cisplatin regimens as salvage therapy for refractory or relapsed AIDS-related non-Hodgkin's lymphoma. J Acquir Immune Defic Syndr. 2001;28:416–21.
20. Gabarre J, Marcelin AG, Azar N, et al. High dose therapy plus autologous hematopoietic stem cell transplantation for human immunodeficiency virus (HIV)-related lymphoma: results and impact on HIV disease. Haematologica. 2004;89:1100–8.
21. Re A, Michieli M, Casari S, et al. High-dose therapy and autologous peripheral blood stem cell transplantation as salvage treatment for AIDS-related lymphoma: long-term results of the Italian Cooperative Group on AIDS and tumors (GICAT) study with analysis of prognostic factors. Blood. 2009;114:1306–13.
22. Spitzer TR, Ambinder RF, Lee JY, et al. Dose-reduced busulfan, cyclophosphamide, and autologous stem cell transplantation for human immunodeficiency virus-associated lymphoma: AIDS malignancy consortium study 020. Biol Blood Marrow Transplant. 2008;14:59–66.
23. Alvarnas J, Rademacher K, Wang Y, et al. Autologous hematopoietic stem cell transplantation for chemotherapy sensitive relapsed/refractory HIV associated lymphoma. Results from the blood and marrow clinical trials network. BMT CTN0803/AIDS malignancy consortium AMC 071 trial. Blood 2014;abstr. 674.
24. Serrano D, Miralles P, Carrion R, et al. Long-term follow-up of autologous stem cell transplant in AIDS-related lymphoma patients. Results of Spanish Cooperative Registry GELTAMO/GESIDA. Bone Marrow Transplant. 2010;45:abstr. 822.

25. Re A, Casari S, Cattaneo C, et al. Hodgkin disease developing in patients infected by human immunodeficiency virus results in clinical features and a prognosis similar to those in patients with human immunodeficiency virus-related non-Hodgkin lymphoma. Cancer. 2001;92:2739–45.
26. Al-Malki MM, Castillo JJ, Sloan JM, Re A. Hematopoietic cell transplantation for plasmablastic lymphoma: a review. Biol Blood Marrow Transplant. 2014;20:1877–84.
27. The International Non-Hodgkin's Lymphoma Prognostic Factors Project. A predictive model for aggressive non-Hodgkin's lymphoma. N Engl J Med. 1993;329:987–94.
28. Rossi G, Donisi A, Casari S, et al. The international prognostic index can be used as a guide to treatment decisions regarding patients with human immunodeficiency virus-related systemic non-Hodgkin lymphoma. Cancer. 1999;86:2391–7.
29. Re A, Cattaneo C, Casari S, et al. Early consolidation with high dose therapy and autologous stem cell transplantation in HIV-associated non Hodgkin lymphoma at high risk (aa-IPI 2-3). Mature results of a multicenter prospective Phase II trial. Blood. 2014;abstr. 2528.
30. Diez-Martin JL, Balsalobre P, Re A, et al. Comparable survival between HIV+ and HIV- non-Hodgkin and Hodgkin lymphoma patients undergoing autologous peripheral blood stem cell transplantation. European group for blood and marrow transplant. Blood. 2009;113:6011–4.
31. Krishnan A, Palmer JM, Zaia JA, Tsai NC, Alvarnas J. HIV status does not affect the outcome of autologous stem cell transplantation (ASCT) for non-Hodgkin lymphoma (NHL). Biol Blood Marrow Transplant. 2010;16:1302–8.
32. Liu R, Paxton WA, Choe S, et al. Homozygous defect in HIV-1 coreceptor accounts for resistance of some multiply-exposed individuals to HIV-1 infection. Cell. 1996;86:367–77.
33. Allers K, Hutter G, Hofmann J, et al. Evidence for the cure of HIV infection by CCR5{Delta}32/{Delta}32 stem cell transplantation. Blood. 2011;117:2791–9.
34. DiGiusto DL, Krishnan A, Li L, et al. RNA-based gene therapy for HIV with lentiviral vector-modified CD34(+) cells in patients undergoing transplantation for AIDS-related lymphoma. Sci Transl Med. 2010;2:1–8.
35. Candotti F, Shaw KL, Muul L, et al. Gene therapy for adenosine deaminase-deficient severe combined immune deficiency: clinical comparison of retroviral vectors and treatment plans. Blood. 2012;120:3635–46.
36. Tebas P, Stein D, Tang WW, et al. Gene editing of CCR5 in autologous CD4 T cells of persons infected with HIV. N Engl J Med. 2014;370:901–10.
37. Morawa E, Martin P, Gergis U, et al. Autologous stem cell transplant in human immunodeficiency virus-positive patients with lymphoid malignancies: focus on infectious complications. Leuk Lymphoma. 2013;54:885–8.

# Allogeneic Stem Cell Transplantation 13

Richard F. Ambinder, Jennifer A. Kanakry,
and Christine Durand

## Contents



## 13.1 AlloBMT in Medicine

Allogeneic bone marrow or hematopoietic stem cell transplantation hereafter referred to as alloBMT is used for the treatment for a variety of malignant hematologic malignancies, especially acute leukemia and lymphoma. Infusion of marrow or hematopoietic stem cells is preceded by a preparative regimen of chemotherapy (and sometimes radiation therapy). When host hematopoiesis is

R.F. Ambinder, MD (✉)
Department of Oncology, Johns Hopkins School of Medicine, Baltimore, MD 21287, USA
e-mail: Rambind1@jhmi.edu

J.A. Kanakry
National Institutes of Health, 10 Center Drive, Building 10/CRC – Rm 4-3132, Bethesda, MD 20892, USA
e-mail: jenkanakry@jhmi.edu

C. Durand
Department of Medicine, Johns Hopkins School of Medicine, Baltimore, MD 21213, USA
e-mail: cdurand2@jhmi.edu



M. Hentrich, S.K. Barta (eds.), *HIV-associated Hematological Malignancies*,
DOI 10.1007/978-3-319-26857-6_13

completely replaced by donor hematopoiesis, it is said that the patient is a complete chimera. Establishment of donor hematopoiesis was originally developed to rescue patients after high-dose cytotoxic therapy for the treatment of malignancy, for the treatment of aplastic anemia, and for the treatment of hemoglobinopathy. With time it was appreciated that in addition to providing a source of hematopoietic stem cells, alloBMT was associated with graft-versus-tumor effects that often helped in the control of hematologic malignancies. This led to the development of transplant strategies for malignancy that focused on preparative regimens that were just sufficient for engraftment of donor cells so as to engender a graft-versus-tumor effect rather than as a method for delivering maximally tolerated cytotoxic therapy. These preparative regimens are known as reduced-dose or non-myeloablative regimens.

## 13.2 Indications for AlloBMT in Patients with HIV

Among the standard indications for alloBMT are acute leukemias and relapsed or primary refractory non-Hodgkin and Hodgkin lymphomas. Although there are some reports that the incidence of acute leukemias may be modestly increased in patients with HIV, the increase if it exists is small [18]. In contrast the incidences of aggressive lymphomas are substantially increased. For AIDS-defining lymphoma types, the standardized incidence ratios are 17-fold increased [3]. Whereas the incidence of primary central nervous system lymphoma has fallen dramatically since the introduction of effective antiretroviral therapy, the incidence of some other lymphoma types such as Burkitt or Hodgkin lymphomas has not been affected by antiretroviral therapy.

## 13.3 Early Experience with AlloBMT in Patients with HIV

Early in the HIV epidemic when it came to be appreciated that CD4+ T cells were the major locus of infection, BMT investigators at Johns Hopkins treating a patient with AIDS lymphoma hypothesized that with the use of zidovudine (the only available antiretroviral at the time), it might be possible to eradicate HIV in parallel with treating the lymphoma [9]. Although the patient's lymphoma relapsed shortly after alloBMT, posttransplant and autopsy studies showed no evidence of HIV (within the limits of detection at the time). Although several more transplants followed, there were no long-term survivors. The use of alloBMT in HIV patients with hematologic malignancies or other indications for transplant was largely abandoned. There was a parallel retreat in the use of aggressive chemotherapy regimens for the upfront treatment of AIDS lymphoma with the demonstration that any benefits in terms of lymphoma control were counterbalanced by the high rates of death associated with opportunistic infections [11].

## 13.4 Improvements in HIV Care

As the management of HIV improved with prophylaxis for opportunistic infections, use of growth factors, and more effective antiretroviral therapy, the outcomes of lymphoma treatment in AIDS patients improved [15, 19]. Many investigators and groups reported success with high-dose therapy with autologous stem cell rescue [12, 16, 20]. This culminated in a trial sponsored by the Bone Marrow Transplant Clinical Trials Network and the AIDS Malignancy Consortium that demonstrated disease-free survival results similar to those achieved in patients with similar malignancies but without HIV.

AlloBMT was also explored [4, 17, 22]. Patients with lymphoma, acute and chronic leukemia, and aplastic anemia underwent alloBMT. Many of the reported transplants involved myeloablative regimens, but an increasing number of reports include patients treated with non-myeloablative regimens [5]. Cord blood was also used as a stem cell source [17]. These reports concluded that alloBMT had a role in the management of HIV patients with standard indications for transplant.

## 13.5 HIV Cure by AlloBMT

AlloBMT results in reconstitution of an immune system that is donor derived, including $CD4^+$ T cells. For over 50 years, alloBMT has successfully been employed as a curative procedure for patients with nonmalignant diseases of the immune system, such as congenital T-cell immunodeficiencies. AlloBMT has the potential to likewise cure *acquired* diseases of T cells, including HIV. Preventing HIV infection of donor cells after alloBMT is an area of active research. Furthermore, given the risks of alloBMT and the availability of other effective, albeit non-curative, therapies, alloBMT for HIV remains at present restricted to those patients who have another indication for transplant, such as a hematologic malignancy.

In Berlin a patient with acute myeloid leukemia was in need of alloBMT [10]. Lacking a related sibling donor, a search of the unrelated donor registries identified many potential matched donors. The astute team caring for the patient screened potential donors for the presence of a CCR5delta32 homozygous polymorphism (Fig. 13.1). Individuals who were homozygous for such mutations had been recognized as being resistant to HIV infection. A donor was identified, myeloablative alloBMT carried out, and antiretroviral therapy stopped. The patient had a complicated course with AML relapse successfully treated with re-induction chemotherapy and second alloBMT. Extensive blood and tissue samplings including gut and brain biopsy have not identified replication-competent HIV [1]. The patient remains alive and apparently HIV-free to date. Although the report attracted a great deal of attention, no subsequent successful matched alloBMT cases with CCR5delta32 homozygous donors have been reported. The CCR5delta32 polymorphism occurs only among Caucasians, and the frequency of homozygosity is approximately 1 %. The chances of finding an HLA-matched donor who is also homozygous for the

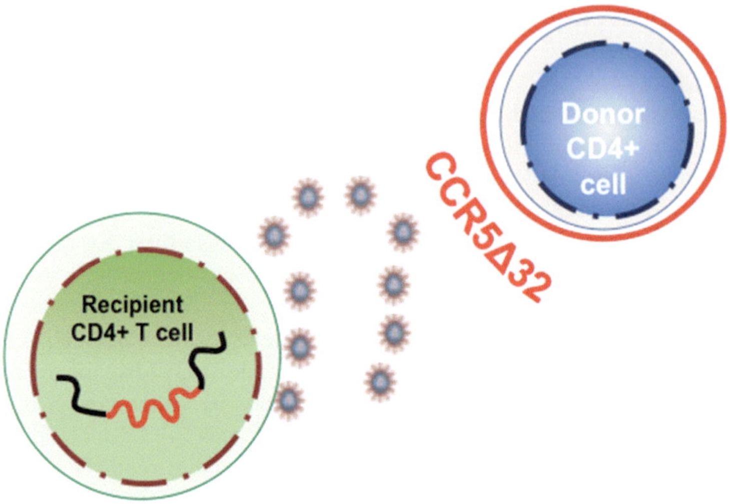


**Fig. 13.1** HIV-resistant donor cells. The "Berlin patient" was cured of HIV with the use of a CCR5delta32 homozygous donor whose cells were resistant to HIV infection

HIV-resistance polymorphism are modest in Caucasian patients and virtually negligible in other groups.

A similar strategy has been envisioned using cord blood banks [14]. Several banks have been screened to identify patients with CCR5delta32 homozygous donors. Because cord blood transplants have not required full HLA matching, identifying appropriate HIV-resistant cord blood units may be easier than identifying matched unrelated HIV-resistant bone marrow donors.

## 13.6 Allotransplantation with Antiretroviral Therapy

In principle, it might also be possible to cure HIV patients of their chronic viral infection with alloBMT if antiretroviral therapy were maintained throughout the peritransplant period [6, 8]. If the only long-term reservoir of HIV is in host resting CD4 cells and antiretroviral therapy protects donor cells from infection, then as donor hematopoietic cells replace host hematopoietic cells, the long-term reservoir should be abolished (Fig. 13.2). Indeed a report from Boston of two individuals who were maintained on antiretroviral therapy indicated that no HIV could be detected several years post-transplant [7]. However, when antiretroviral therapy was discontinued, both patients developed symptomatic HIV rebound, one with HIV meningoencephalitis. Features of rebound were in some ways similar to HIV primary infection syndromes, and it was noted that T-cell response in the donor immune systems was HIV naïve. There are other reports of patients in whom antiretroviral therapy was maintained throughout the transplant period and where HIV immune responses ultimately developed in donor T cells [22]. Concerns with the possibility of symptomatic HIV rebound suggest the

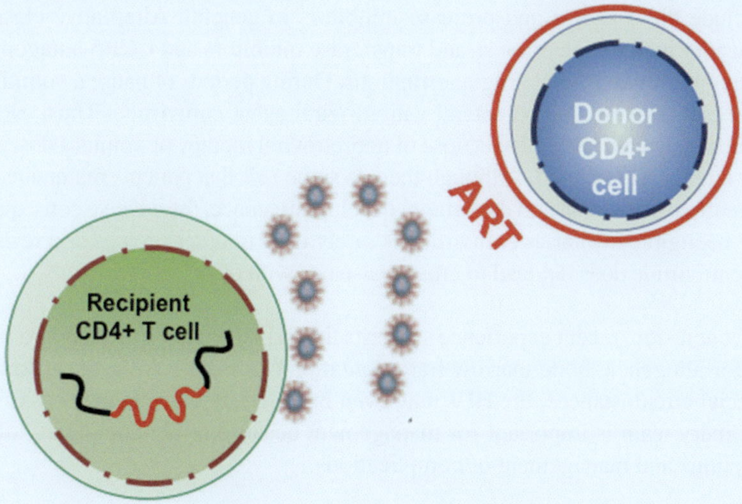


**Fig. 13.2** Antiretroviral protection of donor cells. In principle, antiretroviral therapy may protect donor cells from being infected by HIV in the allogeneic bone marrow transplant process

need for especially close monitoring of patients whose antiretroviral regimen may be interrupted because of noncompliance or other circumstances.

Experience with organ transplantation in HIV patients is also encouraging. Renal and liver transplantation in HIV patients have yielded good results [2, 21]. There is also experience using HIV seropositive kidney donors [13].

## 13.7 Present Status of Allogeneic Bone Marrow Transplantation in Patients with HIV

With increasing acceptance of a role for alloBMT in patients with HIV and hematologic malignancies or other conditions treated with allogeneic transplant, there are some special considerations in management. First it is essential to have a multidisciplinary patient care team with expertise in antiretroviral therapy as well as alloBMT. While some might argue in favor of stopping ART during transplant, with the prolonged immunocompromise that accompanies alloBMT, and evidence that the long-term HIV reservoir can be markedly reduced with continued antiretroviral coverage, we believe that patients will benefit from maintenance antiretroviral therapy throughout the transplant process.

We have identified two special considerations:

1. Minimize drug-drug interactions. Many of the agents used in HIV treatment regimens such as ritonavir and cobicistat are used specifically because they inhibit metabolism of protease inhibitors. They also inhibit and prolong the half-life of immunosuppressive agents and antifungal agents. The ideal regimen will

exclude these agents and protease inhibitors in general. Alternative classes to consider include integrase strand transferase inhibitors and CCR5 antagonists.
2. Minimize antiretroviral drug interruptions. During periods of nausea, vomiting, or mucositis, we use the parenteral antiretroviral agent enfuvirtide. Thus, even if a patient is unable to swallow a dose of antiretroviral therapy or vomits a dose, some coverage is maintained. Although there is some risk that patients maintained only on enfuvirtide for several days might develop resistance, the adverse consequences are negligible insofar as enfuvirtide is rarely used in other settings and resistance to enfuvirtide does not lead to cross-resistance with other antiretrovirals.

In conclusion, recent experience suggests that HIV patients with standard indications for allogeneic bone marrow transplantation can benefit from transplantation. In special circumstances, the HIV may even be cured by transplantation. An interdisciplinary team is important for management because of the complexity of drug interactions and management of complications.

## References

1. Allers K, Hutter G, Hofmann J, Loddenkemper C, Rieger K, Thiel E, Schneider T. Evidence for the cure of HIV infection by CCR5Delta32/Delta32 stem cell transplantation. Blood. 2011;117(10):2791–9. doi:10.1182/blood-2010-09-309591.
2. Cooper C, Kanters S, Klein M, Chaudhury P, Marotta P, Wong P, Kneteman N, Mills EJ. Liver transplant outcomes in HIV-infected patients: a systematic review and meta-analysis with synthetic cohort. AIDS. 2011;25(6):777–86. doi:10.1097/QAD.0b013e328344febb.
3. Gibson TM, Morton LM, Shiels MS, Clarke CA, Engels EA. Risk of non-Hodgkin lymphoma subtypes in HIV-infected people during the HAART era: a population-based study. AIDS. 2014;28(15):2313–8. doi:10.1097/QAD.0000000000000428.
4. Gupta V, Tomblyn M, Pedersen TL, Atkins HL, Battiwalla M, Gress RE, Pollack MS, Storek J, Thompson JC, Tiberghien P, Young JA, Ribaud P, Horowitz MM, Keating A. Allogeneic hematopoietic cell transplantation in human immunodeficiency virus-positive patients with hematologic disorders: a report from the center for international blood and marrow transplant research. Biol Blood Marrow Transplant J Am Soc Blood Marrow Transplant. 2009;15(7):864–71. doi:10.1016/j.bbmt.2009.03.023.
5. Hamadani M, Devine SM. Reduced-intensity conditioning allogeneic stem cell transplantation in HIV patients with hematologic malignancies: yes, we can. Blood. 2009;114(12):2564–6. doi:10.1182/blood-2009-06-229666.
6. Henrich TJ, Gandhi RT. Early treatment and HIV-1 reservoirs: a stitch in time? J Infect Dis. 2013. doi:10.1093/infdis/jit307.
7. Henrich TJ, Hanhauser E, Marty FM, Sirignano MN, Keating S, Lee TH, Robles YP, Davis BT, Li JZ, Heisey A, Hill AL, Busch MP, Armand P, Soiffer RJ, Altfeld M, Kuritzkes DR. Antiretroviral-free HIV-1 remission and viral rebound after allogeneic stem cell transplantation: report of 2 cases. Ann Intern Med. 2014. doi:10.7326/M14-1027.
8. Henrich TJ, Hu Z, Li JZ, Sciaranghella G, Busch MP, Keating SM, Gallien S, Lin NH, Giguel FF, Lavoie L, Ho VT, Armand P, Soiffer RJ, Sagar M, Lacasce AS, Kuritzkes DR. Long-term reduction in peripheral blood HIV type 1 reservoirs following reduced-intensity conditioning allogeneic stem cell transplantation. J Infect Dis. 2013;207(11):1694–702. doi:10.1093/infdis/jit086.
9. Holland HK, Saral R, Rossi JJ, Donnenberg AD, Burns WH, Beschorner WE, Farzadegan H, Jones RJ, Quinnan GV, Vogelsang GB, et al. Allogeneic bone marrow transplantation, zidovudine, and human immunodeficiency virus type 1 (HIV-1) infection. Studies in a patient with non-Hodgkin lymphoma. Ann Intern Med. 1989;111(12):973–81.

10. Hutter G, Nowak D, Mossner M, Ganepola S, Mussig A, Allers K, Schneider T, Hofmann J, Kucherer C, Blau O, Blau IW, Hofmann WK, Thiel E. Long-term control of HIV by CCR5 Delta32/Delta32 stem-cell transplantation. N Engl J Med. 2009;360(7):692–8. doi:10.1056/NEJMoa0802905.
11. Kaplan LD, Straus DJ, Testa MA, Von Roenn J, Dezube BJ, Cooley TP, Herndier B, Northfelt DW, Huang J, Tulpule A, Levine AM. Low-dose compared with standard-dose m-BACOD chemotherapy for non-Hodgkin's lymphoma associated with human immunodeficiency virus infection. National Institute of Allergy and Infectious Diseases AIDS Clinical Trials Group. N Engl J Med. 1997;336(23):1641–8. doi:10.1056/NEJM199706053362304.
12. Krishnan A, Molina A, Zaia J, Smith D, Vasquez D, Kogut N, Falk PM, Rosenthal J, Alvarnas J, Forman SJ. Durable remissions with autologous stem cell transplantation for high-risk HIV-associated lymphomas. Blood. 2005;105(2):874–8. doi:10.1182/blood-2004-04-1532.
13. Muller E, Barday Z, Mendelson M, Kahn D. HIV-positive-to-HIV-positive kidney transplantation–results at 3 to 5 years. N Engl J Med. 2015;372(7):613–20. doi:10.1056/NEJMoa1408896.
14. Petz LD, Redei I, Bryson Y, Regan D, Kurtzberg J, Shpall E, Gutman J, Querol S, Clark P, Tonai R, Santos S, Bravo A, Spellman S, Gragert L, Rossi J, Li S, Li H, Senitzer D, Zaia J, Rosenthal J, Forman S, Chow R. Hematopoietic cell transplantation with cord blood for cure of HIV infections. Biol Blood Marrow Transplant J Am Soc Blood Marrow Transplant. 2013;19(3):393–7. doi:10.1016/j.bbmt.2012.10.017.
15. Ratner L, Lee J, Tang S, Redden D, Hamzeh F, Herndier B, Scadden D, Kaplan L, Ambinder R, Levine A, Harrington W, Grochow L, Flexner C, Tan B, Straus D. Chemotherapy for human immunodeficiency virus-associated non-Hodgkin's lymphoma in combination with highly active antiretroviral therapy. J Clin Oncol Off J Am Soc Clin Oncol. 2001;19(8):2171–8.
16. Re A, Michieli M, Casari S, Allione B, Cattaneo C, Rupolo M, Spina M, Manuele R, Vaccher E, Mazzucato M, Abbruzzese L, Ferremi P, Carosi G, Tirelli U, Rossi G. High-dose therapy and autologous peripheral blood stem cell transplantation as salvage treatment for AIDS-related lymphoma: long-term results of the Italian Cooperative Group on AIDS and Tumors (GICAT) study with analysis of prognostic factors. Blood. 2009;114(7):1306–13. doi:10.1182/blood-2009-02-202762.
17. Serrano D, Miralles P, Balsalobre P, Kwon M, Rodriguez-Macias G, Gayoso J, Anguita J, Buno I, Berenguer J, Diez-Martin JL. Graft-versus-tumor effect after allogeneic stem cell transplantation in HIV-positive patients with high-risk hematologic malignancies. AIDS Res Hum Retroviruses. 2013;29(10):1340–5. doi:10.1089/AID.2013.0001.
18. Shiels MS, Engels EA. Increased risk of histologically defined cancer subtypes in human immunodeficiency virus-infected individuals: clues for possible immunosuppression-related or infectious etiology. Cancer. 2012;118(19):4869–76. doi:10.1002/cncr.27454.
19. Sparano JA, Lee JY, Kaplan LD, Levine AM, Ramos JC, Ambinder RF, Wachsman W, Aboulafia D, Noy A, Henry DH, Von Roenn J, Dezube BJ, Remick SC, Shah MH, Leichman L, Ratner L, Cesarman E, Chadburn A, Mitsuyasu R. Rituximab plus concurrent infusional EPOCH chemotherapy is highly effective in HIV-associated B-cell non-Hodgkin lymphoma. Blood. 2010;115(15):3008–16. doi:10.1182/blood-2009-08-231613.
20. Spitzer TR, Ambinder RF, Lee JY, Kaplan LD, Wachsman W, Straus DJ, Aboulafia DM, Scadden DT. Dose-reduced busulfan, cyclophosphamide, and autologous stem cell transplantation for human immunodeficiency virus-associated lymphoma: AIDS Malignancy Consortium study 020. Biol Blood Marrow Transplant J Am Soc Blood Marrow Transplant. 2008;14(1):59–66. doi:10.1016/j.bbmt.2007.03.014.
21. Stock PG, Barin B, Murphy B, Hanto D, Diego JM, Light J, Davis C, Blumberg E, Simon D, Subramanian A, Millis JM, Lyon GM, Brayman K, Slakey D, Shapiro R, Melancon J, Jacobson JM, Stosor V, Olson JL, Stablein DM, Roland ME. Outcomes of kidney transplantation in HIV-infected recipients. N Engl J Med. 2010;363(21):2004–14. doi:10.1056/NEJMoa1001197.
22. Woolfrey AE, Malhotra U, Harrington RD, McNevin J, Manley TJ, Riddell SR, Coombs RW, Appelbaum FR, Corey L, Storb R. Generation of HIV-1-specific CD8+ cell responses following allogeneic hematopoietic cell transplantation. Blood. 2008;112(8):3484–7. doi:10.1182/blood-2008-05-157511.

# Multiple Myeloma and Monoclonal Gammopathy of Unknown Significance

14

Manfred Hensel

## Contents



HIV-infected individuals have a higher risk to develop both a monoclonal gammopathy (MG) and a multiple myeloma (MM) as compared to the general population. What is the evidence, what could be the reason, and how should it be managed?

The presence of an MG with an M-spike (Fig. 14.1) less than 3 g/dl and without other symptoms and signs, e.g., hypercalcemia, renal insufficiency, anemia, lytic bone lesions (the CRAB criteria), or bone marrow containing more than 10 % plasma cells, is called MG of undetermined significance (MGUS). In individuals without HIV infection, incidence of MGUS is correlated with age. MGUS is prevalent in approximately 5 % of the population above the age of 70, and the proportion is even higher in people older than 80 or 90 [1]. MGUS may progress to MM, other malignant plasma cell disorders, or lymphoma. The risk of progression is

M. Hensel
Mannheimer Onkologie Praxis, Hämatologie, Onkologie, Infektiologie, Palliativmedizin, Mannheim, Germany
e-mail: hensel@mannheimer-onkologie-praxis.de


M. Hentrich, S.K. Barta (eds.), *HIV-associated Hematological Malignancies*,
DOI 10.1007/978-3-319-26857-6_14

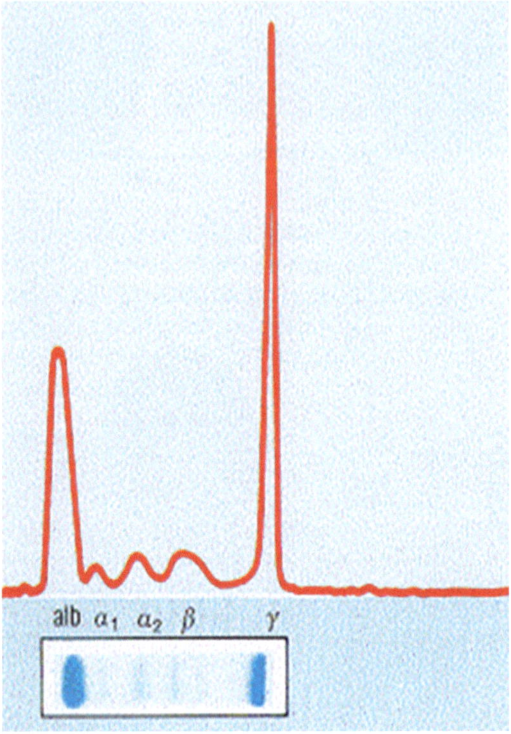


**Fig. 14.1** Electrophoresis with M-spike

approximately 1 % per year. Approximately 25 % of patients with MGUS will develop MM within 20 years of diagnosis [2].

## 14.1 Epidemiology

Few retrospective studies of the prevalence of MG among HIV-infected patients, mostly with small patient numbers, have been published. Older publications from the 1980s have shown a prevalence of 2.5–12 %. Newer publications from the HAART (highly active antiretroviral therapy) era, published after 2000, have shown consistently a prevalence of 3–5 % in HIV-positive individuals. Among 320 consecutive HIV1-infected patients in Boston, many of them taking HAART, oligoclonal banding was detected in 8.1 % and monoclonal bands in 4.4 %. MG correlated with younger age, higher viral load, and higher CD4 cell counts [5]. In Cape Town, blood and urine samples from 368 patients with HIV infections were examined, 326 of them on antiretroviral therapy (ART). Monoclonal bands were found in 12 patients (3.2 %) and oligoclonal bands in 14 (3.8 %). MG was associated with a shorter duration of ART, but not with CD4 count or viral load [6]. In a small retrospective analysis, 3 of 25 HIV-infected patients with MG (12 %) developed a plasma cell malignancy (one MM, two plasmocytomas). In the same series, HAART resulted in a decrease of serum monoclonal protein in 9 (56 %) of 19 HIV-infected patients with MG [7]. In two other small retrospective case series, no progression of MG to a malignant plasma cell disorder could be observed [8, 9].

In contrast, elevated serum free light chains (sFLC) seem to much better predict non-Hodgkin's lymphoma (NHL) and Hodgkin's lymphoma (HL) in HIV-infected individuals, as discovered in two independent retrospective trials with HIV-infected lymphoma patients who had available stored prediagnostic blood samples [10, 11].

The incidence of MM in HIV-infected individuals and patients with AIDS has been evaluated in smaller case series and six large population-based studies (Table 14.1). A meta-analysis of these trials, comprising 444,172 people living with HIV/AIDS (PLWH), revealed a standardized incidence ratio (SIR, which is calculated by dividing the observed number of cases of cancer by the "expected" number of cases in the general population) of MM of 2.71 [18]. In our experience, despite the elevated SIR, the development of MM is still a rare event in HIV-infected individuals, as compared to aggressive NHL and HL. In our own institution, we currently treat only 2 patients with MM out of 1100 patients with HIV infection.

## 14.2 Pathophysiology

The pathophysiology of the development of a monoclonal gammopathy in the context of HIV is complex [3]. The progressive loss of CD4 lymphocytes is the central event in the course of the HIV infection. Additionally, abnormal B-cell function in all stages of the HIV infection is well described and characterized by low antibody levels against specific pathogens and an inadequate response to vaccinations. At the same time, serum immunoglobulin levels, especially IgG levels, are elevated. This reflects a nonspecific polyclonal B-cell activation which is a result of dysregulated T-cell function, high levels of interleukin-6 and interleukin-10, as well as direct interaction of HIV with B-cells. Besides this direct stimulation by HIV, B-cells are also stimulated by other antigens, mitogens, or additional pathogens like HBV, EBV, or HHV-8. The chronic expansion of B-cells results in a follicular hyperplasia in enlarged, reactive lymph nodes, the so-called persistent generalized lymphadenopathy, as well as polyclonal gammopathy. If this condition persists for a long

**Table 14.1** Incidence of multiple myeloma in HIV-infected individuals

| Author | Ref. | Country/ trial | Time period | Population size | SIR of MM |
|---|---|---|---|---|---|
| Frisch M. | *JAMA* 2001 [12] | US | 1978–1996 | 302,834 | 2.6 |
| Engels EA. | *AIDS* 2006 [13] | US | 1996–2002 | 375,933 | 2.2 |
| Grulich AE. | *AIDS* 2002 [14] | Australia | 1995–1999 | 13,067 | 4.17 |
| Dal Maso L. | *Br J Cancer* 2003 [15] | Italy | 1985–1998 | 12,104 | 4.84 |
| Clifford GM. | *J Natl Cancer Inst* 2005 [16] | Switzerland | 1985–2003 | 7304 | 5.0 |
| Newnham A. | *Br J Cancer* 2005 [17] | England | 1985–2001 | 26,080 | 2.7 |

*SIR* standardized incidence ratio, *MM* multiple myeloma

time, clonal selection of abnormal B-cells may result. In the context of reduced immunosurveillance, an oncogenic virus such as EBV may lead to malignant transformation of lymphocytes by different mechanisms. HCV similarly may infect and chronically stimulate B-cells and impair their function. The association of HCV with monoclonal gammopathy, mixed cryoglobulinemia, autoimmune disorders, and lymphomas is well described.

## 14.3 Clinical Presentation

The clinical characteristics of MG in PLWH differ from those of the general population. In a series of 78 patients, the predominant light chain in HIV-related gammopathy was lambda, mostly IgG subtype, with no IgA [4]. Furthermore, the subclass distribution of monoclonal IgG was different from that observed in myeloma.

The correlation of MG in HIV-infected patients with morbidity and mortality as well as the association with the development of myeloma and lymphoma is unclear. Is the rate of transformation to a plasma cell malignancy the same as in the general population? And is a similar risk stratification, utilizing the established factors MG subtype, amount of paraprotein, and serum free light chain ratio, applicable?

Data about clinical presentation, treatment, and prognosis of MM in this population is scarce, and only case reports or small case series have been published. However, there appear to be some important differences as compared to the general population. Plasma cell dyscrasias occur at a younger age, often as solitary bone or extramedullary plasmocytomas, and sometimes as plasma cell leukemia. The M-protein is often low. The aggressiveness is reflected by rapid progression, short overall survival, and histopathology with atypical or anaplastic features [3, 19, 20].

## 14.4 Management

MG in PLWH should be followed up closely. HIV-related myeloma should be treated according to established MM guidelines and treatment recommendations applicable to the general population. Several case reports have described feasibility and effectiveness [3, 21–24]. There are no published trials in this distinct cohort that would support a different treatment strategy.

Once myeloma is diagnosed, symptomatic or not, the initiation of ART should be considered, if not already ongoing. There is evidence, as mentioned above [7], which shows that MG can decrease or even disappear with the onset of ART, and case reports that MM might improve or resolve [25–27]. Protease inhibitors, at least in cell lines, can kill myeloma cells and are synergistic with bortezomib [28–30].

In our experience, currently used treatment protocols for patients with MM in the general population, including bortezomib, thalidomide, lenalidomide, and dexamethasone, are feasible and adequately tolerated in HIV-infected patients. Even high-dose chemotherapy with autologous stem cell transplantation (ASCT) is feasible and should be considered according to the guidelines for MM in the general population [3, 24]. Maintenance therapy with lenalidomide after ASCT has been administered successfully, concurrent with ART [23]. In our center, we have recently treated a 57-year-old HIV-infected patient with newly diagnosed symptomatic MM with three cycles of bortezomib, doxorubicin, and dexamethasone resulting in a partial remission. For stem cell mobilization, he received cyclophosphamide, doxorubicin, and dexamethasone. Nine months after a tandem autologous stem cell transplantation with high-dose melphalan, he remains in a sustained very good partial remission. HAART (tenofovir, emtricitabine, and nevirapine) was administered during the entire period of chemotherapy, without major side effects.

## 14.5 Summary

PLWH have a higher risk to develop both MG and MM as compared to the general population. The pathophysiology is complex and related to the progressive loss of CD4 lymphocytes, abnormal function, and nonspecific polyclonal B-cell activation, T-cell dysregulation, and chronic stimulation of the immune system by several antigens or pathogens. The clinical presentation of MG and MM differs from that in the general population, with a more aggressive course in HIV-infected individuals. In the absence of strong data, MM should be treated according to the guidelines for MM in the general population, including high-dose chemotherapy with autologous stem cell transplantation.

## References


1. Kyle RA, Therneau TM, Rajkumar SV, Larson DR, Plevak MF, Offord JR, Dispenzieri A, Katzmann JA, Melton 3rd LJ. Prevalence of monoclonal gammopathy of undetermined significance. N Engl J Med. 2006;354(13):1362–9.
2. Kyle RA, Therneau TM, Rajkumar SV, Offord JR, Larson DR, Plevak MF, Melton 3rd LJ. A long-term study of prognosis in monoclonal gammopathy of undetermined significance. N Engl J Med. 2002;346(8):564–9.
3. Coker WJ, Jeter A, Schade H, Kang Y. Plasma cell disorders in HIV-infected patients: epidemiology and molecular mechanisms. Biomark Res. 2013;1(1):8.
4. Briault S, Courtois-Capella M, Duarte F, Aucouturier P, Preud'Homme JL. Isotype of serum monoclonal immunoglobulins in human immunodeficiency virus-infected adults. Clin Exp Immunol. 1988;74(2):182–4.
5. Konstantinopoulos PA, Dezube BJ, Pantanowitz L, Horowitz GL, Beckwith BA. Protein electrophoresis and immunoglobulin analysis in HIV-infected patients. Am J Clin Pathol. 2007;128(4):596–603.
6. van Vuuren MJ, Zemlin AE, Germishuys JJ. Monoclonal gammopathy and other serum protein electrophoresis patterns in patients with HIV infection in South Africa. Ann Clin Biochem. 2010;47(Pt 4):366–74.
7. Amara S, Dezube BJ, Cooley TP, Pantanowitz L, Aboulafia DM. HIV -associated monoclonal gammopathy: a retrospective analysis of 25 patients. Clin Infect Dis. 2006;43(9):1198–205.
8. Lefrère JJ, Debbia M, Lambin P. Prospective follow-up of monoclonal gammopathies in HIV-infected individuals. Br J Haematol. 1993;84(1):151–5.

9. Ng VL, Chen KH, Hwang KM, Khayam-Bashi H, McGrath MS. The clinical significance of human immunodeficiency virus type 1-associated paraproteins. Blood. 1989;74(7):2471–5.
10. Landgren O, Goedert JJ, Rabkin CS, Wilson WH, Dunleavy K, Kyle RA, Katzmann JA, Rajkumar SV, Engels EA. Circulating serum free light chains as predictive markers of AIDS-related lymphoma. J Clin Oncol. 2010;28(5):773–9.
11. Bibas M, Trotta MP, Cozzi-Lepri A, Lorenzini P, Pinnetti C, Rizzardini G, Angarano G, Caramello P, Sighinolfi L, Mastroianni CM, Mazzarello G, Di Caro A, Di Giacomo C, d'Arminio Monforte A, Antinori A, ICONA Foundation Study Group. Role of serum free light chains in predicting HIV-associated non-Hodgkin lymphoma and Hodgkin's lymphoma and its correlation with antiretroviral therapy. Am J Hematol. 2012;87(8):749–53.
12. Frisch M, Biggar RJ, Engels EA, Goedert JJ, AIDS-Cancer Match Registry Study Group. Association of cancer with AIDS-related immunosuppression in adults. JAMA. 2001;285(13):1736–45.
13. Engels EA, Pfeiffer RM, Goedert JJ, Virgo P, McNeel TS, Scoppa SM, Biggar RJ, HIV/AIDS Cancer Match Study. Trends in cancer risk among people with AIDS in the United States 1980–2002. AIDS. 2006;20(12):1645–54.
14. Grulich AE, Li Y, McDonald A, Correll PK, Law MG, Kaldor JM. Rates of non-AIDS-defining cancers in people with HIV infection before and after AIDS diagnosis. AIDS. 2002;16(8):1155–61.
15. Dal Maso L, Franceschi S, Polesel J, Braga C, Piselli P, Crocetti E, Falcini F, Guzzinati S, Zanetti R, Vercelli M, Rezza G, Cancer and AIDS Registy Linkage Study. Risk of cancer in persons with AIDS in Italy, 1985–1998. Br J Cancer. 2003;89(1):94–100.
16. Clifford GM, Polesel J, Rickenbach M, Dal Maso L, Keiser O, Kofler A, Rapiti E, Levi F, Jundt G, Fisch T, Bordoni A, De Weck D, Franceschi S, Swiss HIV Cohort. Cancer risk in the Swiss HIV Cohort Study: associations with immunodeficiency, smoking, and highly active antiretroviral therapy. J Natl Cancer Inst. 2005;97(6):425–32.
17. Newnham A, Harris J, Evans HS, Evans BG, Møller H. The risk of cancer in HIV-infected people in southeast England: a cohort study. Br J Cancer. 2005;92(1):194–200.
18. Grulich AE, van Leeuwen MT, Falster MO, Vajdic CM. Incidence of cancers in people with HIV/AIDS compared with immunosuppressed transplant recipients: a meta-analysis. Lancet. 2007;370(9581):59–67.
19. Bladé J, Kyle RA. Multiple myeloma in young patients: clinical presentation and treatment approach. Leuk Lymphoma. 1998;30(5–6):493–501.
20. Feller L, White J, Wood NH, Bouckaert M, Lemmer J, Raubenheimer EJ. Extramedullary myeloma in an HIV-seropositive subject. Literature review and report of an unusual case. Head Face Med. 2009;5:4.
21. Aboulafia DM. Thalidomide-based treatment for HIV-associated multiple myeloma: a case report. AIDS Read. 2003;13(8):383–9.
22. Dezube BJ, Aboulafia DM, Pantanowitz L. Plasma cell disorders in HIV-infected patients: from benign gammopathy to multiple myeloma. AIDS Read. 2004;14(7):372–4, 377–9.
23. Miyagishima T, Tateno T, Kasahara KH, Sawada K, Sogabe S, Oda H. Successful treatment of an HIV-positive multiple myeloma patient with high-dose chemotherapy followed by autologous peripheral blood stem cell transplantation and maintenance therapy with lenalidomide. Rinsho Ketsueki. 2013;54(7):664–9.
24. Kentos A, Vekemans M, Van Vooren JP, Lambermont M, Liesnard C, Feremans W, Farber CM. High-dose chemotherapy and autologous CD34-positive blood stem cell transplantation for multiple myeloma in an HIV carrier. Bone Marrow Transplant. 2002;29(3):273–5.
25. Cauda R, Lucia MB, Marasca G, Rutella S, Petrucci MT, La Verde G, Gastaldi R. Beneficial effect of highly active antiretroviral therapy (HAART) in reducing both HIV viral load and monoclonal gammopathy. Eur J Haematol. 1999;63(2):134–5.
26. Sorli ML, Gimeno E, Abella E, Besses C, Knobel H. Smoldering myeloma in HIV patient: a complete remission after antiretroviral therapy. Leuk Res. 2008;32(9):1482–3.

27. Li G, Lewis RD, Mishra N, Axiotis CA. A retrospective analysis of ten symptomatic multiple myeloma patients with HIV infection: a potential therapeutic effect of HAART in multiple myeloma. Leuk Res. 2014;38(9):1079–84.
28. Kawabata S, Gills JJ, Mercado-Matos JR, Lopiccolo J, Wilson 3rd W, Hollander MC, Dennis PA. Synergistic effects of nelfinavir and bortezomib on proteotoxic death of NSCLC and multiple myeloma cells. Cell Death Dis. 2012;3:e353.
29. Kraus M, Bader J, Overkleeft H, Driessen C. Nelfinavir augments proteasome inhibition by bortezomib in myeloma cells and overcomes bortezomib and carfilzomib resistance. Blood Cancer J. 2013;3:e103.
30. Ikezoe T, Saito T, Bandobashi K, Yang Y, Koeffler HP, Taguchi H. HIV-1 protease inhibitor induces growth arrest and apoptosis of human multiple myeloma cells via inactivation of signal transducer and activator of transcription 3 and extracellular signal-regulated kinase 1/2. Mol Cancer Ther. 2004;3(4):473–9.

# Myeloproliferative Neoplasms

# 15

Ryan C. Fang and David M. Aboulafia

**Contents**



## 15.1 Introduction

Human immunodeficiency virus (HIV) infection is linked to an increased risk of both acquired immunodeficiency syndrome (AIDS)-defining malignancies (ADMs) and non-AIDS-defining malignancies (nADMs). One subset of these nADMs are myeloproliferative neoplasms (MPNs), in which there is an overproduction of red blood cells (RBCs), platelets, or a subset of white blood cells (WBCs). Many patients with MPNs are asymptomatic at the time of medical

R.C. Fang
Section of Hematology and Oncology, Virginia Mason Medical Center, Seattle, WA, USA
e-mail: ryancfang@gmail.com

D.M. Aboulafia, MD (✉)
Section of Hematology and Oncology, Virginia Mason Medical Center, Seattle, WA, USA

Division of Hematology, University of Washington, Seattle, WA, USA
e-mail: hemdma@virginiamason.org



M. Hentrich, S.K. Barta (eds.), *HIV-associated Hematological Malignancies*,
DOI 10.1007/978-3-319-26857-6_15

evaluation, and their diagnosis is established after routine blood testing reveals an anomaly. Others present to medical attention complaining of headache, fatigue, weight loss, and early satiety in the backdrop of splenomegaly, bleeding, and thrombotic complications and clonal evolution.

In this chapter, we will discuss MPNs. Case reports describing MPNs in HIV-infected patients are rare. Subsequently, there is neither ample knowledge regarding the natural history of MPNs in this population nor is there abundant clinical experience in using standard chemotherapies in conjunction with highly active antiretroviral therapy (HAART). Although there is perhaps no inherent reason why people living with HIV/AIDS (PLWHA) should be predisposed to these disorders, we expect more instances of MPNs in this population as these individuals achieve survival rates comparable to the general population.

We focus on the classification of MPNs and the importance of cytogenetics and molecular studies in refining the diagnosis. Chronic myeloid leukemia (CML), which is associated with the Philadelphia chromosome, has been described in only a handful of case reports in the context of HIV infection. We will narrow our discussion to briefly mention the Philadelphia-negative MPNs: polycythemia vera (PV), essential thrombocythemia (ET), and primary myelofibrosis (PMF). For these disorders, even less is known regarding their clinical course and natural history in the backdrop of HIV infection.

## 15.2 Classification

Among the classic MPNs, CML is genetically characterized by the reciprocal chromosomal translocation between chromosomes 9 and 22, t (9; 22). This translocation is associated with a shortened chromosome 22 (the Philadelphia chromosome [Ph]) in 95 % of instances. In the remaining cases, t (9; 22) can be identified by either fluorescence in situ hybridization or reverse transcriptase polymerase chain reaction (PCR) techniques for detection of *BCR-ABL*, a tyrosine kinase protein [1]. While cytogenetic abnormalities are common in PMF and uncommon in ET, no specific cytogenetic abnormality in the MPNs other than CML has yet been established [2].

Janus kinase-2 (JAK-2) mutations are found in virtually all patients with PV and approximately 50 % of those with either ET or PMF. This finding has greatly aided in the diagnosis of MPNs [3]. Further studies identified JAK- signal transducers and activators of transcription (STAT) pathway mutations in the thrombopoietin receptor and the calreticulin gene in JAK-2 non-mutated MPNs [4]. The diagnosis of PV is entertained when there is an unexplained increase in hematocrit/RBC mass in conjunction with presence of a JAK-2 mutation along with a decreased serum erythropoietin level [5].

PMF (agnogenic myeloid metaplasia, chronic idiopathic myelofibrosis) is characterized by the presence of bone marrow fibrosis that cannot be attributed to another myeloid disorder such as CML, PV, ET, or myelodysplastic syndromes

(MDS). ET is a diagnosis of exclusion, representing clonal or autonomous thrombocytosis not classifiable as PV, PMF, CML, or MDS [6].

The MPNs, and PMF in particular, are often accompanied by leukoerythroblastic changes on peripheral blood smear. The characteristic laboratory changes associated with a myelophthisic bone marrow process include nucleated red blood cells and teardrop forms, giant platelets, and immature white blood cells (e.g., myelocytes, metamyelocytes, occasionally promyelocytes and myeloblasts) (Fig. 15.1).

Within the context of the MPNs, an elevated RBC mass is specific for PV. Occasionally, both CML and MDS may present with either isolated thrombocytosis suggesting ET or associated bone marrow fibrosis suggesting PMF [7]. As a result, the diagnostic workup of patients with suspected MPN should always include cytogenetic studies and careful morphologic evaluation to exclude the presence of t (9; 22) and MDS, respectively. The accurate diagnosis and classification of MPNs are prerequisites for appropriate risk-based therapy and should be based on an integrated approach following the World Health Organization (WHO) guidelines that, in addition to clinical, cytogenetic, and molecular evaluation, includes a bone marrow examination [8] (Figs. 15.2, 15.3, and 15.4).

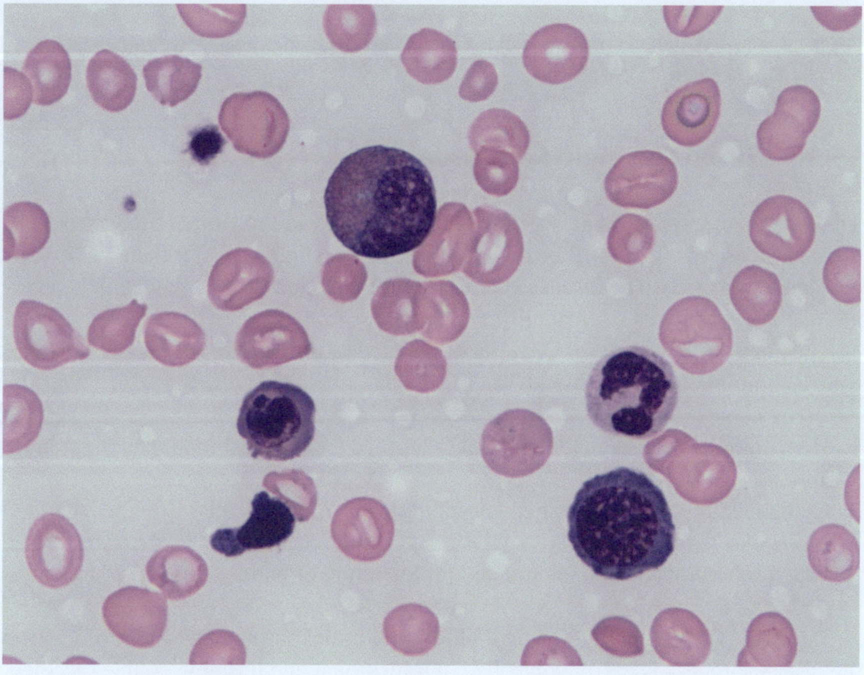

**Fig. 15.1** Leukoerythroblastic peripheral blood smear (Image and description courtesy of Dr. Dick Hwang, Virginia Mason Medical Center)

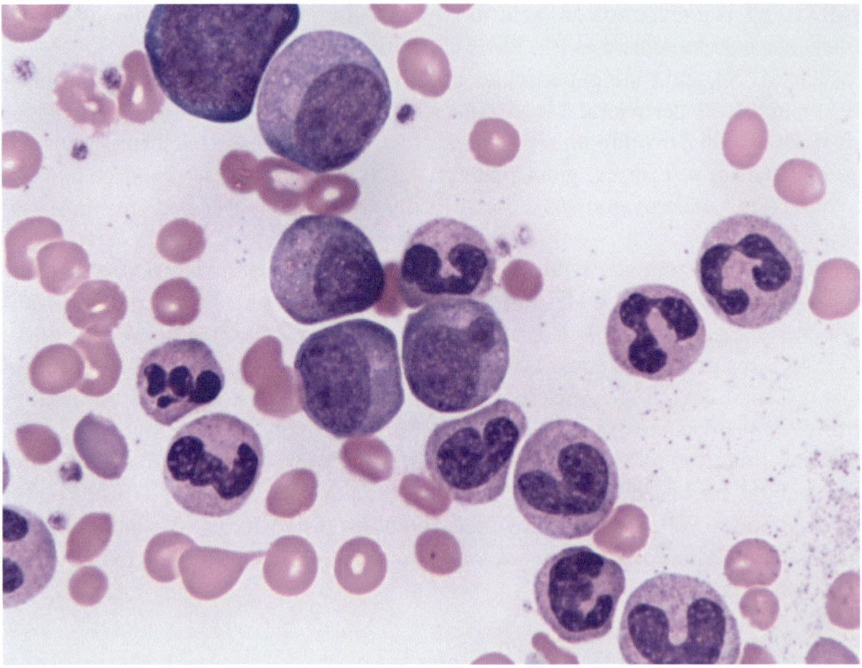

**Fig. 15.2** Chronic myeloid leukemia (CML) (Image and description courtesy of Dr. Dick Hwang, Virginia Mason Medical Center)

## 15.3 Chronic Myeloid Leukemia

The American Cancer Society estimates that in 2015 in the United States, roughly 6600 new cases of CML will be diagnosed, which is slightly higher than 10 % of all new leukemia cases. The disease is more common in men than women and the average age at diagnosis is 64 years [9].

The goals of treatment for CML have changed radically over the past decade and can be summarized as follows [10]:

1. Hematologic remission defined as a normal complete blood count and the absence of splenomegaly
2. Cytogenetic remission (normal karyotype with 0 % Ph+ cells)
3. Molecular remission (negative PCR result for the mutational *BCR/ABL* mRNA), which represents efforts to cure and prolongation of patient survival

Typically, CML has three clinical phases: an initial chronic phase, during which the disease process is easily controlled, a transitional and unstable course (accelerated phase), and finally, a more aggressive course (blast crisis), which is usually fatal. In all three phases, supportive therapy with transfusions of RBCs or platelets may be used to relieve symptoms and improve quality of life.

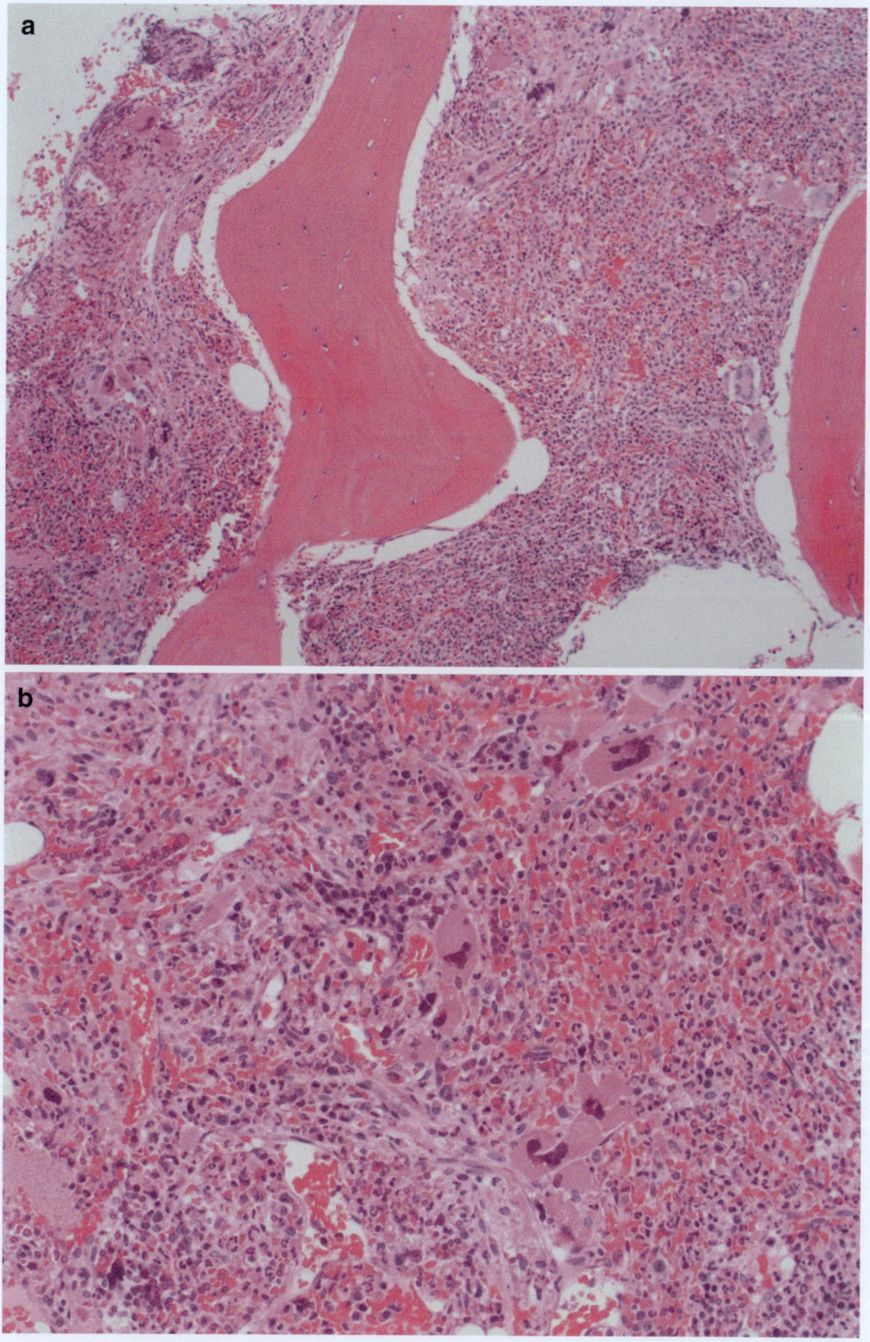


**Fig. 15.3** (**a**) Bone marrow biopsy from a patient with primary myelofibrosis with marrow fibrosis and clusters of atypical megakaryocytes 10×. (**b**) Bone marrow biopsy from a patient with primary myelofibrosis 20×. (**c**) Reticulin stain shows moderate reticulin fibrosis (Images and descriptions courtesy of Dr. Dick Hwang, Virginia Mason Medical Center)

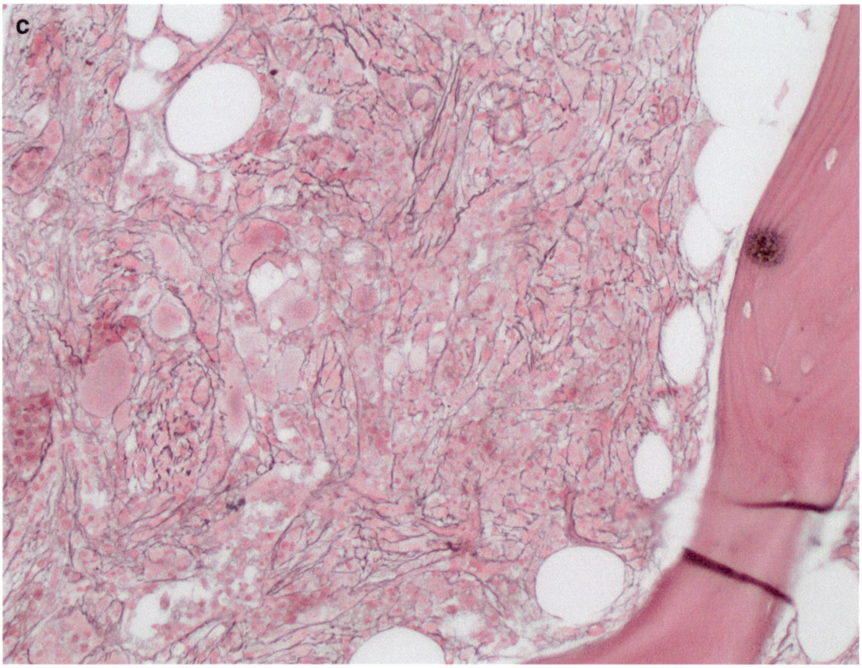


**Fig. 15.3** (Continued)

In Western countries, 90 % of patients with CML are diagnosed in the chronic phase. These patients' WBC count is usually controlled with medication (hematologic remission). The major goal of treatment during this phase is to control symptoms and complications due to anemia, thrombocytopenia, leukocytosis, and splenomegaly. The standard treatment of choice until recently has been imatinib, which is a specific small molecule tyrosine kinase inhibitor (TKI) of *BCR/ABL* and is highly effective in all phases of CML [11, 12].

The chronic phase varies in duration, depending on the maintenance therapy used. It usually lasts 2–3 years with hydroxyurea or busulfan therapy, but it may last for longer than 9.5 years in patients who respond well to interferon alpha therapy. Furthermore, the advent of imatinib and the other TKIs has dramatically improved the duration of hematologic and cytogenetic remissions [13].

Some patients with CML progress to a transitional or accelerated phase which may last for several months. The survival of patients in this phase is 1–1.5 years. This phase is characterized by poor control of blood counts with myelosuppressive medication and the appearance of peripheral blast cells (≥15 %), promyelocytes (≥30 %), basophils (≥20 %), and platelet counts less than 100,000 cells/μL unrelated to therapy.

In a retrospective review of all patients diagnosed with CML at the Chris Hani Baragwanath Academic Hospital (CHBAH) in South Africa between 1991 and 2011, 240 patients were identified with CML 18 of whom (7.5 %) were also infected

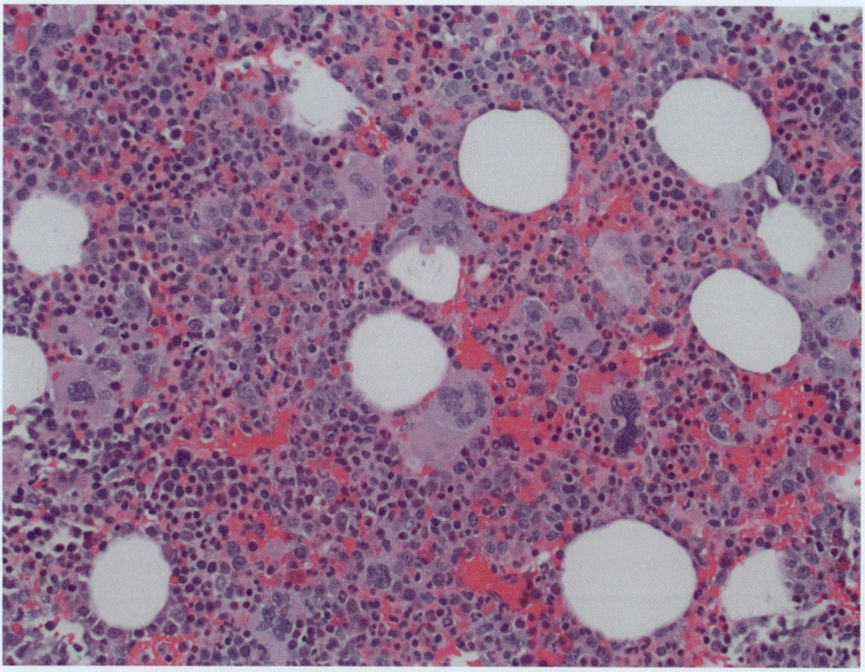

**Fig. 15.4** Bone marrow biopsy from a patient with polycythemia vera showing conspicuous hypercellularity for age with erythroid and megakaryocytic hyperplasia. Megakaryocytes show widely separated nuclear lobes (Image and description courtesy of Dr. Dick Hwang, Virginia Mason Medical Center)

with HIV [14]. This proportion of total CML patients with and without HIV infection was much lower than the HIV seroprevalence in the CHBAH population (25 % in 2004 and 28 % in 2008). Based on this data set, the authors concluded that HIV infection does not increase the prevalence of CML. However, in this same data set, they also noted that the median age of HIV-CML patients was younger (37 years) than that of CML patients not infected with HIV (43 years). Eight out of the 18 (44 %) HIV-CML patients had progressed to accelerated or blast phase CML, while less than 10 % of the seronegative CML patients had been diagnosed with accelerated or blast phase.

Although the incidence of CML might not be augmented in the context of HIV infection, this limited data set from South Africa raises the specter that among PLWHA, CML may have a different natural history. Of the 18 HIV-CML patients, 6 were also treated with imatinib at a standard dose of 400 mg/day [14]. After a median follow-up of 15 months, one patient had died (cause not specified), one (17 %) had achieved a major molecular response (MMR), two (33 %) had achieved a major cytogenetic response (MCR), and two (33 %) had achieved a complete cytogenetic response (CCR). However, the response to imatinib in HIV-CML patients was reported to be inferior to that noted in patients with CML without

HIV. Of 44 HIV-negative patients with CML treated with imatinib, 15 (34 %) had achieved a MCR, 7 (16 %) a CCR, 4 (9 %) a MMR, 15 (34 %) had undetectable ABL-BCR transcripts, and 3 (7 %) had achieved less than a MCR.

In a more recent report, three patients diagnosed with chronic phase CML took imatinib in conjunction with HAART [15]. The first patient had been treated with HAART (nevirapine, abacavir, lamivudine, and zidovudine) and had a CD4+ count of 488 cells/mm$^3$ and a non-detectable HIV viral load when he began imatinib at a dose of 600 mg/day. Three months later, his HIV viral load remained less than 75 copies/mm$^3$, and cytogenetic analysis showed a minor CR. The second patient had also been treated with HAART (lopinavir-ritonavir, abacavir, lamivudine, and zidovudine) for 3 years when he was diagnosed with CML. He had a non-detectable HIV viral load and a CD4+ count of 508 cells/mm$^3$ when he received imatinib at a dose of 400 mg/day. Two weeks later, he began erythropoietin supplementation, but when his anemia worsened imatinib was held for 2 weeks and then resumed at a reduced dose of 300 mg/day. His HAART regimen was also revised and efavirenz was substituted for lopinavir-ritonavir and abacavir, and lamivudine and zidovudine were substituted for emtricitabine and tenofovir. A CCR was attained 13 months later, and at a 20-month follow-up, the patient's HIV viral load remained non-detectable and his CD4+ count was 382 cells/mm$^3$. The third patient had been treated with HAART (nevirapine, abacavir, and lamivudine) for 10 years when he presented to medical attention with isolated leukocytosis and left shifted findings on peripheral blood smear but no overt findings of infection. He had a non-detectable HIV viral load and CD4+ count of 523 cells/mm$^3$ when he began imatinib at a dose of 400 mg/day. Following CML treatment, he developed persistent anemia, alleviated by recombinant erythropoietin and RBC transfusions. Imatinib was subsequently held for 1 month and then restarted at a dose of 200 mg/day. Over a 16-month period, imatinib was gradually increased 400 mg/day. A CCR was achieved 17 months after treatment started and at 69-month follow-up, the patient's HIV viral load remained non-detectable and his CD4+ count was 440 cells/mm$^3$. In each of these three cases, imatinib was taken in conjunction with various HAART options and was generally well tolerated.

In these and other case reports, hydroxyurea was used sparingly and imatinib was the TKI employed most frequently to treat HIV-infected patients with CML [16, 17]. Although details of drug-drug interactions have generally not been reported in this context, it is notable that imatinib is mainly metabolized by cytochrome P450 (CYP) 3A4 isoenzyme and concurrent administration of drugs that affect CYP3A4 may incur similar interactions. Other enzymes which play a minor role in the metabolism of imatinib include CYP1A2, CYP2D6, CYPC9, and CYP2C19 [18, 19]. Taking antiretroviral therapies into consideration, serum imatinib levels are likely affected by certain antiretroviral classes that comprise HAART. Nucleoside reverse transcriptase inhibitors and integrase inhibitors have no effect on the substrate CYP3A4; however, non-nucleoside reverse transcriptase inhibitors induce CYP3A4 and protease inhibitors inhibit CYP3A4 [20]. The US Food and Drug Administration (FDA) recommends dose reduction of imatinib by 50 % if patients are taking a CYP3A4 inhibitor; however, it appears the majority of HIV-infected patients with CML have received full doses of imatinib [18].

Experience with newer agents to treat PLWHA and CML are limited (Table 15.1). In a brief case report, an HIV-infected male received nilotinib *not* for CML but rather for acute myeloid leukemia (AML) [21]. During his hospital course, he began antifungal medication, and serum nilotinib levels were carefully monitored along with electrocardiogram determinants of QT prolongation. Like imatinib, kinetic experiments have shown that CYP3A4 and CYP2C8 enzymes are the main contributors to the metabolism of nilotinib, and coadministration with CYP3A4 inhibitors reduce oxidative metabolism of nilotinib by as much as 95 %. The authors reminded clinicians of this important potential drug-drug interaction and suggested a strategy to minimize sudden cardiac death by QT prolongation.

## 15.4 Polycythemia Vera

PV is a stem cell disorder characterized as a pan-hyperplastic, malignant, and neoplastic marrow disorder. It is most commonly diagnosed in individuals between the ages of 60 and 70 years and is more common in men than women [22, 23]. PV results from uncontrolled blood cell production, especially RBCs, as a result of acquired mutations in an early hematopoietic cell. Because this early cell has the capability to form not only RBCs but also WBCs and platelets, any combination of these cell lines may be affected.

The most prominent feature of PV is an elevated absolute RBC mass because of uncontrolled RBC production. Impaired oxygenation to the tissues as a result of

**Table 15.1** Current treatments for chronic myeloid leukemia

| Treatment | Suggested dosage | Comments |
|---|---|---|
| Imatinib | [a]400 mg/day [b]600 mg/day | First-line TKI treatment for CML approved by the FDA |
| Dasatinib | [a]100 mg/day [b]140 mg/day | First- or second-line TKI for some imatinib-resistant mutants |
| Bosutinib | 500 mg/day | Second-line TKI for some imatinib-resistant mutants |
| Nilotinib | 300 mg twice daily | First- or second-line TKI; slightly modified version of imatinib |
| Omacetaxine | 1.25 mg/m$^2$ via subcutaneous injection twice daily | Alkaloid translation inhibitor for treating T315I-mutant CML |
| Stem cell transplant | Not applicable | Offers curative potential but with greater risks compared to therapy with TKIs; seldom used as initial therapy but considered for patients who have not responded well to other therapies |

Suggested dosages retrieved from US Food and Drug Administration (FDA)
[a]Recommended for chronic phase chronic myelogenous leukemia (CML) specifically
[b]Recommended for accelerated or blast phase CML

changes in serum viscosity and sludging of RBCs may lead to headaches, visual impairment, dizziness, vertigo, and claudication [24]. Bleeding complications, seen in approximately 1 % of patients with PV, include epistaxis, gum bleeding, ecchymosis, and gastrointestinal bleeding.

Underlying vascular disease, common in older persons with PV as well as in the aging population of PLWHA, can increase the risk of clotting complications [25]. Blood clots occur in about 30 % of patients even before the PV diagnosis is made. During the first 10 years after a diagnosis of PV, 40–60 % of untreated PV patients may develop blood clots. This is particularly relevant in the context of HIV infection as this may be the first manifestation of a clotting disorder in the backdrop of HIV infection [26]. Roughly three-fourths of PV patients will have splenomegaly and one-third will have hepatomegaly at time of diagnosis. A large proportion will also have plethora, hypertension, fatigue, and pruritus. In addition to the signs and symptoms above, people with PV are at slightly greater risk than the general population for developing leukemia as a result of the disease and/or certain drug treatments.

According to the 2008 revised WHO guidelines, diagnosis of PV requires the presence of both major criteria and one minor criterion or the presence of the first major criterion together with two minor criteria [27].

WHO criteria are described in the following bullets, with major criteria in 1–2 and minor in 3–5:

1. Hemoglobin >18.5 g/dL in men and >16.5 g/dL in women or other evidence of increased RBC volume
2. The presence of JAK2617V F or other functionally similar mutation, such as *JAK2* exon 12 mutation
3. Bone marrow biopsy showing hypercellularity for age with tri-lineage growth (pan-myelosis) with prominent erythroid, granulocytic, and megakaryocytic proliferation
4. Serum erythropoietin level below the reference range for normal
5. Endogenous erythroid colony formation in vitro

In reviewing HIV literature, it is often a challenge to discern instances of true PV from secondary causes of elevated RBC mass. In a number of instances, patients were presumed to have PV but secondary causes including testosterone replacement therapy, sleep apnea, chronic dehydration, and smoking were not excluded [28, 29].

There have been very few studies on the impact of HIV infection on the development of PV [30]. In one instance, an HIV-infected male with hemophilia and a 10-year history of PV presented to medical attention with an elevated WBC and was diagnosed with AML. He died from respiratory complications 2 days later [31]. In a second report, a 45-year-old nonsmoking male presented with a hemoglobin of 15.7 g/dl and was subsequently diagnosed with HIV infection [32]. The patient was initially treated with zidovudine and later with didanosine, lamivudine, and saquinavir. Seven years later, he appeared plethoric and with splenomegaly, had an erythrocyte mass of 71 ml/kg, and had an oxygen saturation of 94 %. His hematocrit was 63 %, leukocytes 12,400, erythropoietin <5 nmol/ml, CD4+ count was 321 cells/mm$^3$, and his HIV viral load was non-detectable. After a diagnosis of PV, he was treated with a series of phlebotomies to achieve an iron-deficient state coupled with hydroxyurea at a dose of 1 g/day. Despite the potentially myelosuppressive effect of hydroxyurea, his CD4+ count gradually rose to 474 cells/mm$^3$ and HIV viral load remained non-detectable. At 12-month follow-up, there was no discernible change in CD4+ cell count or HIV viral load, and PV was well controlled.

Therapeutic approaches to PV focus on the following: controlling and maintaining hematocrit levels at <45 % in men and <42 % in women, treating complications of thrombosis and hemorrhage, reducing thrombotic risk and minimizing the risk of leukemogenic transformation, and managing splenomegaly and other disease-related symptoms [33]. If not otherwise contraindicated because of a history of major bleeding or intolerance, aspirin should be given to all patients in a low dose of 75–100 mg/day [34, 35].

To date, no drug has been shown to improve survival or lower risk of leukemic transformation in PV. Whether or not the demonstration of mutant JAK-2 allele burden reduction associated with treatment with interferon alpha or busulfan translates into a survival advantage is currently unclear and cannot be used as a rationale to choose these drugs over hydroxyurea as first-line therapy for high-risk patients. Until new data emerges, hydroxyurea continues to be widely used in response to PV (Table 15.2).

Ruxolitinib is a Janus kinase inhibitor (JKI) with selectivity for subtypes JAK-1 and JAK-2 of this enzyme. Ruxolitinib inhibits deregulated JAK-STAT signaling associated with myelofibrosis leading to modulation of cytokine gene expression. Data regarding the use of ruxolitinib in PV come from a phase II trial and an

**Table 15.2** Clinical properties of hydroxyurea

| Characteristic | Hydroxyurea |
|---|---|
| Drug class | Antimetabolite |
| Mechanism of action | Impairs DNA repair by inhibiting ribonucleotide reductase |
| Specificity | Affects all cell lines |
| Pharmacology | Half-life 4 h, renal excretion |
| Starting dose | 15 mg/kg per day orally |
| Onset of action | Three to 5 days when the usual starting dose is employed (15 mg/kg per day) |
| Side effects observed in >10 % of patients | Neutropenia, anemia, oral ulcers, hyperpigmentation, rash, nail changes |
| Side effects observed in ≤10 % of patients | Ankle ulcers, lichen planus-like lesions of the mouth and skin, nausea, diarrhea |
| Rare side effects | Fever, liver function test abnormalities |
| Contraindications | Neutropenia, pregnancy, childbearing potential, breast feeding |
| Annual cost | $1700.00, for 500 mg three times daily dose |

Adapted from Tefferi [50] up to date. Accessed May 28, 2015

open-label phase III trial in patients with hydroxyurea-related toxicities or with uncontrolled disease despite hydroxyurea [36]. Based on these studies, ruxolitinib is approved by the US FDA for the treatment of patients with intolerance or resistance to hydroxyurea.

While clinical experience with ruxolitinib for PV patients infected with HIV is lacking, in vitro it does block T-cell activation-mediated HIV replication [37]. Immunologic side effects relevant to PLWHA and who might be considered for ruxolitinib include herpes zoster (shingles; 1.9 %) and opportunistic infections [38]. Metabolic side effects have included weight gain (7.1 %). Laboratory abnormalities have included alanine transaminase (ALT) abnormalities (25.2 %), aspartate transaminase (AST) abnormalities (17.4 %), and elevated cholesterol levels (16.8 %) [39]. Other common adverse events are grade 3–4 anemia (45 %) and thrombocytopenia (10–15 %).

## 15.5 Essential Thrombocythemia

ET is a MPN in which the body produces too many platelets. ET is the most nondescript of MPNs and the one that can most easily be confused with other entities, since isolated thrombocytosis can be seen in PV, PMF, CML, and more commonly as a complication of many other illnesses. Persistence of thrombocytosis is central to establish an ET diagnosis, along with the exclusion of reactive causes such as iron deficiency and inflammatory states and conditions that frequently comingle with HIV infection [40].

ET can present with headache, visual disturbance, erythromelalgia, or transient ischemic attack. Low-risk ET patients who are asymptomatic often do not need treatment [41]. While most patients with ET enjoy a normal life expectancy, treatment with low-dose aspirin is required for those with vasomotor symptoms. Thrombotic events in low-risk patients with ET are too infrequent to justify the long-term use of potentially harmful agents. The risk may be higher, however, in the presence of cardiovascular risk factors and/or extreme uncontrolled thrombocytosis. Whether or not drug therapy is indicated in this situation remains controversial. On the other hand, approximately 20 % of patients with ET present with major thrombotic events and another 15 % may experience recurrent thrombosis. This complication is most common in patients older than 60. Therefore, cytoreductive therapy in the form of hydroxyurea (and less commonly, anagrelide and interferon alpha) is indicated in these high-risk patients (i.e., age >60 years or history of prior thrombosis); bleeding complications are less frequent and may be prevented by avoiding doses of aspirin greater than 100 mg/day and nonsteroidal anti-inflammatory agents [42].

## 15.6 Primary Myelofibrosis

PMF is the least common of the MPNs and is characterized by the proliferation of an abnormal clone of hematopoietic stem cells in the bone marrow resulting in fibrosis or the replacement of bone marrow with collagenous connective tissue fibers. Symptoms include splenomegaly, bone pain, bruising and easy bleeding, fatigue, increased susceptibility to infection, and anemia.

Currently, there are no therapies approved specifically for PMF. However, hematopoietic stem cell transplantation (SCT) is potentially curative and is increasingly being utilized for HIV-infected patients with chemosensitive lymphoid and plasma cell malignancies [43–45]. Allogeneic SCT is associated with high treatment-related mortality and may not be appropriate for older patients with several comorbidities; however, studies utilizing reduced intensity conditioning resulted in a reduction of transplant-related mortality and morbidity [46].

Treatment of PMF is dependent on the individual case and is usually withheld until development of symptoms of disease progression. Cytoreductive therapies such as hydroxyurea, low-dose interferon alpha, and busulfan are effective for hyper-proliferation such as leukocytosis, splenomegaly, and thrombocytosis [42]. Corticosteroids can be given for constitutional symptoms and are also effective for treating PMF-related anemia along with androgens or recombinant erythropoietin [47, 48]. Low-dose thalidomide in conjunction with prednisone has also been shown to be effective treatment for anemia, thrombocytopenia, and splenomegaly in approximately 20–60 % of PMF patients [49]. Experiences treating patients with PMF and HIV infection have not been reported.

## Conclusion

There are few cases of MPNs (CML, PV, ET, and PMF) in HIV-infected patients reported in the literature. We briefly review the epidemiology and clinical characteristics associated with these conditions, and we emphasize the importance of cytogenetic and molecular studies when classifying these disorders. CML is characterized by the Philadelphia chromosome, present in 95 % of cases. JAK-2 mutations are found in essentially all patients with PV and approximately 50 % of those with either ET or PMF. Accurate classification and diagnosis are paramount in assigning appropriate risk-based therapy.

Current treatment goals for CML include hematologic remission defined as a CBC which returns to normal values, the absence of splenomegaly, and cytogenetic and molecular remission. Standard treatment is imatinib, which is highly effective in all phases of CML. Available data sets suggest that HIV infection does not increase the prevalence of CML; however, response to imatinib in HIV-CML patients was reported to be inferior to that noted in patients with CML without HIV. Imatinib is metabolized by CYP3A4, and certain antiretroviral classes such as non-nucleoside reverse transcriptase inhibitors and protease inhibitors are known to affect CYP3A4; despite this, imatinib taken in conjunction with various HAART regimens appears to be well tolerated and without significant drug interactions.

The most prominent feature of PV is an elevated absolute RBC mass. There are very few cases that present or study the effect of HIV infection on the development of PV. Hydroxyurea is widely used in response to PV, while alternative treatments include phlebotomy, interferon alpha, or busulfan. Ruxolitinib has also been used for the treatment of patients with intolerance or resistance to hydroxyurea and has also been demonstrated in vitro to block T-cell activation mediated HIV replication.

ET can easily be confused with other entities since isolated thrombocytosis can be seen in the other MPNs and, more commonly, as a complication of many other illnesses. Most patients with ET maintain normal life expectancy, and only those with vasomotor symptoms or high-risk disease require treatment with low-dose aspirin and hydroxyurea.

PMF is the least common of the MPNs. Treatment of PMF depends on each individual case and can include cytoreductive therapies, corticosteroids, androgens, recombinant erythropoietin, and, rarely, hematopoietic SCT. Accounts of treating patients with PMF and HIV infection have not been reported in the literature.

## References


1. Konopka JB, Witte ON. Detection of c-abl tyrosine kinase activity in vitro permits direct comparison of normal and altered abl gene products. Mol Cell Biol. 1985;5(11):3116–23.
2. Reilly JT. Pathogenetic insight and prognostic information from standard and molecular cytogenetic studies in the BCR-ABL-negative myeloproliferative neoplasms (MPNs). Leukemia. 2008;22(10):1818–27.
3. Bench AJ, et al. Molecular diagnosis of the myeloproliferative neoplasms: UK guidelines for the detection of JAK2 V617F and other relevant mutations. Br J Haematol. 2013;160(1):25–34.
4. Kleppe M, et al. JAK-STAT pathway activation in malignant and nonmalignant cells contributes to MPN pathogenesis and therapeutic response. Cancer Discov. 2015;5(3):316–31.
5. Tefferi A, et al. Survival and prognosis among 1545 patients with contemporary polycythemia vera: an international study. Leukemia. 2013;27(9):1874–81.
6. Tefferi A, et al. Proposals and rationale for revision of the World Health Organization diagnostic criteria for polycythemia vera, essential thrombocythemia, and primary myelofibrosis: recommendations from an ad hoc international expert panel. Blood. 2007;110(4):1092–7.
7. Cervantes F, et al. Chronic myeloid leukemia of thrombocythemic onset: a CML subtype with distinct hematological and molecular features? Leukemia. 1996;10(7):1241–3.
8. Pozdnyakova O, et al. Impact of bone marrow pathology on the clinical management of Philadelphia chromosome-negative myeloproliferative neoplasms. Clin Lymphoma Myeloma Leuk. 2015;15(5):253–61.
9. What are the key statistics about chronic myeloid leukemia? www.cancer.org/cancer/leukemia-chronicmyeloidcml/detailedguide/leukemia-chronic-myeloidmyelogenous-key-statistics. Accessed Nov. 29, 2015.
10. Bacarani M. International Journal of Hematologic Oncology Treatment of chronic myeloid leukemia, which drugs? How long? How much? Intern J Hematol Oncol. 2015;4(3):93–102.
11. NCCN. Clinical practice guidelines in oncology: chronic myelogenous leukemia. J Natl Compr Canc Netw. 2013;11:1327–40.
12. Gambacorti-Passerini C, Piazza R. Imatinib-a new tyrosine kinase inhibitor for first-line treatment of chronic myeloid leukemia in 2015. JAMA Oncol. 2015;1(2):143–4.
13. Hughes T, White D. Which TKI? An embarrassment of riches for chronic myeloid leukemia patients. Hematol Am Soc Hematol Educ Prog. 2013;2013:168–75.
14. Patel M, et al. Human immunodeficiency virus infection and chronic myeloid leukemia. Leuk Res. 2012;36(11):1334–8.

15. Schlaberg R, et al. Chronic myeloid leukemia and HIV-infection. Leuk Lymphoma. 2008;49(6):1155–60.
16. Tuljipurkar V, Phatak U. Human immunodeficiency virus infection in a patient with chronic myeloid leukemia. Indian J Med Paediatr Oncol. 2013;34:323–6.
17. Hagiwara S, et al. Non-AIDS-defining hematological malignancies in HIV-infected patients: an epidemiological study in Japan. AIDS. 2013;27(2):279–83.
18. Gleevec package insert. http://www.accessdata.fda.gov/drugsatfda_docs/label/2006/021588s009lbl.pdf.
19. Peng B, Lloyd P, Schran H. Clinical pharmacokinetics of imatinib. Clin Pharmacokinet. 2005;44(9):879–94.
20. Inoue T, et al. Lifetime treatment of mice with azidothymidine (AZT) produces myelodysplasia. Leukemia. 1997;11 Suppl 3:123–7.
21. Ahmed M, Begum T, Iroegbu N. Serum nilotinib level monitoring during concomitant use of CYP3A4 inhibitors. J Invest Med. 2015;63(156):369.
22. Berlin N. Diagnosis and classification of polycythemias. Semin Hematol. 1975;12:339.
23. Ania BJ, et al. Trends in the incidence of polycythemia vera among Olmsted County, Minnesota residents, 1935–1989. Am J Hematol. 1994;47(2):89–93.
24. Polycythemia vera facts. Leukemia & Lymphoma Society. www.lls.org/sites/default/files/file_assets/FS13_PolycythemiaVera_FactSheet_final5.1.15.pdf. Accessed Nov. 29, 2015.
25. Krsak M, et al. Myocardial infarction, stroke, and mortality in cART-treated HIV patients on statins. AIDS Patient Care STDS. 2015;29(6):307–13.
26. Crum-Cianflone NF, Weekes J, Bavaro M. Review: thromboses among HIV-infected patients during the highly active antiretroviral therapy era. AIDS Patient Care STDS. 2008;22(10):771–8.
27. Spivak JL, Silver RT. The revised World Health Organization diagnostic criteria for polycythemia vera, essential thrombocytosis, and primary myelofibrosis: an alternative proposal. Blood. 2008;112(2):231–9.
28. Vorkas CK, Vaamonde CM, Glesby MJ. Testosterone replacement therapy and polycythemia in HIV-infected patients. AIDS. 2012;26(2):243–5.
29. Rose SR, et al. Etiology of thrombocytosis in a general medicine population: analysis of 801 cases with emphasis on infectious causes. J Clin Med Res. 2012;4(6):415–23.
30. Battian R, Ottaviano Porcelli M, Distenfeld A. Polycythemia in patients with AIDS. Lancet. 1990;335:1342–3.
31. Hentrich M, et al. Acute myelogenous leukaemia and myelomonocytic blast crisis following polycythemia vera in HIV positive patients: report of cases and review of the literature. Ann Oncol. 2000;11(2):195–200.
32. Sassaki MG, et al. Polycythemia vera in a patient with the human immunodeficiency virus: a case report. Braz J Infect Dis. 2000;4(4):204–7.
33. Streiff MB, Smith B, Spivak JL. The diagnosis and management of polycythemia vera in the era since the Polycythemia Vera Study Group: a survey of American Society of Hematology members' practice patterns. Blood. 2002;99(4):1144–9.
34. Landolfi R, Marchioli R. European collaboration on low-dose aspirin in polycythemia vera (ECLAP): a randomized trial. Semin Thromb Hemost. 1997;23(5):473–8.
35. Landolfi R, et al. Efficacy and safety of low-dose aspirin in polycythemia vera. N Engl J Med. 2004;350(2):114–24.
36. Cervantes F, et al. Three-year efficacy, safety, and survival findings from COMFORT-II, a phase 3 study comparing ruxolitinib with best available therapy for myelofibrosis. Blood. 2013;122(25):4047–53.
37. Dupuy F, et al. JAK inhibitors tofacitinib and ruxolitinib block T-cell activation mediated HIV replication. Top Antivir Med. 2014;22(e-1):182–3.
38. Wysham NG, Sullivan DR, Allada G. An opportunistic infection associated with ruxolitinib, a novel janus kinase 1, 2 inhibitor. Chest. 2013;143(5):1478–9.

39. Vannucchi AM, et al. Ruxolitinib versus standard therapy for the treatment of polycythemia vera. N Engl J Med. 2015;372(5):426–35.
40. Ruggeri M, et al. The rate of progression to polycythemia vera or essential thrombocythemia in patients with erythrocytosis or thrombocytosis. Ann Intern Med. 2003;139(6):470–5.
41. Ruggeri M, et al. No treatment for low-risk thrombocythaemia: results from a prospective study. Br J Haematol. 1998;103(3):772–7.
42. Zhan H, Spivak JL. The diagnosis and management of polycythemia vera, essential thrombocythemia, and primary myelofibrosis in the JAK2 V617F era. Clin Adv Hematol Oncol. 2009;7(5):334–42.
43. Santos FP, et al. Phase 2 study of CEP-701, an orally available JAK2 inhibitor, in patients with primary or post-polycythemia vera/essential thrombocythemia myelofibrosis. Blood. 2010;115(6):1131–6.
44. Deeg HJ, et al. Allogeneic hematopoietic stem cell transplantation for myelofibrosis. Blood. 2003;102(12):3912–8.
45. Guardiola P, et al. Allogeneic stem cell transplantation for agnogenic myeloid metaplasia: a European Group for Blood and Marrow Transplantation, Societe Francaise de Greffe de Moelle, Gruppo Italiano per il Trapianto del Midollo Osseo, and Fred Hutchinson Cancer Research Center Collaborative Study. Blood. 1999;93(9):2831–8.
46. Rondelli D, et al. Allogeneic hematopoietic stem-cell transplantation with reduced-intensity conditioning in intermediate- or high-risk patients with myelofibrosis with myeloid metaplasia. Blood. 2005;105(10):4115–9.
47. Cervantes F, et al. Danazol treatment of idiopathic myelofibrosis with severe anemia. Haematologica. 2000;85(6):595–9.
48. Cervantes F, et al. Erythropoietin treatment of the anaemia of myelofibrosis with myeloid metaplasia: results in 20 patients and review of the literature. Br J Haematol. 2004;127(4): 399–403.
49. Mesa RA, et al. A phase 2 trial of combination low-dose thalidomide and prednisone for the treatment of myelofibrosis with myeloid metaplasia. Blood. 2003;101(7):2534–41.
50. Tefferri A. Polycythemia vera and essential thrombocythemia: 2015 update on diagnosis, risk-stratification and management. Am J Hematol. 2015;90(2):162–73. doi: 10.1002/ajh.23895.

# HIV-Associated Multicentric Castleman's Disease

# 16

Christian Hoffmann, Eric Oksenhendler, and Laurence Gérard

## Contents



Multicentric Castleman's disease (MCD) is a polyclonal B-cell lymphoproliferative disorder presenting with various clinical features. In HIV-infected patients, almost all MCD cases are associated with human herpesvirus 8 (HHV-8) coinfection [38]. In comparison to the benign localized mediastinal masses composed of follicular hyperplasia initially described by Benjamin Castleman in 1954, HIV-MCD is a severe disease [8, 9, 31, 41]. Although considered to be nonmalignant, HIV-MCD can be life-threatening, either through multiple organ failure or the development of non-Hodgkin lymphoma (NHL).

C. Hoffmann, MD (✉)
Infektionsmedizinisches Centrum Hamburg (ICH), Hamburg, Germany
e-mail: hoffmann@ich-hamburg.de

E. Oksenhendler • L. Gérard
Hôpital Saint-Louis, AP-HP, and EA3963, University Paris Diderot, Paris, France
e-mail: eric.oksenhendler@sls.aphp.fr; laurence.gerard@sls.aphp.fr



M. Hentrich, S.K. Barta (eds.), *HIV-associated Hematological Malignancies*,
DOI 10.1007/978-3-319-26857-6_16

## 16.1 Epidemiology

HIV-MCD is a rare disease. In a prospective HIV database with 56,202 patient-years of follow-up in the UK, the incidence was 4.3/10,000 patient-years [35]. Because of its nonspecific symptoms and remitting and relapsing course, MCD is probably underrecognized and underreported. The disease appears to occur more frequently in patients with suppressed HIV RNA and with a relatively preserved immune function. Almost half of the patients display CD4 T-cell counts above $200 \times 10^6$/L at the time of MCD diagnosis [16, 24, 35]. In contrast to Kaposi sarcoma (KS), HIV-MCD is not associated with a lack of HHV-8-specific CD8 T cells or a limitation of their functional profile [15].

## 16.2 Pathogenesis

The pathogenesis of the disease is not completely understood. There is a close association with HHV-8, a double-stranded DNA virus that encodes several homologues of cellular proteins. By contrast to KS and primary effusion lymphoma, two other HHV-8-associated diseases, lytically active HHV-8 is found in a substantial proportion of infected cells. HHV-8 encodes a homologue of IL-6 (viral IL-6) that has been shown to be biologically active in several assays and whose activities mirror those of its mammalian counterparts [10, 23]. Lytic activation and the production of viral IL-6 are thought to underlie its pathogenesis. Viral IL-6 mediates its effects by forming a tetrameric complex with the IL-6 receptor superfamily gp130 component, which is widely expressed in human tissues, without requiring binding to the classical gp80 IL-6 receptor. Hence, signaling does not depend on the structurally related IL-6 receptor subunit [21]. As a result, viral IL-6 may be able to initiate signaling in a wider variety of cell types compared to human IL-6, contributing to MCD disease manifestations. However, both viral and human IL-6 can independently or together lead to MCD flares, suggesting that they may jointly contribute to disease severity [33]. Viral and human IL-6 overexpression in mouse models can each produce phenotypes resembling that of HHV-8-MCD [7]. There are some reports of an IL-6-related systemic inflammatory syndrome in HIV-infected patients with HHV-8 infection but without MCD [45]. It may be possible that at least some of these cases may just present prodromal symptoms to frank HHV-8-associated MCD.

It remains unclear why only such a small proportion of HIV-infected patients with active HHV-8 coinfection develop MCD. Unlike idiopathic HIV-negative MCD in which IL-6 polymorphisms have been shown to contribute to the activation of the IL-6 signaling pathway [40], there is currently no data suggesting a genetic predisposition for MCD in HIV-infected patients.

## 16.3 Clinical Presentation and Natural Course

The main signs are significant lymph node and spleen enlargements, which are usually combined with severe B symptoms, weakness, and malaise. Heterogeneous symptoms can be associated, the most common being nonspecific respiratory and gastrointestinal disorders. Nasal obstruction is frequently reported. Hepatomegaly, edema, and effusions are also seen in many cases. Laboratory tests show elevated serum C-reactive protein (CRP) level, polyclonal hypergammaglobulinemia, cytopenia, and low serum albumin level. The disease is characterized by episodic exacerbations ("Castleman flares") with subsequent spontaneous remissions. In some patients, a life-threatening acute illness may occur with a rapid fatal course through multiple organ failure, hemophagocytic syndrome, or evolution toward lymphoma.

The prognosis of MCD has dramatically improved in recent years, mainly due to the widespread use of combination antiretroviral therapy (cART) and targeted therapies [4, 14, 16, 24]. Unlike earlier series in which the median survival was about 12 months [31], 1-year survival now exceeds 85 %, and sustained responses are often seen. According to a review on 84 cases, life expectancy has significantly improved in the era of cART with a mortality rate of only 29 %, compared to 75 % in the pre-cART era [24]. Before the introduction of rituximab, progression to malignant non-Hodgkin lymphoma, mainly HHV-8-associated entities such as primary effusion lymphoma or plasmablastic subtypes, was frequent and was the major cause of death [12, 29]. There is evidence that rituximab decreases the risk of subsequent development of NHL [14].

## 16.4 Diagnosis and Monitoring

The diagnosis of MCD is based on clinical features and lymph node biopsy. The classical pathological features include angiofollicular hyperplasia, hypocellular germinal centers with hyalinization, and mantle zone hyperplasia. In the mantle zone, concentric layers of small lymphocytes constitute the so-called onion-skin feature, associated with an intense interfollicular plasmacytic hyperplasia (Figs. 16.1 and 16.2). A subset of B cells, namely plasmablasts, is infected with HHV-8, as demonstrated by expression of the HHV-8 latency-associated nuclear antigen (LANA-1). Plasmablasts are located in the mantle zone (Fig. 16.3) and may express the CD20 surface antigen [12]. They have a mature phenotype and express high levels of λ-light chain restricted immunoglobulin (Ig)M but are polyclonal and do not harbor somatic mutations in the rearranged Ig genes, indicating an origination from naive B lymphocytes [10, 12]. Some of these typical features are often missing, and pathological diagnosis can be difficult with atypical or incomplete MCD histological features. Foci of KS can be observed in lymph nodes in addition to MCD lesions and argue for the diagnosis of HHV-8-associated disorder [26].

Although the diagnosis is based primarily on histopathologic features, clinical features should be present to confirm a diagnosis of active disease. The diagnosis of HIV-MCD must be considered in every case of an HIV-infected patient presenting with episodic flares of B symptoms, splenomegaly, lymphadenopathy, severe cytopenia, and elevated CRP. Association with KS, which is present in up to 70 % at the time of MCD diagnosis, should alert for this disease [24]. A high level of HHV-8 DNA copies in the blood is an important diagnosis tool, with a high negative predictive value [30, 39]. Numerous studies have shown that HHV-8 DNA is almost always detectable in active MCD and that levels correlate with symptomatic disease

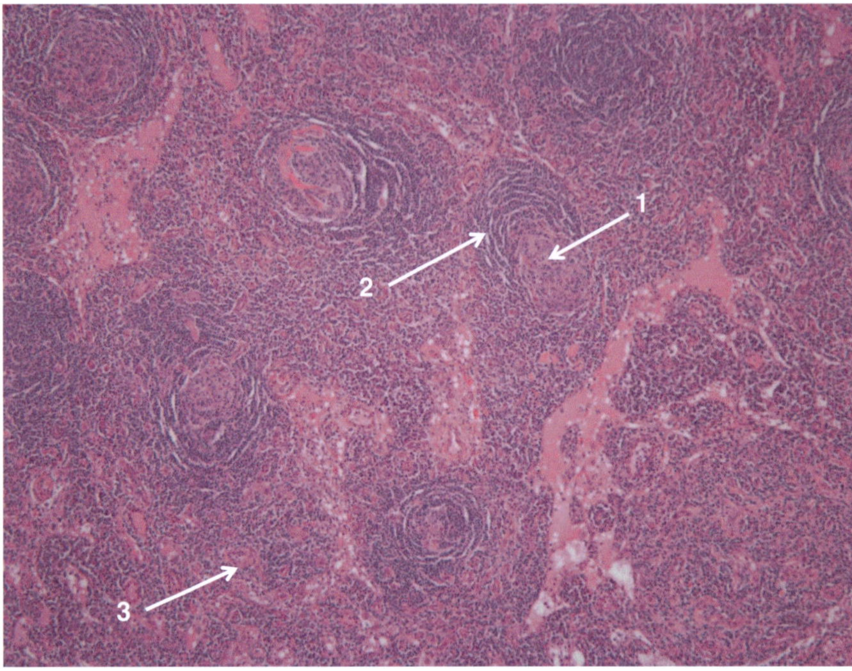


**Fig. 16.1** Lymph node of a patient with HIV-MCD (hematoxylin and eosin staining, ×100). Germinal centers are atrophic and depleted of lymphocytes (*1*). The lymphocytes in the surrounding mantle zone are expanded and arranged in multiple concentric layers, imparting an "onion-skin" appearance (*2*). Angioproliferation and expansion of plasma cells in the interfollicular zones (*3*) (Courtesy of Véronique Meignin)

[11, 30, 34]. In contrast, only a minority of patients with KS has detectable HHV-8 DNA, and levels are significantly lower than seen in MCD patients [22, 42].

In the context of HIV infection, a typical clinical presentation associated with an intense plasmacytosis in the lymph node or in the bone marrow, a high serum CRP, and a high HHV-8 DNA level in the blood are highly suggestive for MCD diagnosis. In critically ill patients, these findings may be sufficient to initiate MCD treatment [32].

## 16.5 Treatment

MCD often arises in patients with undetectable HIV RNA, and clinical observations do not support the effectiveness of cART in the treatment of MCD [1]. MCD can even occur or worsen after initiation of cART [47]. However, the control of HIV infection is mandatory in all HIV-MCD patients, and cART should always be initiated or optimized [6, 32, 34].

Specific treatment of MCD should be reserved for symptomatic disease. Due to the rarity of HIV-MCD, no option has been tested in randomized controlled trials,

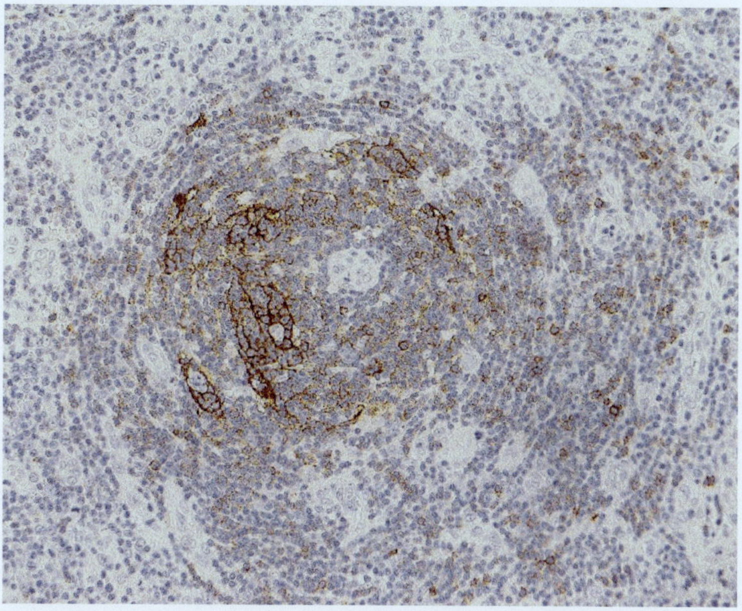

**Fig. 16.2** Lymph node of another patient with HIV-MCD (CD23 staining). A hyalinized germinal center showing hyalinized areas. The "onion-skin" arrangement in the mantle zone is partially destroyed (Courtesy of Markus Tiemann)

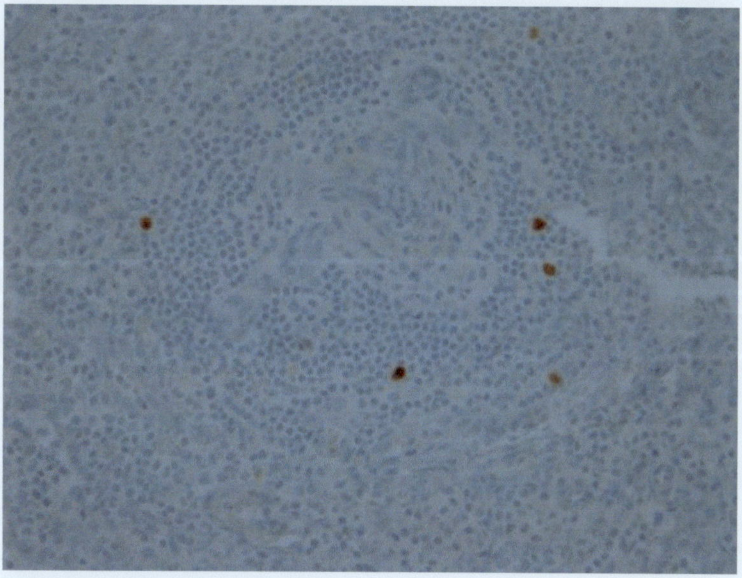

**Fig. 16.3** Immunohistochemistry using monoclonal antibodies to LANA-1 (Clone 13B10, Novocastra) shows nuclear staining (*brown*) of plasmablasts in the mantle zone (×400) (Courtesy of Véronique Meignin)

and there is no widely accepted standard of care. A wide variety of strategies have been reported, including cytotoxic elimination of cells responsible for hypercytokinemia, antiherpesvirus therapies, and anti-inflammatory and immunosuppressive therapies. More recently, blockade of IL-6 signaling with monoclonal antibodies (mAb) has been discussed.

Rituximab, a mAb against CD20-expressing cells, has demonstrated its efficacy in HIV-MCD patients in two prospective trials. Used as first-line therapy in 21 patients, a 2-year overall and disease-free survival of 95 % and 79 % was achieved, respectively [5]. In a second study on 24 patients with severe disease, in which rituximab was given after initial control of MCD by single-agent chemotherapy, 1-year overall and disease-free survival was 92 % and 71 %, respectively [13]. These results were confirmed in a retrospective cohort on 52 patients, in which rituximab markedly improved prognosis in HIV-MCD compared to patients receiving chemotherapy only [16]. Sustained remissions are frequently seen (Fig. 16.4). Rituximab is also effective as retreatment in rituximab-pretreated HIV-MCD [36]. The mechanism of action of rituximab remains poorly understood. The main limitation of rituximab use is exacerbation of KS, which was observed in 35–67 % of the cases [5, 13]. A recent study suggested that KS progression can be prevented by combination of rituximab with liposomal doxorubicin [43].

Cytotoxic chemotherapy, used as single-agent or in combination regimens, including etoposide, vincristine, vinblastine, or doxorubicin are promptly effective and remain the first-line therapy in patients with severe disease or with contraindication to rituximab [19, 37]. In severe life-threatening flares, treatment with intravenous etoposide (120–150 mg/m$^2$) should be initiated. Clinical remission is usually

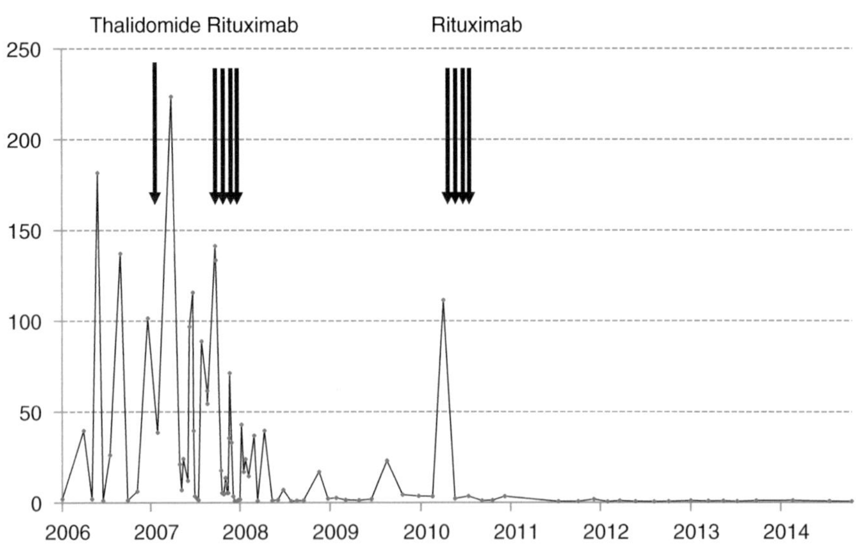


**Fig. 16.4** C-reactive protein over time in a patient with HIV-MCD: durable remission (also clinically) after two cycles of rituximab, HHV-8-PCR negative since July 2010

promptly achieved and is often seen after a single infusion. In the absence of a response, an alternate diagnosis should be considered, particularly NHL. With clinical improvement, oral etoposide (100–120 mg/m$^2$ weekly) can be started. Within a few weeks, etoposide dosage can be progressively tapered and stopped. Despite its rapid effectiveness, some patients experienced relapse after discontinuation, and the toxicity is of concern with prolonged use [3, 32]. In cases with severe refractory cytopenia or if lymphoma is suspected without histologic evidence, splenectomy could be considered.

Active lytic viral replication is highest in MCD compared to other HHV-8-associated diseases, and disease flares are associated with an increase in HHV-8 viremia. Although antiherpesvirus agents show activity against HHV-8 in vitro [18], clinical data are controversial. Recently, one study suggested that valganciclovir (combined with high-dose zidovudine) was active in HIV-MCD [44]. However, others were unable to confirm these findings [16], and antiviral therapy with foscarnet or cidofovir had no benefit [2]. Thus, the role of valganciclovir as maintenance therapy remains to be demonstrated.

Anti-inflammatory agents have been used in MCD with only moderate success. Thalidomide has been noted to have some activity against MCD [17, 20], but neurologic and venous thromboembolic toxicities limit its use in this indication. In contrast to HIV-negative MCD, steroids are not effective in HIV-MCD. For interferon, positive as well as negative cases were reported [28].

An attractive approach seems to be targeting IL-6 and IL-6 receptor using monoclonal antibodies. In HIV-negative patients, encouraging data from Japan have been published with tocilizumab, a humanized anti-IL-6 receptor antibody [27]. Recently, the two first cases of HIV- and HHV-8-positive MCD treated with tocilizumab were reported. In both cases, a significant and rapid clinical improvement was observed, but remissions were not sustained, and recurrence was observed after 15 and 22 weeks on treatment [25]. IL-6 blockade with siltuximab has been approved for symptomatic HIV-negative MCD [46] and may also be an important new treatment option for HIV-MCD. However, data in HIV- and HHV-8 patients are lacking.

In conclusion, experts propose treatment according to the severity of the disease. In patients with good performance status and without organ involvement or active KS, most experts advocate rituximab monotherapy [4, 32]. In severe life-threatening flares, treatment with intravenous etoposide should be initiated. Some experts recommend the initial use of rituximab in association with chemotherapy in these patients [4], and others reserve it to patients who relapsed after discontinuation of chemotherapy [32].

## References

1. Alzahrani M, Hull MC, Sherlock C, Griswold D, Leger CS, Leitch HA. Human immunodeficiency virus-associated multicentric Castleman disease refractory to antiretroviral therapy: clinical features, treatment and outcome. Leuk Lymphoma. 2015;56:1246–51.
2. Bérezné A, Agbalika F, Oksenhendler E. Failure of cidofovir in HIV-associated multicentric Castleman disease. Blood. 2004;103:4368–9.

3. Boshoff C, Begent RH, Oliver RT, et al. Secondary tumours following etoposide containing therapy for germ cell cancer. Ann Oncol. 1995;6:35–40.
4. Bower M, Newsom-Davis T, Naresh K, et al. Clinical features and outcome in HIV-associated multicentric Castleman's disease. J Clin Oncol. 2011;29:2481–6.
5. Bower M, Powles T, Williams S, et al. Brief communication: rituximab in HIV-associated multicentric Castleman disease. Ann Int Med. 2007;147:836–9.
6. Bower M. How I, treat HIV-associated multicentric Castleman disease. Blood. 2010;116:4415–21.
7. Brandt SJ, Bodine DM, Dunbar CE, Nienhuis AW. Retroviral-mediated transfer of interleukin-6 into hematopoietic cells of mice results in a syndrome resembling Castleman's disease. Curr Top Microbiol Immunol. 1990;166:37–41.
8. Castleman B, Towne VW. Case records of the Massachusetts General Hospital: case no. 40231. N Eng J Med. 1954;250:1001–5.
9. Castleman B, Iverson L, Menendez VP. Localized mediastinal lymph-node hyperplasia resembling lymphoma. Cancer. 1956;9:822–30.
10. Du MQ, Liu H, Diss TC, et al. Kaposi sarcoma-associated herpesvirus infects monotypic (IgM lambda) but polyclonal naive B cells in Castleman disease and associated lymphoproliferative disorders. Blood. 2001;97:2130–6.
11. Du MQ, Bacon CM, Isaacson PG. Kaposi sarcoma-associated herpesvirus/human herpesvirus 8 and lymphoproliferative disorders. J Clin Pathol. 2007;60:1350–7.
12. Dupin N, Diss TL, Kellam P, et al. HHV-8 is associated with a plasmablastic variant of Castleman disease that is linked to HHV-8-positive plasmablastic lymphoma. Blood. 2000;95:1406–12.
13. Gérard L, Bérezné A, Galicier L, et al. Prospective study of rituximab in chemotherapy-dependent human immunodeficiency virus associated multicentric Castleman's disease: ANRS 117 CastlemaB trial. J Clin Oncol. 2007;25:3350–6.
14. Gérard L, Michot JM, Burcheri S, et al. Rituximab decreases the risk of lymphoma in patients with HIV-associated multicentric Castleman disease. Blood. 2012;119:2228–33.
15. Guihot A, Oksenhendler E, Galicier L, et al. Multicentric Castleman disease is associated with polyfunctional effector memory HHV-8 – specific CD8+ T cells. Blood. 2008;111:1387–95.
16. Hoffmann C, Schmid H, Müller M, et al. Improved outcome with rituximab in patients with HIV-associated multicentric Castleman disease. Blood. 2011;118:3499–503.
17. Jung CP, Emmerich B, Goebel FD, Bogner JR. Successful treatment of a patient with HIV-associated multicentric Castleman disease (MCD) with thalidomide. Am J Hematol. 2004;75:176–7.
18. Klass CM, Offermann MK. Targeting human herpesvirus-8 for treatment of Kaposi's sarcoma and primary effusion lymphoma. Curr Opin Oncol. 2005;17:447–55.
19. Kotb R, Vincent I, Dulioust A, et al. Life-threatening interaction between antiretroviral therapy and vinblastine in HIV-associated multicentric Castleman's disease. Eur J Haematol. 2006;76:269–71.
20. Lee FC, Merchant SH. Alleviation of systemic manifestations of multicentric Castleman's disease by thalidomide. Am J Hematol. 2003;73:48–53.
21. Li H, Wang H, Nicholas J. Detection of direct binding of human herpesvirus 8-encoded interleukin-6 (vIL-6) to both gp130 and IL-6 receptor (IL-6R) and identification of amino acid residues of vIL-6 important for IL-6R-dependent and -independent signaling. J Virol. 2001;75:3325–34.
22. Marcelin A-G, Motol J, Guihot A, et al. Relationship between the quantity of Kaposi sarcoma-associated herpesvirus (KSHV) in peripheral blood and effusion fluid samples and KSHV-associated disease. J Infect Dis. 2007;196:1163–6.
23. Moore PS, Boshoff C, Weiss RA, Chang Y. Molecular mimicry of human cytokine and cytokine response pathway genes by KSHV. Science. 1996;274:1739–44.
24. Mylona EE, Baraboutis IG, Lekakis LJ, et al. Multicentric Castleman's disease in HIV infection: a systematic review of the literature. AIDS Rev. 2008;10:25–35.
25. Nagao A, Nakazawa S, Hanabusa H. Short-term efficacy of the IL6 receptor antibody tocilizumab in patients with HIV-associated multicentric Castleman disease: report of two cases. J Hematol Oncol. 2014;7:10.

26. Naresh KN, Rice AJ, Bower M. Lymph nodes involved by multicentric Castleman disease among HIV-positive individuals are often involved by Kaposi sarcoma. Am J Surg Pathol. 2008;32:1006–12.
27. Nishimoto N, Kanakura Y, Aozasa K, et al. Humanized anti-interleukin-6 receptor antibody treatment of multicentric Castleman disease. Blood. 2005;106:2627–32.
28. Nord JA, Karter D. Low dose interferon-alpha therapy for HIV-associated multicentric Castleman's disease. Int J STD AIDS. 2003;14:61–2.
29. Oksenhendler E, Boulanger E, Galicier L, et al. High incidence of Kaposi sarcoma-associated herpesvirus-related non-Hodgkin lymphoma in patients with HIV infection and multicentric Castleman disease. Blood. 2002;99:2331–6.
30. Oksenhendler E, Carcelain G, Aoki Y, et al. High levels of human herpesvirus 8 viral load, human interleukin-6, interleukin-10, and C reactive protein correlate with exacerbation of multicentric castleman disease in HIV-infected patients. Blood. 2000;96:2069–73.
31. Oksenhendler E, Duarte M, Soulier J, et al. Multicentric Castleman's disease in HIV infection: a clinical and pathological study of 20 patients. AIDS. 1996;10:61–7.
32. Oksenhendler E. HIV-associated multicentric Castleman disease. Curr Opin HIV AIDS. 2009;4:16–21.
33. Polizzotto MN, Uldrick TS, Wang V, et al. Human and viral interleukin-6 and other cytokines in Kaposi sarcoma herpesvirus-associated multicentric Castleman disease. Blood. 2013;122:4189–98.
34. Polizzotto MN, Uldrick TS, Hu D, Yarchoan R. Clinical manifestations of Kaposi sarcoma herpesvirus lytic activation: multicentric Castleman disease (KSHV-MCD) and the KSHV inflammatory cytokine syndrome. Front Microbiol. 2012;3:73.
35. Powles T, Stebbing J, Bazeos A, et al. The role of immune suppression and HHV-8 in the increasing incidence of HIV-associated multicentric Castleman's disease. Ann Oncol. 2009;20:775–9.
36. Powles T, Stebbing J, Montoto S, et al. Rituximab as retreatment for rituximab pretreated HIV-associated multicentric Castleman disease. Blood. 2007;110:4132–3.
37. Scott D, Cabral L, Harrington Jr WJ. Treatment of HIV-associated multicentric Castleman's disease with oral etoposide. Am J Hematol. 2001;66:148–50.
38. Soulier J, Grollet L, Oksenhendler E, et al. Kaposi's sarcoma-associated herpesvirus-like DNA sequences in multicentric Castleman's disease. Blood. 1995;86:1276–80.
39. Stebbing J, Adams C, Sanitt A, et al. Plasma HHV8 DNA predicts relapse in individuals with HIV-associated multicentric Castleman disease. Blood. 2011;118:271–5.
40. Stone K, Woods E, Szmania SM, et al. Interleukin-6 receptor polymorphism is prevalent in HIV-negative Castleman disease and is associated with increased soluble interleukin-6 receptor levels. PLoS One. 2013;8:e54610.
41. Talat N, Schulte KM. Castleman's disease: systematic analysis of 416 patients from the literature. Oncologist. 2011;16:1316–24.
42. Tedeschi R, Marus A, Bidoli E, Simonelli C, De Paoli P. Human herpesvirus 8 DNA quantification in matched plasma and PBMCs samples of patients with HHV8-related lymphoproliferative diseases. J Clin Virol. 2008;43:255–9.
43. Uldrick TS, Polizzotto MN, Aleman K, et al. Rituximab plus liposomal doxorubicin in HIV-infected patients with KSHV-associated multicentric Castleman disease. Blood. 2014;124:3544–52.
44. Uldrick TS, Polizzotto MN, Aleman K, et al. High-dose zidovudine plus valganciclovir for Kaposi sarcoma herpesvirus-associated multicentric Castleman disease: a pilot study of virus-activated cytotoxic therapy. Blood. 2011;117(26):6977–86.
45. Uldrick TS, Wang V, O'Mahony D, et al. An interleukin-6-related systemic inflammatory syndrome in patients co-infected with Kaposi sarcoma-associated herpesvirus and HIV but without Multicentric Castleman disease. Clin Infect Dis. 2010;51:350–8.
46. van Rhee F, Wong RS, Munshi N, et al. Siltuximab for multicentric Castleman's disease: a randomised, double-blind, placebo-controlled trial. Lancet Oncol. 2014;15:966–74.
47. Zietz C, Bogner JR, Goebel FD, Lohrs U. An unusual cluster of cases of Castleman's disease during HAART for AIDS. N Engl J Med. 1999;340:1923–4.

# Chemotherapy and Interactions with Combination Antiretroviral Therapy

17

Nicolas Mounier and Michelle A. Rudek

## Contents



N. Mounier (✉)
Department of Onco-Hematology, Archet Hospital, Nice, France
e-mail: mounier.n@chu-nice.fr

M.A. Rudek
The Sidney Kimmel Comprehensive Cancer Center, Johns Hopkins University, Baltimore, MD, USA
e-mail: mrudek2@jhmi.edu



M. Hentrich, S.K. Barta (eds.), *HIV-associated Hematological Malignancies*,
DOI 10.1007/978-3-319-26857-6_17

## 17.1 Combination of Antiretroviral Therapy (cART) and Chemotherapy

### 17.1.1 Main cART Regimens

Since its introduction in the 1990s, combination antiretroviral therapy (cART) has markedly improved the clinical management of HIV infection. HIV-infected patients are often on combination regimens that include antiretroviral drugs from different categories to prevent resistance. Initial regimens in a newly diagnosed patient with HIV include combinations of two nucleoside/nucleotide reverse transcriptase inhibitors (NRTIs for nucleoside, NtRTI for nucleotide) combined with a third drug from one of the following classes: a non-NRTI (NNRTI), a protease inhibitor (PI) boosted with ritonavir, or an integrase strand transfer inhibitor (INSTI) [1]. The presence of multiple drugs in cART regimens enhances the risk of drug-drug interactions and drug toxicity. While involvement of common metabolic pathways primarily involves the CYP450 enzymes, changes in expression of drug efflux transporters are also possible (i.e., ABCB1 or ABCG2).

### 17.1.2 Impact of cART with Chemotherapy

Survival in HIV-infected patients suffering from hematologic malignancies (HM) has greatly increased in recent years [2]. cART contributed to improving CD4 counts thus reducing the risk of opportunistic infections and relapse [3]. Furthermore, recent improvements in supportive care (e.g., use of granulocyte colony-stimulating factor (G-CSF)) reduce hematological toxicity and positively impact survival and quality of life. cART is administered with conventional chemotherapy regimens with promising results [4, 5]. The best example is Hodgkin's lymphoma (HL) where a significant improvement in overall survival (OS) is observed in patients with HIV who responded to cART, are less than 45 years at the time of diagnosis, and achieved a complete remission (CR) status [6]. Similarly, the Spanish group GESIDA noted in HIV-related HL that the only variable independently associated with OS was the achievement of CR under adequate chemotherapy and cART [7].

### 17.1.3 The Issue of Timing

To administer cART concurrently with chemotherapy versus after treatment is still a matter of debate and may be guided by the time of diagnosis. The recommendations should be different if a patient is diagnosed with a hematological malignancy with a known HIV status who is on cART versus if the diagnosis of AIDS is made concurrently. In the case where a patient who has HIV is already on cART, and presents at a curable stage of cancer, the intent should be to maintain dose intensity and adherence to the schedule of the anticancer regimen [8]. If a co-diagnosis is made, then it may be prudent to either select a cART with minimal chances of drug interactions or delay the initiation of cART until tolerance to the anticancer regimen is known. In all cases, the intent is to maximize the likelihood of response to the cancer.

Initial experience suggests that cART can be used concomitantly in lymphoma even with dose-intense regimens [9]. This was associated with a decreased risk of opportunistic infections during antineoplastic treatment secondary to an effective cART regimen (i.e., CD4 cell levels are restored and viral load reduced). The benefit may not occur when the toxicities are too severe. As noted in one such HL trial reports, high incidences of bone marrow suppression and neurotoxicity were observed in patients treated concomitantly with a Stanford V regimen and cART, in particular if the myelotoxic drug zidovudine and neurotoxic antiretrovirals such as didanosine, zalcitabine or stavudine were used (i.e., didanosine, zalcitabine, or stavudine) [10].

When considering whether cART should be omitted during chemotherapy, the degree of immunosuppression present (which would in turn affect the risk of death from bacterial and opportunistic infections) combined with the benefit of viral suppression for survival and tumor response should be weighed against the possible overlapping toxicities from cART and chemotherapy. Sparano et al. omitted cART during the administration of the intensive EPOCH regimen in non-Hodgkin's lymphoma patients who were never previously treated with cART [11]. Systematic administration of hematopoietic growth factors may improve survival by making allowance for higher dose intensity chemotherapy and long-term use of cART. On the other hand, given the relatively preserved immune response of HIV-HL patients, as seen in the Italian cohort, clinical outcome is not influenced by the initiation time of cART [12].

Overall, infection prophylaxis and prompt diagnosis and treatment of bacterial, parasitic, fungal, and viral infections are needed to improve treatment outcomes.

## 17.2 Addition of Toxicities due to Pharmacodynamic Interactions

Depending on the exact combination, cART may be associated with a variety of side effects. Drug-drug interactions can occur when the pharmacological effect of one drug is changed by another through action on the same physiological process. In combining cART and anticancer drug therapy, overlapping toxicity profiles should be avoided.

### 17.2.1 Focus on Hepatotoxicity

Anticancer drugs may have dose adjustment recommendations based on the degree of hepatic impairment, most commonly measured by the bilirubin alterations or the Child-Pugh Score. Unconjugated hyperbilirubinemia, which has been observed with the PIs atazanavir and indinavir, may be overlooked when assessing if dose modifications of anticancer drugs are needed if there are no other signs of liver dysfunction. Lactic acidosis is a hepatotoxicity which cannot be ignored and has been associated with the NRTIs didanosine, stavudine, and zidovudine. However, the preferred NRTIs (i.e., abacavir, emtricitabine, lamivudine, and tenofovir) are less hepatotoxic.

### 17.2.2 Focus on Cytotoxics

Zidovudine is a myelotoxic antiretroviral, which should be avoided when combining with traditional cytotoxic chemotherapy regimens. Neuropathy is another toxicity which has been associated with both chemotherapy (i.e., platinums, taxanes, and vinca alkaloids) and with selected NRTIs (i.e., didanosine and stavudine). If a patient with HIV develops a malignancy and is receiving one of the above cART, the clinical management should be to (1) substitute with a different antiretroviral, (2) select an alternative chemotherapy regimen with no overlapping toxic effects, or (3) temporarily discontinue antiretroviral therapy.

### 17.2.3 Focus on Targeted Drugs

As our understanding of the molecular mechanisms of cancer has increased, the trend in anticancer drug development has been to move away from indiscriminate cytotoxic agents. Molecularly targeted agents tend to have a different toxicity profile than the classic side effects associated with cytotoxics (i.e., diarrhea, myelosuppression, or peripheral neuropathy).

However, a side effect that has emerged as concerning is the overlapping cardiac toxicity risk from QT prolongation. QT prolongation has been associated with atazanavir, ritonavir-boosted lopinavir, and saquinavir. QT prolongation is increasingly common with the tyrosine kinase inhibitors (e.g., nilotinib) and other molecularly targeted agents. Due to the potential for arrhythmias and sudden death, combinations of agents that can prolong the QT interval should be avoided.

## 17.3 Pharmacokinetic Interactions

### 17.3.1 Focus on Antiretrovirals

Bidirectional drug interactions could be anticipated in case of cART since the majority are substrates of and inhibit or induce CYP450s. CYP3A4 is the major CYP450 isozyme which metabolizes all NNRTIs and PIs and some INSTIs and entry inhibitors (e.g., chemokine coreceptor 5 (CCR5) antagonists). However, while several NNRTIs are CYP450 inducers, all PIs are known CYP450 inhibitors, and the INSTIs and entry inhibitors tend not to induce or inhibit CYP450 isozymes (see Table 17.1).

**Table 17.1** Table of interaction between HAART and CYP450

| Drug class | Route of elimination | Effect on CYP450 | Drug interaction potential as a perpetrator[a] | Drug interaction potential as a victim[a] |
|---|---|---|---|---|
| NRTIs | Renal | None/insignificant | 1 | 2 |
| NtRTIs | Renal | CYP450 inhibitor | 2 | 2 |
| NNRTIs | Hepatic (CYP450) | CYP450 inducer or inhibitor | 4 | 2 |
| Protease inhibitors | Hepatic (CYP450) | CYP450 inducer or inhibitor | 3 | 2 |
| Ritonavir- or cobicistat-boosted PI | Hepatic (CYP450) | CYP450 inducer or inhibitor | 5 (inhibitor) | 2 |
| Fusion inhibitors | Catabolism | None | 1 | 1 |
| Entry inhibitor | Hepatic (CYP450) | None | 1 | 3 |
| Integrase inhibitor | Hepatic (UGT) | None | 1 | 3 |

[a]DDI potential code and clinical relevance:

(1) Interaction unlikely or known minor interaction not requiring modification to therapy

(2) Possible interaction based on pharmacology of the drug. No modification to therapy but monitor closely for signs of toxicity

(3) Potential for significant interaction based on pharmacology of the drug. No modification to therapy but monitor closely for signs of toxicity. Consider therapy modification if unable to monitor closely

(4) Potential for clinically significant interaction based on pharmacology of the drug or known interaction. Need for dose adjustment or consideration of therapy modification

(5) Major clinically significant interaction or potential critical interaction. Coadministration is contraindicated

Broadly, drug-mediated induction or inhibition of CYP enzymes can lead to different scenarios which may cause inappropriate drug-drug interactions leading to suboptimal response. The pharmacological effect of these interactions will depend on whether the parent drug or the metabolite causes the majority of the effect. Indeed, toxicity would be anticipated with increased concentrations, while decreased efficacy would be anticipated with decreased concentrations.

- When a drug is an inducer of a CYP450 isozyme, it will result in the substrate drug having decreased parent drug concentrations but increased metabolites.
- When a drug is an inhibitor of a CYP450 isozyme, it will result in the substrate drug having increased parent drug concentrations but decreased metabolites.

Therefore, it is critical to examine the possible involvement of each CYP450 isozyme when combining anticancer and cART drugs, which would help adjust drug dose and drug regimens. Tables 17.1 and 17.2 are intentionally broad since information regarding drug interactions is constantly evolving and would be out of date when this chapter is published. Therefore, the prudent approach would be to assess each drug's interaction potential utilizing a current resource [13].

**Table 17.2** Table of interaction between anticancer agents an CYP450

| Drug class | Route of elimination | Effect on CYP450 | Drug interaction potential as a perpetrator[a] | Drug interaction potential as a victim[a] |
|---|---|---|---|---|
| *Cytotoxic agents* | | | | |
| Alkylating agents | Hepatic (CYP450) | CYP450 inducer or inhibitor | 1 | 3 |
| Anthracyclines | Hepatic (non-CYP450) | CYP450 inhibitor; transporter, inducer | 2 | 2 |
| Antimicrotubular (taxanes) | Hepatic (CYP450) | CYP450 inducer or inhibitor, transporter, inhibitor | 2 | 3 |
| Antitumor antibiotic | Nonenzymatic | None | 1 | 1 |
| Antimetabolite | Renal and hepatic (non-CYP450) | None | 1 | 1 |
| Camptothecins | Non-enzymatic and hepatic (CYP450/UGT) | None | 1 | 4 |
| DNA methyltransferase inhibitors | Cytidine deaminase | None | 1 | 1 |
| Epipodophyllotoxin | Hepatic (CYP450) | CYP450 inhibitor | 2 | 3 |
| Histone deacetylase inhibitors | Hepatic (CYP450/UGT) | Transporter inhibitor | 1 | 2 |
| Platinums | Nonenzymatic and renal | None | 1 | 2 |
| Vinca alkaloids | Hepatic (CYP450) | CYP450 inhibitor, transporter, inducer | 2 | 3 |
| *Molecularly targeted agents* | | | | |
| Immunomodulators | | | 1 | 3 |
| mTOR inhibitors | Hepatic (CYP450) | CYP450 inhibitor | 2 | 4 |
| Proteasome inhibitor | Hepatic (CYP450) | CYP450 inducer and inhibitor | 2 | 3 |
| Tyrosine kinase inhibitor | Hepatic (CYP450) | CYP450 inhibitor (1°), transporter, inhibitor | 3 | 4 |

[a]DDI potential code and clinical relevance:
(1) Interaction unlikely or known minor interaction not requiring modification to therapy
(2) Possible interaction based on pharmacology of the drug. No modification to therapy but monitor closely for signs of toxicity
(3) Potential for significant interaction based on pharmacology of the drug. No modification to therapy but monitor closely for signs of toxicity. Consider therapy modification if unable to monitor closely
(4) Potential for clinically significant interaction based on pharmacology of the drug or known interaction. Need for dose adjustment or consideration of therapy modification
(5) Major clinically significant interaction or potential critical interaction. Coadministration is contraindicated

If a patient with HIV develops a malignancy and is receiving cART, the clinical management should be to assess the regimen for drug interaction potential and if one exists to (1) substitute a different antiretroviral with less drug interaction potential, (2) select an alternative chemotherapy regimen with less drug interaction potential, or (3) temporarily discontinue antiretroviral therapy.

### 17.3.2 Focus on Cytotoxics

Drug interactions with the following classes of anticancer drugs are unlikely since the primary route of elimination is via non-CYP450-mediated routes: anthracyclines, antimetabolite agents, antitumor antibiotics, and platinums. A unidirectional drug interaction could be anticipated with camptothecins which are substrates of but do not alter CYP450 isozymes and are therefore likely to be victims of ART-mediated interactions. In addition, bidirectional drug interactions could be anticipated with taxanes, vinca alkaloids, alkylating agents, and epipodophyllotoxins, which are substrates of and inhibit or induce CYP450 isozymes [14–16].

### 17.3.3 Focus on Targeted Drugs

Monoclonal antibodies (mAb) are metabolized into small peptides and are unlikely to elicit a direct effect on the metabolic pathways for small molecular therapeutics. However, new small molecules targeted anticancer agents are highly likely to be involved in drug interactions. Proteasome inhibitors are substrates of but not inhibitors or inducers of CYP450 isozymes and are likely to have unidirectional drug interactions with cART. Bidirectional drug interactions could be anticipated with tyrosine kinase inhibitors and mTOR inhibitors, which are substrates of and inhibit or induce CYPs [17–19].

### 17.3.4 Perspectives

Current literature is lacking from definitive clinical guidance on how best to combine cART and anticancer agents in patients with HIV and hematological malignancies [20–22]. However, as patients with HIV live longer, it is becoming critical to have dosing recommendations. Therefore, clinical trials are being conducted to provide more definitive recommendation. Until this information is available, communication among oncologists, infectious disease physicians, and pharmacologists will be crucial to guide treatment decisions.

## References

1. Panel on Antiretroviral Guidelines for Adults and Adolescents. Guidelines for the use of antiretroviral agents in HIV-1-infected adults and adolescents. Department of Health and Human Services. Available at http://www.aidsinfo.nih.gov/ContentFiles/AdultandAdolescentGL.pdf. Accessed 27 Nov 2014.

2. Montoto S, Shaw K, Okosun J, et al. HIV status does not influence outcome in patients with classical Hodgkin lymphoma treated with chemotherapy using doxorubicin, bleomycin, vinblastine, and dacarbazine in the highly active antiretroviral therapy era. J Clin Oncol. 2012;30:4111–6.
3. Montoto S, Wilson J, Shaw K, et al. Excellent immunological recovery following CODOX-M/IVAC, an effective intensive chemotherapy for HIV-associated Burkitt's lymphoma. AIDS. 2010;24:851–6.
4. Xicoy B, Ribera JM, Miralles P, et al. Results of treatment with doxorubicin, bleomycin, vinblastine and dacarbazine and highly active antiretroviral therapy in advanced stage, human immunodeficiency virus-related Hodgkin's lymphoma. Haematologica. 2007;92:191–8.
5. Barta SK, Xue X, Wang D, et al. Treatment factors affecting outcomes in HIV-associated non-Hodgkin lymphomas: a pooled analysis of 1546 patients. Blood. 2013;122:3251–62.
6. Hoffmann C, Chow KU, Wolf E, et al. Strong impact of highly active antiretroviral therapy on survival in patients with human immunodeficiency virus-associated Hodgkin's disease. Br J Haematol. 2004;125:455–62.
7. Berenguer J, Miralles P, Ribera JM, et al. Characteristics and outcome of AIDS-related Hodgkin lymphoma before and after the introduction of highly active antiretroviral therapy. J Acquir Immune Defic Syndr. 2008;47:422–8.
8. Hentrich M, Berger M, Wyen C, et al. Stage-adapted treatment of HIV-associated Hodgkin lymphoma: results of a prospective multicenter study. J Clin Oncol. 2012;30:4117–23.
9. Mounier N, Spina M, Gabarre J, et al. AIDS-related non-Hodgkin lymphoma: final analysis of 485 patients treated with risk-adapted intensive chemotherapy. Blood. 2006;107:3832–40.
10. Spina M, Gabarre J, Rossi G, et al. Stanford V regimen and concomitant HAART in 59 patients with Hodgkin disease and HIV infection. Blood. 2002;100:1984–8.
11. Sparano JA, Lee JY, Kaplan LD, et al. Rituximab plus concurrent infusional EPOCH chemotherapy is highly effective in HIV-associated B-cell non-Hodgkin lymphoma. Blood. 2010;115:3008–16.
12. Martis N, Mounier N. Hodgkin lymphoma in patients with HIV infection: a review. Curr Hematol Malig Rep. 2012;7:228–34.
13. Ezzat HM, Cheung MC, Hicks LK, et al. Incidence, predictors and significance of severe toxicity in patients with human immunodeficiency virus-associated Hodgkin lymphoma. Leuk Lymphoma. 2012;53:2390–6.
14. Cingolani A, Torti L, Pinnetti C, et al. Detrimental clinical interaction between ritonavir-boosted protease inhibitors and vinblastine in HIV-infected patients with Hodgkin's lymphoma. AIDS. 2010;24:2408–12.
15. Cianfrocca M, Lee S, Von Roenn J, et al. Pilot study evaluating the interaction between paclitaxel and protease inhibitors in patients with human immunodeficiency virus-associated Kaposi's sarcoma: an Eastern Cooperative Oncology Group (ECOG) and AIDS Malignancy Consortium (AMC) trial. Cancer Chemother Pharmacol. 2011;68:827–33.
16. Rudek MA, Chang CY, Steadman K, et al. Combination antiretroviral therapy (cART) component ritonavir significantly alters docetaxel exposure. Cancer Chemother Pharmacol. 2014;73:729–36.
17. Koon HB, Krown SE, Lee JY, et al. Phase II trial of imatinib in AIDS-associated Kaposi's sarcoma: AIDS Malignancy Consortium Protocol 042. J Clin Oncol. 2014;32:402–8.
18. Rudek MA, Moore PC, Mitsuyasu RT, et al. A phase 1/pharmacokinetic study of sunitinib in combination with highly active antiretroviral therapy in human immunodeficiency virus-positive patients with cancer: AIDS Malignancy Consortium trial AMC 061. Cancer. 2014;120:1194–1202.
19. Pillai VC, Venkataramanan R, Parise RA, et al. Ritonavir and efavirenz significantly alter the metabolism of erlotinib–an observation in primary cultures of human hepatocytes that is relevant to HIV patients with cancer. Drug Metab Dispos. 2013;41:1843–51.
20. Pillai VC, Parise RA, Christner SM, et al. Potential interactions between HIV drugs, ritonavir and efavirenz and anticancer drug, nilotinib–a study in primary cultures of human hepatocytes that is applicable to HIV patients with cancer. J Clin Pharmacol. 2014;54:1272–9.
21. Rudek MA, Flexner C, Ambinder RF. Use of antineoplastic agents in patients with cancer who have HIV/AIDS. Lancet Oncol. 2011;12:905–12.
22. Beumer JH, Venkataramanan R, Rudek MA. Pharmacotherapy in cancer patients with HIV/AIDS. Clin Pharmacol Ther. 2014;95:370–2.

# 18 Diagnosis, Prophylaxis and Treatment of Central Nervous System Involvement by Non-Hodgkin Lymphoma in HIV-Infected Patients

Michele Spina

## Contents



With the widespread use of highly active antiretroviral therapy (HAART), the incidence of systemic non-Hodgkin lymphoma (NHL) in patients infected with the human immunodeficiency virus (HIV) has declined [1]. HAART has also modified the clinical manifestations of these tumours, with a lower frequency of involvement of the central nervous system (CNS) [2]. Before the introduction of HAART, up to 25 % of patients showed CNS involvement; currently, the frequency of meningeal involvement at the time of diagnosis of NHL in HIV-infected patients varies between 3 and 5 %, and its frequency is related to histological subtype, ranging from uncommon in indolent lymphomas to more frequent in aggressive lymphomas such as diffuse large B-cell lymphoma (DLBCL), lymphoblastic lymphoma, blastoid variant of mantle cell lymphoma and Burkitt's lymphoma (BL) [3]. Clinical criteria, such as involvement of the paranasal sinus, testes, orbital cavities or bone marrow, advanced stage, high International Prognostic Index, elevated LDH levels and the involvement of multiple extranodal sites all help to better identify the risk factors in patients for whom the administration of prophylaxis is strongly recommended. Prophylactic treatment is necessary to reduce the incidence of CNS relapse in

M. Spina, MD
Division of Medical Oncology A, National Cancer Institute, Aviano, PN, Italy
e-mail: mspina@cro.it



M. Hentrich, S.K. Barta (eds.), *HIV-associated Hematological Malignancies*,
DOI 10.1007/978-3-319-26857-6_18

aggressive NHL but also increases the toxicity of systemic chemotherapy; therefore, clinical risk paradigms lead to the identification of patients who may benefit from CNS prophylaxis [4]. Unfortunately, because the cohort of patients characterized by risk factors could be four- to fivefold larger than the subgroup that will actually develop CNS disease, more sensitive and specific laboratory methods are needed to detect occult CNS infiltration and to ensure optimal treatment while avoiding unnecessary therapies.

Considering the high risk of progression during the treatment or recurrence during the remission, the use of intrathecal prophylaxis has been considered a mandatory part of the systemic treatment of HIV-NHLs. However, despite the use of standard treatment including methotrexate and/or cytarabine, the CNS recurrence remains a challenge in the outcome of these patients.

## 18.1 Diagnostic Procedures

The diagnosis of meningeal lymphoma relies in clinical findings, imaging techniques and cerebrospinal fluid (CSF) examination.

Magnetic resonance imaging (MRI) with gadolinium is the preferred neuroimaging method to investigate patients with clinical findings that are suggestive of neoplastic meningitis [5, 6] and is reported to be of high diagnostic accuracy in patients with solid tumours. However, several studies have demonstrated that MRI is of limited utility in detecting meningeal infiltration by haematological diseases [7–9]; therefore, light microscopic examination of cytospin preparations is still considered the gold standard for detecting neoplastic cells in the CSF in haematological malignancies.

Among patients who develop CNS disease, only a small fraction have cytologically detectable malignant cells in the CSF on initial staging. This observation raised the question of whether cytology was unable to detect low-volume disease or if leptomeningeal spread was a late event. Cytology of the CSF, the diagnostic gold standard, however, has a low sensitivity with a reported false-negative rate of 20–60 %, suggesting pretreatment leptomeningeal involvement is probably greater than initially reported [10, 11].

Recently, several studies have shown that flow cytometry (FCM) is a diagnostic technique with a higher sensitivity and specificity than conventional cytology for the diagnosis of meningeal lymphoma. All studies showed up to 50 % detection improvement in comparison with cytology with a significant correlation with the outcome of these patients. In other words, those patients with cytology negative and FCM positive have a worse outcome in comparison with both cytology- and FCM-negative patients raising the question whether these patients should be intensively treated as cytology positive patients [12–17]. In particular, in our study, we demonstrated that FCM analysis detected a clonal population in 18 of 174 patients (10 %), whereas CC detected abnormal cells only in 7 patients (4 %; $P = 0.001$). Therefore, procedure results were concordant (FCM+/CC+) in 7 (4 %) cases and discordant (FCM+/CC−) in 11 (6 %) cases. Moreover, the 2-year progression-free and overall survival were significantly higher in patients with FCM- CSF (62 % and 72 %) compared with those FCM+ CSF (39 % and 50 %, respectively), with a 2-year CNS relapse cumulative incidence of 3 % (95 % confidence interval [CI], 0–7) versus 17 % (95 % CI, 0–34; $P=0.004$), respectively. The risk of CNS progression was significantly higher in FMC+/CC− versus FCM−/CC− patients (hazard ratio = 8.16, 95 % CI, 1.45–46) [16]. However, flow cytometry is not yet considered to be the gold standard for this purpose because of several limitations in the standardization of methods and interpretation of the results (i.e. fresh analysis vs fixation, limited vs adequate sample volume, limited number of antibodies used) [18, 19].

Molecular biology techniques have also been applied to the CSF in an attempt to improve the diagnostic accuracy of CNS involvement in haematological malignancies. The morphological distinction between reactive mononuclear and neoplastic lymphoma cells can be difficult to discern because mitotic activity and atypical features present in lymphocytes may be observed in normal CSF samples, contributing to false-positive results. DNA-based molecular techniques identify tumour-specific DNA and do not require intact cells. DNA is stable and can be recovered from the CSF even after tumour cell lysis, potentially making it a more sensitive indicator of malignancy than tests requiring the presence of intact tumour cells. In this issue, different studies have reported the usefulness of DNA-based techniques for the diagnosis of CNS involvement in lymphoproliferative disorders. These studies have shown that polymerase chain reaction (PCR) analysis of clonal IgH genes in CSF is practical and may serve as a complementary test to conventional cytology [20–22].

Finally, despite the wide array of biomarkers that have been tested for the detection of CNS involvement in haematological malignancies, their use has not become widespread in clinical practice. To date, several soluble tumour-related markers have been proposed as diagnostic tools for leptomeningeal involvement of haematological tumours, including LDH, beta-2-microglobulin, fibronectin and various interleukins [23–27]. Unfortunately, none of these have proved to be useful for diagnostic purposes due to their low sensitivity and, even worse, modest specificity [24, 28, 29].

## 18.2 Prophylaxis

Until recently, most experts recommended neuromeningeal prophylaxis for all HIV-infected patients with aggressive NHL. However, at present, this prophylaxis is recommended only in patients with higher risk of CNS relapse according to different sites of involvement, stage and histological subtype.

We can suggest the following parameters for using a prophylaxis in these patients:

(a) Aggressive histological subtypes (i.e. Burkitt's lymphoma, primary effusion lymphoma, plasmoblastic lymphoma for oral cavity)
(b) Patients unable to receive an effective HAART and/or with CD4<50/dl
(c) Involvement of specific extranodal sites such as the testes, paranasal sinuses, hard palate, orbit paravertebral masses

**Table 18.1** CNS prophylaxis in NHL-HIV: schedules of intrathecal injections in phase II and III studies

| Regimen | Drug | Schedule | Study (Ref) |
|---|---|---|---|
| CODOX-M | Cytarabine 70 mg methotrexate 12 mg | Days 1, 3 | Magrath [35] |
| | | Day 15 | |
| IVAC | Methotrexate 12 mg | Day 5 | Magrath [35] |
| Stanford | Methotrexate 12 mg | Days 1, 10 | Bernstein [36] |
| M-BACOD | Cytarabine 50 mg | Days 1, 8, 15, 22 | Kaplan [37] |
| | | Cycle 1 only | |
| CDE | Cytarabine 50 mg | Days 1 and 4 | Sparano [38] |
| | | Cycles 1 and 2 | |
| EPOCH | Methotrexate12 mg | Days 1 and 5 | Little [39] |
| | | Cycles 3, 4, 5, 6 | |
| R-CDE | Methotrexate 12 mg | Day 1 | Spina [40] |
| R-CHOP | Cytarabine 50 mg or methotrexate 12 mg | Days 1, 8, 15, 22 | Kaplan [41] |
| | | Cycle 1 only | |
| ACVBP | Methotrexate 12 mg | Day 1 | Mounier [42] |
| SC-EPOCH-RR | Methotrexate 12 mg | Days 1, 5 | Dunleavy [43] |
| | | Cycles 3, 4, 5 | |

(d) High – intermediate/high IPI score (particularly reflecting the presence of high level of LDH and involvement of more than one extranodal site)

The introduction of rituximab had significantly improved the outcome of lymphomas also in HIV patients prolonging survival and reducing the risk of progression or relapse. The analysis of all published studies in the general population seem to show a significant reduction of CNS progression or relapse in favour of those patients treated with the combination of rituximab plus chemotherapy [30–34].

Different regimens have been used for prophylaxis and treatment for meningeal lymphoma. The most common drugs used for this purpose are methotrexate and cytosine arabinoside with no studies showing a superiority of one drug over each other. Table 18.1 summarized the most common drugs and schedules reported in phase II and III studies [35–43]. However, there are other alternatives such as liposomal cytosine arabinoside that requires fewer spinal taps for drug administration and whose results are very promising [44–46].

One promising alternative might be the use of i.v. MTX, although the high doses necessary to reach effective doses in the CNS will cause additional toxicity and effectiveness has not been formally demonstrated. The low incidence of CNS disease reported by the GELA with AVCBP regimen [47] after implementation of consolidative therapy with high-dose MTX, etoposide, ifosfamide and cytosine arabinoside is remarkable and lends some interest to this approach. Similar data have been reported combining the classical R-CHOP to high-dose MTX [48].

Because CNS disease tends to occur early in most patients with DLBCL and frequently is associated with other lymphoma manifestations, systemic MTX should be administered as early as possible after diagnosis. The advantage of this approach over intrathecal therapy is related to a more uniform distribution of the drug throughout the neuroaxis with therapeutic concentrations gained in brain and spinal cord tissues and deep perivascular spaces [49].

In summary, in the context of an effective HAART, HIV-infected patients with NHL have a frequency of CNS involvement by lymphoma similar to that found among immunocompetent hosts. Consequently, indications and regimens for CNS prophylaxis in HIV-infected patients with NHL should not be different than those employed in the general population.

## References


1. Robbins HA, Pfeiffer RM, Shiels MS, et al. Excess cancers among HIV-infected people in the United States. J Natl Cancer Inst. 2015;107(4):1–8.
2. Vaccher E, Spina M, Talamini R, et al. Improvement of systemic human immunodeficiency virus-related non-Hodgkin lymphoma outcome in the era of highly active antiretroviral therapy. Clin Infect Dis. 2003;37(11):1556–64.
3. Navarro JT, Vall-Llovera F, Mate JL, et al. Decrease in the frequency of meningeal involvement in AIDS-related systemic lymphoma in patients receiving HAART. Haematologica. 2008;93(1):149–50.
4. Hollender A, Kvaloy S, Nome O, et al. Central nervous system involvement following diagnosis of non-Hodgkin's lymphoma: a risk model. Ann Oncol. 2002;13:1099–107.
5. Kaplan JG, DeSouza TG, Farkash A, et al. Leptomeningeal metastases: comparison of clinical features and laboratory data of solid tumors, lymphomas and leukemias. J Neurooncol. 1990;9:225–9.
6. Chamberlain MC, Sandy A, Press GA, et al. Leptomeningeal metastasis: a comparison of gadolinium-enhanced MR and contrast-enhanced CT of the brain. Neurology. 1990;40:435–8.
7. Zeiser R, Burger JA, Bley TA, et al. Clinical follow-up indicates differential accuracy of magnetic resonance imaging and immunocytology of the cerebral spinal fluid for the diagnosis of neoplastic meningitis – a single centre experience. Br J Haematol. 2004;124:762–8.
8. Freilich RJ, Krol G, De Angelis LM. Neuroimaging and cerebrospinal fluid cytology in the diagnosis of leptomeningeal metastases. Ann Neurol. 1995;38:51–7.
9. Pauls S, Fischer AC, Brambs HJ, Fetscher S, Höche W, Bommer M. Use of magnetic resonance imaging to detect neoplastic meningitis: limited use in leukemia and lymphoma but convincing results in solid tumors. Eur J Radiol. 2012;81(5):974–8.
10. De Angelis LM, Cairncross JG. A better way to find tumor in the CSF? Neurology. 2002;58:339–40.
11. Perske C, Nagel I, Nagel H, Strik H. CSF cytology—the ongoing dilemma to distinguish neoplastic and inflammatory lymphocytes. Diagn Cytopathol. 2011;39:621–6.
12. Bromberg JE, Breems DA, Kraan J, et al. CSF flow cytometry greatly improves diagnostic accuracy in CNS hematologic malignancies. Neurology. 2007;68(20):1674–9.
13. Quijano S, López A, Manuel Sancho J, et al. Identification of leptomeningeal disease in aggressive B-cell non-Hodgkin's lymphoma: improved sensitivity of flow cytometry. J Clin Oncol. 2009;27(9):1462–9.
14. Hegde U, Filie A, Little RF, et al. High incidence of occult leptomeningeal disease detected by flow cytometry in newly diagnosed aggressive B-cell lymphomas at risk for central nervous system involvement: the role of flow cytometry versus cytology. Blood. 2005;105(2):496–502.

15. Sancho JM, Orfao A, Quijano S, et al. Clinical significance of occult cerebrospinal fluid involvement assessed by flow cytometry in non-Hodgkin's lymphoma patients at high risk of central nervous system disease in the rituximab era. Eur J Haematol. 2010;85(4):321–8.
16. Benevolo G, Stacchini A, Spina M, et al. Final results of a multicenter trial addressing role of CSF flow cytometric analysis in NHL patients at high risk for CNS dissemination. Blood. 2012;120(16):3222–8.
17. Wilson WH, Bromberg JE, Stetler-Stevenson M, et al. Detection and outcome of occult leptomeningeal disease in diffuse large B-cell lymphoma and Burkitt lymphoma. Haematologica. 2014;99(7):1228–35.
18. Moriarty AT, Wiersema L, Snyder W, et al. Immunophenotyping of cytologic specimens by flow cytometry. Diagn Cytopathol. 1993;9:252–8.
19. Craig FE, Ohori NP, Gorrill TS, et al. Flow cytometric immunophenotyping of cerebrospinal fluid specimens. Am J Clin Pathol. 2011;135(1):22–34.
20. Sayed D, Badrawy H, Ali AM, et al. Immunophenotyping and immunoglobulin heavy chain gene rearrangement analysis in cerebrospinal fluid of pediatric patients with acute lymphoblastic leukemia. Leuk Res. 2009;33:655–61.
21. de Haas V, Vet RJWM, Verhagen OJHM, et al. Early detection of central nervous system relapse by polymerase chain reaction in children with B-precursor acute lymphoblastic leukemia. Ann Hematol. 2002;81:59–61.
22. Ekstein D, Ben-Yehuda D, Slyusarevsky E, et al. CSF analysis of IgH gene rearrangement in CNS lymphoma: relationship to the disease course. J Neurol Sci. 2006;247:39–46.
23. Chamberlain MC. Neoplastic, meningitis. Neurologist. 2006;12(4):179–87.
24. Ernerudh J, Olsson T, Berlin G, et al. Cell surface markers for diagnosis of central nervous system involvement in lymphoproliferative disease. Ann Neurol. 1986;20:610–5.
25. Mavligit GM, Stuckey SE, Cabanillas FF, et al. Diagnosis of leukemia or lymphoma in the central nervous system by Beta-2-microglobulin determination. N Engl J Med. 1980;303: 718–22.
26. Rajantie J, Koskiniemia M, Siimes MA, et al. CSF fibronectin in Burkitt's lymphoma: an early marker for CNS involvement. Eur J Haematol. 1989;42:313–4.
27. Weller M, Stevens A, Sommer N, et al. Comparative analysis of cytokine patterns in immunological, infectious and oncological neurological disorders. J Neurol Sci. 1991;104:215–21.
28. Ernerudh J, Olsson T, Berlin G, et al. Cerebrospinal fluid immunoglobulins and Beta-2-microglobulin in lymphoproliferative and other neoplastic disease of the central nervous system. Arch Neurol. 1987;44:915–20.
29. Weller M, Stevens A, Sommer N, Schabet M, Wiethölter H, Humoral CSF. Parameters in the differential diagnosis of hematologic CNS neoplasia. Acta Neurol Scand. 1992;86:129–33.
30. Feugier P, Virion JM, Tilly H, et al. Incidence and risk factors for central nervous system occurrence in elderly patients with diffuse large-B-cell lymphoma: influence of rituximab. Ann Oncol. 2004;15(1):129–33.
31. Villa D, Connors JM, Shenkier TN, et al. Incidence and risk factors for central nervous system relapse in patients with diffuse large B-cell lymphoma: the impact of the addition of rituximab to CHOP chemotherapy. Ann Oncol. 2010;21(5):1046–52.
32. Boehme V, Schmitz N, Zeynalova S, et al. CNS events in elderly patients with aggressive lymphoma treated with modern chemotherapy (CHOP-14) with or without rituximab: an analysis of patients treated in the RICOVER-60 trial of the German High-Grade Non-Hodgkin Lymphoma Study Group (DSHNHL). Blood. 2009;113(17):3896–902.
33. Schmitz N, Zeynalova S, Glass B, et al. CNS disease in younger patients with aggressive B-cell lymphoma: an analysis of patients treated on the Mabthera International Trial and trials of the German High-Grade Non-Hodgkin Lymphoma Study Group. Ann Oncol. 2012;23: 1267–73.
34. Shimazu Y, Notohara K, Ueda Y. Diffuse large B-cell lymphoma with central nervous system relapse: prognosis and risk factors according to retrospective analysis from a single-center experience. Int J Hematol. 2009;89(5):577–83.

35. Magrath I, Adde M, Shad A, et al. Adults and children with small non-cleaved-cell lymphoma have a similar excellent outcome when treated with the same chemotherapy regimen. J Clin Oncol. 1996;14:925–34.
36. Bernstein JI, Coleman CN, Strickler JG, et al. Combined modality therapy for adults with small noncleaved cell lymphoma (Burkitt's and non-Burkitt's types). J Clin Oncol. 1986;4:847–58.
37. Kaplan LD, Straus DJ, Testa MA, et al. Low-dose compared with standard-dose m-BACOD chemotherapy for non-Hodgkin's lymphoma associated with human immunodeficiency virus infection. National Institute of Allergy and Infectious Diseases AIDS Clinical Trials Group. N Engl J Med. 1997;336:1641–8.
38. Sparano JA, Wiernik PH, Strack M, et al. Infusional cyclophosphamide, doxorubicin, and etoposide in human immunodeficiency virus- and human T-cell leukemia virus type I-related non-Hodgkin's lymphoma: a highly active regimen. Blood. 1993;81(10):2810–5.
39. Little RF, Pittaluga S, Grant N, et al. Highly effective treatment of acquired immunodeficiency syndrome-related lymphoma with dose-adjusted EPOCH: impact of antiretroviral therapy suspension and tumor biology. Blood. 2003;101:4653–9.
40. Spina M, Jaeger U, Sparano JA, et al. Rituximab plus infusional cyclophosphamide, doxorubicin, and etoposide (RCDE) in HIV-associated non-Hodgkin's lymphoma: pooled results from 3 phase II trials. Blood. 2005;105:1891–7.
41. Kaplan LD, Lee JY, Ambider RF, et al. Rituximab does not improve clinical outcome in a randomized phase 3 trial of CHOP with or without rituximab in patients with HIV-associated non-Hodgkin lymphoma: AIDS-Malignancies Consortium Trial 010. Blood. 2005;106(5):1538–43.
42. Mounier N, Spina M, Gabarre J, et al. AIDS-related non-Hodgkin lymphoma: final analysis of 485 patients treated with risk-adapted intensive chemotherapy. Blood. 2006;107:3832–40.
43. Dunleavy K, Little RF, Pittaluga S, et al. The role of tumor histogenesis, FDG-PET, and short-course EPOCH with dose-dense rituximab (SC-EPOCH-RR) in HIV-associated diffuse large B-cell lymphoma. Blood. 2010;115(15):3017–24.
44. Spina M, Chimienti E, Martellotta F, et al. Phase 2 study of intrathecal, long-acting liposomal cytarabine in the prophylaxis of lymphomatous meningitis in human immunodeficiency virus-related non-Hodgkin lymphoma. Cancer. 2010;116:1495–501.
45. Mazhar D, Stebbing J, Lewis R, et al. The management of meningeal lymphoma in patients with HIV in the era of HAART: intrathecal depot cytarabine is effective and safe. Blood. 2006;107:3412–4.
46. Garcia-Marco JA, Panizo C, Garcia ES, et al. Efficacy and safety of liposomal cytarabine in lymphoma patients with central nervous system involvement from lymphoma. Cancer. 2009;115(9):1892–8.
47. Tilly H, Lepage E, Coiffier B, et al. Intensive conventional chemotherapy (ACVBP regimen) compared with standard CHOP for poor-prognosis aggressive non-Hodgkin lymphoma. Blood. 2003;102(13):4284–9.
48. Abramson JS, Hellmann M, Barnes JA, et al. Intravenous methotrexate as central nervous system (CNS) prophylaxis is associated with a low risk of CNS recurrence in high-risk patients with diffuse large B-cell lymphoma. Cancer. 2010;116:4283–90.
49. Siegal T, Zylber-Katz E. Strategies for increasing drug delivery to the brain: focus on brain lymphoma. Clin Pharmacokinet. 2002;41:171–86.

# Infection Prophylaxis 19

Marcus Hentrich

## Contents



Chemotherapy for HIV-related hematological malignancies is associated with an increased risk of infection due to myelosuppression and additional CD4 lymphocyte count loss. The risk of infection may be further increased by the presence of central venous catheters or by neutropenia associated with HIV infection [1, 2].

Guidelines are available for both, the prevention of opportunistic infections in HIV-positive individuals [3–6] and for infection prophylaxis in HIV-negative patients with hematological malignancies [7–10]. However, to our knowledge, there is only one guideline available for opportunistic infection prophylaxis in HIV-associated malignancy [11]. The evidence some of the recommendations on infection prophylaxis in HIV-associated malignancies are based on is limited as randomized controlled trials or comparative studies with historical controls have not been published. Nevertheless, based on the available literature, the following recommendations can be made for patients with HIV-associated hematological malignancies:

M. Hentrich, MD
Department of Hematology and Oncology, Red Cross Hospital, University of Munich, Munich, Germany
e-mail: marcus.hentrich@swmbrk.de



M. Hentrich, S.K. Barta (eds.), *HIV-associated Hematological Malignancies*,
DOI 10.1007/978-3-319-26857-6_19

## 19.1 Pneumocystis Carinii Pneumonia (PcP) Prophylaxis

Prophylaxis against *PcP* is strongly recommended when the CD4 cell count falls below 200 cells/μl [3–6]. This recommendation is based on results from randomized controlled trials [12, 13]. However, prophylaxis should also be offered at higher CD4 counts in patients with HIV-associated hematological malignancies as chemotherapy usually causes profound falls in CD4 cell counts. Trimethoprim-sulfamethoxazole (cotrimoxazole) is the agent of choice [3, 5, 6, 14]. Given potential myelosuppressive effects of a daily double-strength regimen, the preferred regimen is one double-strength tablet (800/160 mg) three times weekly or one single-strength tablet daily. Cotrimoxazole provides cross-protection against toxoplasmosis and certain bacterial infections [6, 7, 13].

## 19.2 Prophylaxis for Enteric Bacteria

Prophylactic fluoroquinolones cannot be generally recommended. However, their use may be advocated for patients undergoing intensive chemotherapy who are likely to have prolonged (>8 days) and profound (ANC <500 cells/μl) neutropenia [7].

## 19.3 Prophylaxis for Mycobacterium Avium Complex (MAC) Disease

Prophylaxis against MAC is recommended for individuals with a CD4 cell count less than 50 cells/μl [3–6]. Azithromycin (1,200 mg once weekly) or clarithromycin (2×500 mg daily) is preferred with rifabutin being considered as an alternative [3, 5, 15, 16].

## 19.4 Antifungal Prophylaxis

Systemic antifungal prophylaxis may be given to patients with CD4 counts <100 cells/μl [6]. Secondary prophylaxis following mucosal candidiasis is strongly recommended [17]. Given potential drug interactions of itraconazole, posaconazole, and voriconazole, fluconazole should be considered agent of choice [6]. However, for patients with acute myeloid leukemia, undergoing induction chemotherapy posaconazole may be preferred as it proved superior to itraconazole/fluconazole in terms of overall survival in a randomized trial [18].

## 19.5 Antiviral Prophylaxis

Herpes simplex prophylaxis should be generally offered only to patients with a history of HSV infection [3, 11]. However, patients receiving bortezomib are at increased risk of herpes zoster and should, thus, receive prophylaxis with acyclovir [19].

## References


1. Tacconelli E, Tumbarello M, de Gaetano DK, et al. Morbidity associated with central venous catheter-use in a cohort of 212 hospitalized subjects with HIV infection. J Hosp Infect. 2000;44:186–92.
2. Levine AM, Karim R, Mack W, et al. Neutropenia in human immunodeficiency virus infection: data from the women's interagency HIV study. Arch Intern Med. 2006;166:405–10.
3. European AIDS Clinical Society guidelines Version 7.1 Nov 2014. Part V: opportunistic infections. p. 76–81. http://www.eacsociety.org/files/guidelines-7.1-english.pdf.
4. Masur H, Brooks JT, Benson CA, et al. Prevention and treatment of opportunistic infections in HIV-infected adults and adolescents: updated guidelines from the centers for disease control and prevention, National Institutes of Health, and HIV Medicine Association of the Infectious Diseases Society of America. Clin Infect Dis. 2014;58:1308–11.
5. Panel on Opportunistic Infections in HIV-Infected Adults and Adolescents. Guidelines for the prevention and treatment of opportunistic infections in HIV-infected adults and adolescents: recommendations from the Centers for Disease Control and Prevention, the National Institutes of Health, and the HIV Medicine Association of the Infectious Diseases Society of America. Available at http://aidsinfo.nih.gov/contentfiles/lvguidelines/adult_oi.pdf. Accessed 06 Apr 2015.
6. Nelson M, Dockrell D, Edwards S, et al. British HIV Association and British Infection Association guidelines for the treatment of opportunistic infection in HIV seropositive individuals 2011. HIV Med. 2011;12 Suppl 2:1–140.
7. Freifeld AG, Bow EJ, Sepkowitz KA, et al. Clinical practice guideline for the use of antimicrobial agents in neutropenic patients with cancer: 2010 update by the Infectious Diseases Society of America. Clin Infect Dis. 2011;52:e56–93.
8. Flowers CR, Seidenfeld J, Bow EJ, et al. Antimicrobial prophylaxis and outpatient management of fever and neutropenia in adults treated for malignancy: American Society of Clinical Oncology clinical practice guideline. J Clin Oncol. 2013;31:794–810.
9. Sandherr M, Hentrich M, von Lilienfeld-Toal M, et al. Antiviral prophylaxis in patients with solid tumours and haematological malignancies – update of the Guidelines of the Infectious Diseases Working Party (AGIHO) of the German Society for Hematology and Medical Oncology (DGHO). Ann Hematol. 2015;94:1441–50.
10. Cornely OA, Böhme A, Buchheidt D, et al. Primary prophylaxis of invasive fungal infections in patients with hematologic malignancies. Recommendations of the Infectious Diseases Working Party of the German Society for Haematology and Oncology. Haematologica. 2009;94:113–22.
11. Bower M, Palfreeman A, Alfa-Wali M, et al. British HIV association guidelines for HIV-associated malignancies 2014. HIV Med. 2014;15 Suppl 2:85–90.
12. Schneider MM, Hoepelman AI, Eeftinck Schattenkerk JK, et al. A controlled trial of aerosolized pentamidine or trimethoprim-sulfamethoxazole as primary prophylaxis against Pneumocystis carinii pneumonia in patients with human immunodeficiency virus infection. The Dutch AIDS Treatment Group. N Engl J Med. 1992;327:1836–41.
13. Hardy WD, Feinberg J, Finkelstein DM, et al. A controlled trial of trimethoprim-sulfamethoxazole or aerosolized pentamidine for secondary prophylaxis of Pneumocystis carinii pneumonia in patients with the acquired immunodeficiency syndrome. AIDS Clinical Trials Group Protocol 021. N Engl J Med. 1992;327:1842–8.
14. El-Sadr WM, Luskin-Hawk R, Yurik TM, with Terry Beirn Community Programs for Clinical Research on AIDS (CPCRA), et al. A randomized trial of daily and thrice-weekly trimethoprim-sulfamethoxazole for the prevention of Pneumocystis carinii pneumonia in human immunodeficiency virus-infected persons. Clin Infect Dis. 1999;29:775–83.
15. Pierce M, Crampton S, Henry D, et al. A randomized trial of clarithromycin as prophylaxis against disseminated mycobacterium avium complex infection in patients with advanced acquired immunodeficiency syndrome. N Engl J Med. 1996;335:384–91.

16. Havlir DV, Dube MP, Sattler FR, et al. Prophylaxis against disseminated Mycobacterium avium complex with weekly azithromycin, daily rifabutin, or both. California Collaborative Treatment Group. N Engl J Med. 1996;335:392–8.
17. Goldman M, Cloud GA, Wade KD, et al. A randomized study of the use of fluconazole in continuous versus episodic therapy in patients with advanced HIV infection and a history of oropharyngeal candidiasis: AIDS Clinical Trials Group Study 323/Mycoses Study Group Study 40. Clin Infect Dis. 2005;41:1473–80.
18. Cornely OA, Maertens J, Winston DJ, et al. Posaconazole vs. fluconazole or itraconazole prophylaxis in patients with neutropenia. N Engl J Med. 2007;356:348–59.
19. Swaika A, Paulus A, Miller KC, et al. Acyclovir prophylaxis against varicella zoster virus reactivation in multiple myeloma patients treated with bortezomib-based therapies: a retrospective analysis of 100 patients. J Support Oncol. 2012;10:155–9.

# Coinfection with Hepatitis B or C in People Living with HIV Undergoing Immunosuppressive Therapy

# 20

Stefan K. Barta

## Contents



## 20.1 Epidemiology

HIV and both the hepatitis B virus (HBV) and hepatitis C virus (HCV) share similar forms of transmission (unprotected sexual intercourse, injection drug use (IDU), and transfusion of blood products), which explains why coinfection with HIV and either HBV, HCV, or even both is not uncommon. Additionally, patients coinfected with HIV and hepatitis B or C are at a higher risk of decompensation of liver disease and development of cirrhosis [1–5]. Therefore, screening of all patients diagnosed with HIV for hepatitis infection is critical to identify coinfection and prevent excess morbidity and mortality.

The coinfection rate of people living with HIV or AIDS (PLWHA) with HBV as defined by persistent positivity for the hepatitis B surface antigen (HBsAg) varies with geographical distribution and ranges between 5 % and 10 % in Western Europe and North America. The prevalence of HBV coinfection in PLWHA is highest if there is also a history of IDU or in men who have sex with men (MSM) [4, 6–8].

S.K. Barta, MD, MS, MRCP (UK) (✉)
Fox Chase Cancer Center, Temple BMT Program, Temple University Health System, Philadelphia, PA, USA
e-mail: Stefan.Barta@fccc.edu



M. Hentrich, S.K. Barta (eds.), *HIV-associated Hematological Malignancies*,
DOI 10.1007/978-3-319-26857-6_20

Patients who are HBsAg negative, but have detectable hepatitis B DNA, with or without positive hepatitis B core total antibody (HBcAb), have occult HBV infection (OBI). The prevalence of occult HBV infection in Europe and North America in coinfected patients is probably higher than chronic active hepatitis B infection, and estimates for OBI vary depending on definition and geographical region between 1 and 45% [9–12].

The prevalence of HCV coinfection in PLWHA ranges between 6 % and 25 %, but is much higher in patients with a history of IDU or men who have sex with men (MSM) [13–17]. The prevalence in Europe and North America might be declining, possibly reflecting the declining HCV burden in the general population owing to the screening of blood products, increased patient screening, and more effective HCV treatment [18].

## 20.2 Management of Chronic HBV Infection and Prevention of HBV Reactivation

As mentioned above, PLWHA coinfected with hepatitis B and/or C have at baseline a higher risk of liver-related morbidity and mortality. This is further exacerbated in patients receiving immunosuppressive therapy (IST), including chemotherapy or immunotherapy (e.g., CD20-directed antibodies like rituximab or ofatumumab), which can lead to exacerbation of chronic viral hepatitis or reactivation of OBI. Reactivation of HepB is defined as either detection of HBV DNA in a patient with previously undetectable HBV DNA or an at least tenfold rise in HBV DNA [19, 20].

HBV reactivation occurs in 40–50 % of patients undergoing chemotherapy for hematological malignancies [20, 21] and can lead to lethal liver failure in up to 16 % [22, 23]. Additionally, interruption of chemotherapy due to transaminitis can result in treatment delays and thereby impair cancer-related outcomes [24].

Risk factors for HBV reactivation include high baseline HBV DNA levels, treatment with B-cell-depleting drugs such as the CD20 antibodies rituximab or ofatumumab, and positivity for HepBsAg [19, 21, 25–27]. However, even in anti-HepB core antibody-positive patients with clinically resolved hepatitis B, who have detectable HepBsAb levels and no detectable HBV DNA, reactivation occurs in up to 35 % and can be seen up to 2 years after completion of chemotherapy [21].

Two different strategies have been applied to lower the reactivation rates in HBV-infected patients without HIV treated with IST: (1) prophylaxis with antiviral agents or (2) close monitoring for reactivation and on-demand initiation of antiviral therapy. Antiviral agents against HBV most extensively studied include lamivudine, tenofovir and entecavir, which are nucleoside/nucleotide reverse transcriptase inhibitors (NRTIs) that suppress HBV DNA. Lamivudine, an antiviral agent with activity also against HIV and a component of several combination antiretroviral therapy (cART) regimens, has been shown to reduce the risk of HBV reactivation and HBV-related deaths in patients treated for hematological malignancies by at least 80 % [20, 22, 23, 28–30]. However, there is concern about emergence of HBV

**Table 20.1** Constellation of serological markers for HBV infection and risk of HBV reactivation with immunosuppressive therapy

| Interpretation of results | HBsAg | HBsAb | HBcAb | HB DNA | HBV reactivation risk[a] |
|---|---|---|---|---|---|
| H/o HBV vaccination | – | + | – | – | None |
| Resolved HBV | – | + | + | – | Moderate to high |
| OBI | – | – | – | + | Moderate to high |
| | – | – | + | + | Moderate to high |
| Isolated positive HBcAb | – | – | + | – | Moderate to high |
| Chronic active HBV | + | – | + | + | High |

*HBsAg* hepatitis B surface antigen, *HBsAb* hepatitis B surface antibody, *HBcAb* hepatitis B core antibody, *H/o* history of, *OBI* occult HBV infection

[a]Risk deemed low if risk of reactivation <1 %, moderate if risk 1–10 %, and high if risk >10% [39]

resistance to lamivudine [24, 31, 32]. Entecavir has been shown to be superior to lamivudine in a direct comparison and appears to lack the risk of resistance, but is not used in cART [24]. Tenofovir has shown activity even against lamivudine-resistant HBV with no reports of resistance and is furthermore active against HIV [33–36]. Chemotherapy does not need to be delayed for the start of these prophylactic antiviral medications in most cases, but patients should initiate them as soon as possible and continue up to 6–12 months after completion of chemotherapy, depending on the type of IST.

In PLWHA with HBV coinfection who are at any risk of HBV reactivation (see Table 20.1) and who are being treated for hematological malignancies, we therefore recommend using or switching to a cART regimen that contains tenofovir +/– lamivudine or emtricitabine. Antiretroviral-naïve patients should be started on tenofovir based cART ideally prior to initiating IST. Using tenofovir alone is strongly discouraged out of concern for emergence of HIV resistance. This recommendation is supported by several guidelines concerned with the management of patients coinfected with HIV and HBV [37, 38].

It should be noted that the risk of reactivation is truly an interplay between patients' serological profiles (see Table 20.1) and IST. For example, the risk of HBV reactivation is high for B-cell depleting therapies with any serological profile except for a history of vaccination, and probably only moderate for other chemotherapy regimens even in patients who are positive for HBcAB +/-HBsAg [39].

## 20.3 Hepatitis C and Immunosuppressive Therapy

While HBV reactivation with IST is well studied, less is known about HCV reactivation. An HCV flare is usually defined as greater than threefold increase in serum level of alanine aminotransferase (ALT) and HCV reactivation as ~1 log10 IU/ml increase in the HCV viral load [40]. In HIV-negative patients treated for hematological malignancies, elevation of transaminases is commonly seen during or even months after completion of chemotherapy (11–55 %); however, liver failure only occurs very rarely [40–45]. The CD20-directed monoclonal antibody rituximab specifically appears to impart an increased risk for HCV reactivation [40, 46, 47].

Rates of HCV flares, severe liver dysfunction, and liver failure during lymphoma treatment in HIV and HCV-coinfected patients appear similar to those in non-HIV-infected patients. In the largest retrospective study published on behalf of the Fondazione Italiana Linfomi (FIL), which analyzed 535 HIV-/HCV-coinfected patients with DLBCL who were consecutively treated between 1995 and 2010, severe hepatotoxicity was seen in 14 % of patients; of these 28 % had to hold or discontinue chemotherapy [48]. Nevertheless, only one patient died of liver failure, and overall survival was the same between patients who had to interrupt therapy and those who did not. Risk factors for severe liver dysfunction were low albumin levels (which may be indicative of already advanced underlying liver disease) and poor performance status, but not the use of rituximab or baseline HCV RNA levels. Other uncontrolled retrospective studies of HCV-coinfected HIV+ patients with lymphoma described similar findings, with some degree of liver toxicity occurring in 27–33 %, treatment interruption in 12–15 %, and discontinuation because of liver toxicity in only 4–5 %. Less than 1 % of patients died of liver failure. Event-free survival (EFS) and overall survival (OS) were similar to matched controls. Interestingly, HCV viral load appears not to be associated with outcome [49–51]. In contrast, Besson and colleagues on behalf of the Groupe d'Etude des Lymphomes del'Adulte Programs (GELA) reported characteristics and outcomes of 26 patients with HIV and HCV coinfection treated on two French protocols for DLBCL. In this much smaller series, grade 1–4 hepatotoxicity was seen in 65 % (29 % grade 3 or 4) of the treated patients, and one died of liver failure. Although lymphoma treatment was frequently interrupted for liver toxicity, complete response rate and EFS were similar in HCV+ patients compared to matched controls. However, OS was worse in HCV+ patients (56 % vs. 80 %; $p=0.02$) [52].

Currently there are no strategies to prevent reactivation in HCV-infected patients undergoing IST. While with current novel antiviral drug combinations, eradication of HCV is achievable for the majority of patients, the vast majority of patients with hematological malignancies cannot wait to complete treatment for HCV prior to initiating chemo(immuno)therapy. Nevertheless, should it be possible to delay treatment, there are several guidelines by international professional organizations to guide HCV treatment for patients infected with HCV [53–55]. Similarly good outcomes can be achieved in HIV- and HCV-coinfected patients as compared to HCV mono-infected patients [56–58]. In essence, HCV treatment recommendations for mono-infected and for HIV- and HCV-coinfected patients are identical, although consideration should be given to possible drug-drug interactions with cART. Several international guidelines exist that guide the management of PLWHA coinfected with HCV [37, 59–62]. In addition, it should be noted that treatment of HCV can lead to lymphoma regression in some indolent non-Hodgkin lymphomas [63–67].

For the majority of patients, for whom cancer treatment trumps HCV treatment, we recommend frequent monitoring (two to four weekly) of liver tests, especially the ALT, during and after completion of cancer therapy. If abnormal liver tests preclude the use of certain chemotherapy drugs, treatment should be interrupted until resolution to baseline or discontinued with severe hepatotoxicity or in the event of decompensated liver failure. While monitoring HCV RNA levels might be informative, cancer treatment interruption or discontinuation should not be based on the HCV viral load. After patients enter a complete remission, HCV treatment should be strongly considered for all patients. In general it is strongly recommended that a hepatologist is involved in the care of HIV- and HCV-coinfected patients undergoing treatment for hematological malignancies.

**Acknowledgement** I would like to thank Dr. Minhhuyen T. Nguyen for critically reviewing this chapter.

## References

1. Deng LP, Gui XE, Zhang YX, et al. Impact of human immunodeficiency virus infection on the course of hepatitis C virus infection: a meta-analysis. World J Gastroenterol. 2009;15:996–1003.
2. Graham CS, Baden LR, Yu E, et al. Influence of human immunodeficiency virus infection on the course of hepatitis C virus infection: a meta-analysis. Clin Infect Dis. 2001;33:562–9.
3. Greub G, Ledergerber B, Battegay M, et al. Clinical progression, survival, and immune recovery during antiretroviral therapy in patients with HIV-1 and hepatitis C virus coinfection: the Swiss HIV Cohort Study. Lancet. 2000;356:1800–5.
4. Konopnicki D, Mocroft A, de Wit S, et al. Hepatitis B and HIV: prevalence, AIDS progression, response to highly active antiretroviral therapy and increased mortality in the EuroSIDA cohort. AIDS. 2005;19:593–601.
5. Nikolopoulos GK, Paraskevis D, Hatzitheodorou E, et al. Impact of hepatitis B virus infection on the progression of AIDS and mortality in HIV-infected individuals: a cohort study and meta-analysis. Clin Infect Dis. 2009;48:1763–71.
6. Price H, Bansi L, Sabin CA, et al. Hepatitis B virus infection in HIV-positive individuals in the UK collaborative HIV cohort (UK CHIC) study. PLoS One. 2012;7:e49314.
7. Pittman C, Plitt S, Birse T, et al. Prevalence and correlates of HIV and hepatitis B virus coinfection in Northern Alberta. Can J Infect Dis Med Microbiol. 2014;25:e8–13.
8. Spradling PR, Richardson JT, Buchacz K, et al. Prevalence of chronic hepatitis B virus infection among patients in the HIV Outpatient Study, 1996–2007. J Viral Hepat. 2010;17:879–86.
9. Morsica G, Ancarani F, Bagaglio S, et al. Occult hepatitis B virus infection in a cohort of HIV-positive patients: correlation with hepatitis C virus coinfection, virological and immunological features. Infection. 2009;37:445–9.
10. Coffin CS, Mulrooney-Cousins PM, Osiowy C, et al. Virological characteristics of occult hepatitis B virus in a North American cohort of human immunodeficiency virus type 1-positive patients on dual active anti-HBV/HIV therapy. J Clin Virol. 2014;60:347–53.
11. Maldonado-Rodriguez A, Cevallos AM, Rojas-Montes O, et al. Occult hepatitis B virus co-infection in human immunodeficiency virus-positive patients: a review of prevalence, diagnosis and clinical significance. World J Hepatol. 2015;7:253–60.
12. Chadwick D, Doyle T, Ellis S, et al. Occult hepatitis B virus coinfection in HIV-positive African migrants to the UK: a point prevalence study. HIV Med. 2014;15:189–92.
13. Petty LA, Steinbeck JL, Pursell K, et al. Human immunodeficiency virus and coinfection with hepatitis B and C. Infect Dis Clin N Am. 2014;28:477–99.
14. Marcellin F, Lorente N, Demoulin B, et al. Comparison of risk factors in HIV-infected men who have sex with men, coinfected or not with hepatitis C virus (ANRS VESPA2 French cross-sectional national survey). Sex Transm Infect. 2015;91:21–3.

15. Kouyos RD, Rauch A, Braun DL, et al. Higher risk of incident hepatitis C virus coinfection among men who have sex with men, in whom the HIV genetic bottleneck at transmission was wide. J Infect Dis. 2014;210:1555–61.
16. Akselrod H, Grau LE, Barbour R, et al. Seroprevalence of HIV, hepatitis B virus, and HCV among injection drug users in Connecticut: understanding infection and coinfection risks in a nonurban population. Am J Public Health. 2014;104:1713–21.
17. Sanchez MA, Scheer S, Shallow S, et al. Epidemiology of the viral hepatitis-HIV syndemic in San Francisco: a collaborative surveillance approach. Public Health Rep. 2014;129 Suppl 1:95–101.
18. Serrano-Villar S, Sobrino-Vegas P, Monge S, et al. Decreasing prevalence of HCV coinfection in all risk groups for HIV infection between 2004 and 2011 in Spain. J Viral Hepat. 2015;22:496–503.
19. Perrillo RP, Gish R, Falck-Ytter YT. American Gastroenterological Association Institute technical review on prevention and treatment of hepatitis B virus reactivation during immunosuppressive drug therapy. Gastroenterology. 2015;148:221–44.e3.
20. Lau GK, Yiu HH, Fong DY, et al. Early is superior to deferred preemptive lamivudine therapy for hepatitis B patients undergoing chemotherapy. Gastroenterology. 2003;125:1742–9.
21. Seto WK, Chan TS, Hwang YY, et al. Hepatitis B reactivation in patients with previous hepatitis B virus exposure undergoing rituximab-containing chemotherapy for lymphoma: a prospective study. J Clin Oncol. 2014;32:3736–43.
22. Loomba R, Rowley A, Wesley R, et al. Systematic review: the effect of preventive lamivudine on hepatitis B reactivation during chemotherapy. Ann Intern Med. 2008;148:519–28.
23. Leaw SJ, Yen CJ, Huang WT, et al. Preemptive use of interferon or lamivudine for hepatitis B reactivation in patients with aggressive lymphoma receiving chemotherapy. Ann Hematol. 2004;83:270–5.
24. Huang H, Li X, Zhu J, et al. Entecavir vs lamivudine for prevention of hepatitis B virus reactivation among patients with untreated diffuse large B-cell lymphoma receiving R-CHOP chemotherapy: a randomized clinical trial. JAMA. 2014;312:2521–30.
25. Zhong S, Yeo W, Schroder C, et al. High hepatitis B virus (HBV) DNA viral load is an important risk factor for HBV reactivation in breast cancer patients undergoing cytotoxic chemotherapy. J Viral Hepat. 2004;11:55–9.
26. Di Bisceglie AM, Lok AS, Martin P, et al. Recent US Food and Drug Administration warnings on hepatitis B reactivation with immune-suppressing and anticancer drugs: just the tip of the iceberg? Hepatology. 2015;61:703–11.
27. Yeo W, Zee B, Zhong S, et al. Comprehensive analysis of risk factors associating with hepatitis B virus (HBV) reactivation in cancer patients undergoing cytotoxic chemotherapy. Br J Cancer. 2004;90:1306–11.
28. Li YH, He YF, Jiang WQ, et al. Lamivudine prophylaxis reduces the incidence and severity of hepatitis in hepatitis B virus carriers who receive chemotherapy for lymphoma. Cancer. 2006;106:1320–5.
29. Rossi G, Pelizzari A, Motta M, et al. Primary prophylaxis with lamivudine of hepatitis B virus reactivation in chronic HbsAg carriers with lymphoid malignancies treated with chemotherapy. Br J Haematol. 2001;115:58–62.
30. Yeo W, Chan PK, Ho WM, et al. Lamivudine for the prevention of hepatitis B virus reactivation in hepatitis B s-antigen seropositive cancer patients undergoing cytotoxic chemotherapy. J Clin Oncol. 2004;22:927–34.
31. Lai CL, Chien RN, Leung NW, et al. A one-year trial of lamivudine for chronic hepatitis B. Asia Hepatitis Lamivudine Study Group. N Engl J Med. 1998;339:61–8.
32. Lok AS, Lai CL, Leung N, et al. Long-term safety of lamivudine treatment in patients with chronic hepatitis B. Gastroenterology. 2003;125:1714–22.
33. Benhamou Y, Tubiana R, Thibault V. Tenofovir disoproxil fumarate in patients with HIV and lamivudine-resistant hepatitis B virus. N Engl J Med. 2003;348:177–8.
34. Dore GJ, Cooper DA, Pozniak AL, et al. Efficacy of tenofovir disoproxil fumarate in antiretroviral therapy-naive and -experienced patients coinfected with HIV-1 and hepatitis B virus. J Infect Dis. 2004;189:1185–92.

35. Boyd A, Lasnier E, Molina JM, et al. Liver fibrosis changes in HIV-HBV-coinfected patients: clinical, biochemical and histological effect of long-term tenofovir disoproxil fumarate use. Antivir Ther. 2010;15:963–74.
36. Martin-Carbonero L, Teixeira T, Poveda E, et al. Clinical and virological outcomes in HIV-infected patients with chronic hepatitis B on long-term nucleos(t)ide analogues. AIDS. 2011;25:73–9.
37. Wilkins E, Nelson M, Agarwal K, et al. British HIV Association guidelines for the management of hepatitis viruses in adults infected with HIV 2013. HIV Med. 2013;14 Suppl 4:1–71.
38. Lok AS, McMahon BJ. Chronic hepatitis B: update 2009. Hepatology. 2009;50:661–2.
39. Reddy KR, Beavers KL, Hammond SP, et al. American Gastroenterological Association Institute guideline on the prevention and treatment of hepatitis B virus reactivation during immunosuppressive drug therapy. Gastroenterology. 2015;148:215–9; quiz e16–7.
40. Mahale P, Kontoyiannis DP, Chemaly RF, et al. Acute exacerbation and reactivation of chronic hepatitis C virus infection in cancer patients. J Hepatol. 2012;57:1177–85.
41. Markovic S, Drozina G, Vovk M, et al. Reactivation of hepatitis B but not hepatitis C in patients with malignant lymphoma and immunosuppressive therapy. A prospective study in 305 patients. Hepatogastroenterology. 1999;46:2925–30.
42. Kawatani T, Suou T, Tajima F, et al. Incidence of hepatitis virus infection and severe liver dysfunction in patients receiving chemotherapy for hematologic malignancies. Eur J Haematol. 2001;67:45–50.
43. Faggioli P, De Paschale M, Tocci A, et al. Acute hepatic toxicity during cyclic chemotherapy in non Hodgkin's lymphoma. Haematologica. 1997;82:38–42.
44. Takai S, Tsurumi H, Ando K, et al. Prevalence of hepatitis B and C virus infection in haematological malignancies and liver injury following chemotherapy. Eur J Haematol. 2005;74:158–65.
45. Zuckerman E, Zuckerman T, Douer D, et al. Liver dysfunction in patients infected with hepatitis C virus undergoing chemotherapy for hematologic malignancies. Cancer. 1998;83: 1224–30.
46. Torres HA, Davila M. Reactivation of hepatitis B virus and hepatitis C virus in patients with cancer. Nat Rev Clin Oncol. 2012;9:156–66.
47. Zaky AH, Bakry R, El-Sayed MI, et al. Impact of treatment-related toxicity on outcome of HCV-positive diffuse large B-cell lymphoma in rituximab era. Hematology. 2014; 19:412–6.
48. Merli M, Visco C, Spina M, et al. Outcome prediction of diffuse large B-cell lymphomas associated with hepatitis C virus infection: a study on behalf of the Fondazione Italiana Linfomi. Haematologica. 2014;99:489–96.
49. Visco C, Arcaini L, Brusamolino E, et al. Distinctive natural history in hepatitis C virus positive diffuse large B-cell lymphoma: analysis of 156 patients from northern Italy. Ann Oncol. 2006;17:1434–40.
50. Ennishi D, Maeda Y, Niitsu N, et al. Hepatic toxicity and prognosis in hepatitis C virus–infected patients with diffuse large B-cell lymphoma treated with rituximab-containing chemotherapy regimens: a Japanese multicenter analysis. Blood. 2010;116:5119–25.
51. Sridharan A, Curtis SA, Kaner JD, et al. Hepatitis C co-infection in HIV-positive patients treated for lymphoma. ASCO Meet Abstr. 2014;32:8578.
52. Besson C, Canioni D, Lepage E, et al. Characteristics and outcome of diffuse large B-cell lymphoma in hepatitis C virus–positive patients in LNH 93 and LNH 98 Groupe d'Etude des Lymphomes de l'Adulte Programs. J Clin Oncol. 2006;24:953–60.
53. European Association for the Study of the Liver. EASL recommendations on treatment of hepatitis C 2014. J Hepatol. 2014;61:373–95.
54. Miller MH, Agarwal K, Austin A, et al. Review article: 2014 UK consensus guidelines – hepatitis C management and direct-acting anti-viral therapy. Aliment Pharmacol Ther. 2014;39:1363–75.
55. WHO Guidelines Approved by the Guidelines Review Committee. Guidelines for the screening, care and treatment of persons with hepatitis C infection. Geneva: World Health Organization; 2014. Copyright (c) World Health Organization 2014.

56. Sulkowski MS, Eron JJ, Wyles D, et al. Ombitasvir, paritaprevir co-dosed with ritonavir, dasabuvir, and ribavirin for hepatitis C in patients co-infected with HIV-1: a randomized trial. JAMA. 2015;313(12):1223–31.
57. Osinusi A, Townsend K, Kohli A, et al. Virologic response following combined ledipasvir and sofosbuvir administration in patients with HCV genotype 1 and HIV co-infection. JAMA. 2015;313:1232–9.
58. Graham CS. Hepatitis C and HIV: closing the gaps. JAMA. 2015;313:1217–8.
59. Hull M, Klein M, Shafran S, et al. CIHR Canadian HIV trials network coinfection and concurrent diseases core: Canadian guidelines for management and treatment of HIV/hepatitis C coinfection in adults. Can J Infect Dis Med Microbiol. 2013;24:217–38.
60. European AIDS Clinical Society (EACS) guidelines. 22 Apr 2015. http://www.eacsociety.org/files/guidelines-7.1-english.pdf.
61. Panel on Antiretroviral Guidelines for Adults and Adolescents. Guidelines for the use of antiretroviral agents in HIV-1-infected adults and adolescents. Department of Health and Human Services. 22 Apr 2015. http://aidsinfo.nih.gov/contentfiles/lvguidelines/AdultandAdolescentGL.pdf.
62. Ghany MG, Nelson DR, Strader DB, et al. An update on treatment of genotype 1 chronic hepatitis C virus infection: 2011 practice guideline by the American Association for the Study of Liver Diseases. Hepatology. 2011;54:1433–44.
63. Hermine O, Lefrere F, Bronowicki JP, et al. Regression of splenic lymphoma with villous lymphocytes after treatment of hepatitis C virus infection. N Engl J Med. 2002;347:89–94.
64. Kelaidi C, Rollot F, Park S, et al. Response to antiviral treatment in hepatitis C virus-associated marginal zone lymphomas. Leukemia. 2004;18:1711–6.
65. Gisbert JP, Garcia-Buey L, Pajares JM, et al. Systematic review: regression of lymphoproliferative disorders after treatment for hepatitis C infection. Aliment Pharmacol Ther. 2005;21:653–62.
66. Vallisa D, Bernuzzi P, Arcaini L, et al. Role of anti-hepatitis C virus (HCV) treatment in HCV-related, low-grade, B-cell, non-Hodgkin's lymphoma: a multicenter Italian experience. J Clin Oncol. 2005;23:468–73.
67. La Mura V, De Renzo A, Perna F, et al. Antiviral therapy after complete response to chemotherapy could be efficacious in HCV-positive non-Hodgkin's lymphoma. J Hepatol. 2008;49:557–63.

# Second Malignancies

# 21

Josep-Maria Ribera

## Contents



The incidence and spectrum of neoplasms among persons infected with HIV have risen with the increasing survival in the era of combined antiretroviral therapy (cART) [1, 2] and have contributed as a significant cause of death in this population [2, 3]. The specific neoplasms developed include anal cancer, liver cancer, lung cancer, head and neck carcinomas, and carcinomas of the skin, including penile and vulvar/vaginal cancer, among others.

Epidemiologic studies have shown that these neoplasms occur with higher frequency than in non-HIV-infected persons and, in general, tend to occur in patients who are younger than their HIV-negative counterparts. On the other hand, these cancers tend to show atypical pathology (e.g., poorly differentiated neoplasms and high tumor grade) and have a more aggressive behavior (e.g., higher probability of local progression and metastasis), resulting in poorer response to therapy and outcome [2].

In addition to a true increased prevalence of these tumors in HIV-infected patients, other factors can explain the higher frequency observed in recent times.

J.-M. Ribera, MD, PhD
Clinical Hematology Department,
ICO-Hospital Germans Trias i Pujol. Jose Carreras Research Institute,
Badalona, Spain

Universitat Autònoma de Barcelona, Barcelona, Spain
e-mail: jribera@iconcologia.net



M. Hentrich, S.K. Barta (eds.), *HIV-associated Hematological Malignancies*,
DOI 10.1007/978-3-319-26857-6_21

There may be the greater screening of some groups (e.g., Papanicolaou test for anal cancer), more frequent detection of incidental lesions during controls of HIV infection and treatment, and longevity in the presence of chronic immunodeficiency. In this regard, the role of a low CD4+ cell count in the development of AIDS-defining cancers is well established. Other contributing factors may include the increased aging of the HIV-infected population, certain lifestyle habits (e.g., sexual behavior) and increased exposure to carcinogens (e.g., tobacco and alcohol), and coinfection with oncogenic viruses (e.g., human papillomavirus, Epstein-Barr virus, hepatitis C virus, hepatitis B virus), among others [2–4]. No association has been demonstrated between long-term exposure to antiretroviral agents and occurrence of malignancies [5]. Some studies on structured antiretroviral treatment interruptions have resulted in an increase of AIDS-defining and non-AIDS-defining cancers, but this finding needs further evaluation. Finally, long-term follow-up should be performed in patients cured of AIDS-defining cancers (e.g., lymphomas), in whom the development of second cancers is not infrequent [6, 7].

The timing of cancer diagnoses among patients initiating cART is different for AIDS-defining and non-AIDS-defining neoplasms. While the former cancers decrease over time, the incidence of the latter group increases especially when CD4+ cell counts remain low after 12 months of cART. These results indicate the crucial importance of early HIV diagnosis followed by prompt cART initiation along with aggressive cancer screening and prevention efforts throughout the course of HIV care.

Clinicians should attempt to adhere to standard screening recommendations established for the non-HIV-infected population [8] and should promote risk-reduction behaviors (e.g., safe sexual practices and smoking cessation, among others). Further research is needed for additional cancer-specific screening (e.g., screening for human papillomavirus in the squamous epithelium of the oral cavity and anus).

The management of non-AIDS-defining cancers is challenging for several reasons [9]. Tumor staging may be affected by the presence of reactive lymphadenopathy or other imaging abnormalities unrelated to cancer. On the other hand, the comorbidities associated with the HIV infection may result in a poor performance status. Prophylaxis against opportunistic infections and hematopoietic growth factor support are often needed [10–12]. Finally, the combination of cytotoxic chemotherapy with antiretrovirals may result in additive cytotoxicity or other drug-drug interactions that may further enhance immunosuppression [13]. Nonetheless, the general recommendation is to treat HIV-infected patients with cancer with the same strategies employed in noninfected patients, whenever possible.

**Funding** Supported in part by grants from the Red Temática de Investigación Cooperativa en Cáncer (RTICC, FEDER) (RD12/0036/0029); 2014 SGR225 (GRE) Generalitat de Catalunya; PI14/01971 from Fondo de Investigaciones Sanitarias, Instituto de Salud Carlos III; and Fundació Internacional Josep Carreras i Obra Social "la Caixa," Spain.

## References

1. Stebbing J, Duru O, Bower M. Non-AIDS-defining cancers. Curr Opin Infect Dis. 2009;22: 7–10.
2. Pantanowitz L, Dezube BJ. Evolving spectrum and incidence of non-AIDS-defining malignancies. Curr Opin HIV AIDS. 2009;4:27–34.
3. Ingle SM, May MT, Gill MJ, Mugavero MJ, Lewden C, Abgrall S, et al. Impact of risk factors for specific causes of death in the first and subsequent years of antiretroviral therapy among HIV-infected patients. Clin Infect Dis. 2014;59:287–97.
4. Shiels MS, Pfeiffer RM, Gail MH, Hall HI, Li J, Chaturvedi AK, et al. Cancer burden in the HIV-infected population in the United States. J Natl Cancer Inst. 2011;103:753–62.
5. Chao C, Leyden WA, Xu L, Horberg MA, Klein D, Towner WJ, et al. Exposure to antiretroviral therapy and risk of cancer in HIV-infected persons. AIDS. 2012;26:2223–31.
6. Ribera JM, Morgades M, González-Barca E, Miralles P, López-Guillermo A, Gardella S, et al. Long-term follow-up of patients with HIV-related diffuse large B-cell lymphomas treated in a phase II study with rituximab and CHOP. Br J Haematol. 2012;157:637–9.
7. Xicoy B, Miralles P, Morgades M, Rubio R, Valencia ME, Ribera JM. Long-term follow-up of patients with human immunodeficiency virus infection and advanced stage Hodgkin's lymphoma treated with doxorubicin, bleomycin, vinblastine and dacarbazine. Haematologica. 2013;98:e85–6.
8. Mani D, Aboulafia DM. Screening guidelines for non-AIDS defining cancers in HIV-infected individuals. Curr Opin Oncol. 2013;25:518–25.
9. Vaccher E, Serraino D, Carbone A, De Paoli P. The evolving scenario of non-AIDS-defining cancers: challenges and opportunities of care. Oncologist. 2014;19:860–7.
10. Panel on Opportunistic Infections in HIV-Infected Adults and Adolescents. Guidelines for the prevention and treatment of opportunistic infections in HIV-infected adults and adolescents: recommendations from the Centers for Disease Control and Prevention, the National Institutes of Health, and the HIV Medicine Association of the Infectious Diseases Society of America. Available at: http://aidsinfo.nih.gov/contentfiles/lvguidelines/adult_oi.pdf.
11. Smith TJ, Khatcheressian J, Lyman GH, Ozer H, Armitage JO, Balducci L, et al. 2006 recommendations for the use of white blood cell growth factors: an evidence-based clinical practice guidelines. J Clin Oncol. 2006;24:3187–205.
12. Rizzo JD, Brouwers M, Hurley P, Seidenfeld J, Arcasoy MO, Spivak JL, et al. American Society of Clinical Oncology/American Society of Hematology clinical practice guideline update on the use of epoetin and darbepoetin in adult patients with cancer. J Clin Oncol. 2010;28:4996–5009.
13. Rudek MA, Flexner C, Ambinder RF. Use of antineoplastic agents in patients with cancer who have HIV/AIDS. Lancet Oncol. 2011;12:905–12.

MIX
Papier aus verantwortungsvollen Quellen
Paper from responsible sources
FSC® C105338

If you have any concerns about our products,
you can contact us on
**ProductSafety@springernature.com**

In case Publisher is established outside the EU,
the EU authorized representative is:
**Springer Nature Customer Service Center GmbH**
**Europaplatz 3, 69115 Heidelberg, Germany**

Printed by Libri Plureos GmbH
in Hamburg, Germany